MW01200341

Implementation Science 3.0

Bianca Albers • Aron Shlonsky • Robyn Mildon
Editors

Implementation Science 3.0

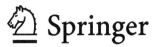 Springer

Editors
Bianca Albers
European Implementation Collaborative
Copenhagen, Denmark

Aron Shlonsky
Monash University
Clayton, Australia

Robyn Mildon
Centre for Evidence and Implementation
Melbourne, Australia

ISBN 978-3-030-03873-1 ISBN 978-3-030-03874-8 (eBook)
https://doi.org/10.1007/978-3-030-03874-8

This Springer imprint is published by the registered company Springer Nature Switzerland AG
The registered company address is: Gewerbestrasse 11, 6330 Cham, Switzerland

Preface

The word *implementation* is in the air. You can hear it whispered and shouted across academia, government, and providers of health and social services. That includes us. No doubt, the three of us have been infected by the implementation bug – and have lived with it for a while. We belong to a continuously growing group of applied researchers interested in developing the field of implementation science, which – and we should stress this from the beginning – always includes practice.

Robyn Mildon has been a powerful voice in the human service sector for some time, continually pointing out to academics, service agencies, and governments that producing and translating evidence would amount to nothing if nobody actually used it; Aron Shlonsky, an evidence-based academic by training and by heart, has far too often experienced just how little evidence matters when governments fail to make effective services available; and Bianca Albers, after having led the dissemination and implementation of multiple research-informed programs in both government and nongovernment organizations, has learned that the "importation" of manualized interventions into real-world settings requires far more than you'd think and often exceeds what you have.

One could therefore say that frustration brought us together – close to a decade ago – frustration about the many things that appeared to be in the way of getting evidence into practice. Since then, we have had numerous discussions about this new kid on the block – implementation science. These centered on how to teach it, how to make it accessible to decision-makers, and how to integrate it into practice. Simultaneously, Robyn established the Southern Hemisphere's first implementation-focused conference, now in its 10th year of operation, and Bianca the European Implementation Collaborative, and together, they co-founded the Centre for Evidence and Implementation, now operating from offices in Melbourne, Sydney, and Singapore. Simultaneously, Aron laid the foundation for moving two different university departments of social work toward a stronger focus on evidence-based and implementation-informed practice – first at the University of Melbourne and since 2018 at Monash University. Hence, both the organizations we work in, and we, as leaders in these organizations, have a considerable interest in continuously building a better understanding of what implementation science is, where it is heading and how it can be of use in human service practice.

Together, the three of us also began applying for and receiving a large number of government and service provider contracts aimed at helping to improve services through the use of evidence and implementation. This work has formed our understanding of how implementation processes unfold and how to best support and research them. It has also connected us to a network of international colleagues – implementation scientists as well as intermediaries and implementation practitioners – whose valuable work and thinking have influenced our own. Near the end of one decade of collaborating around implementation, it was only natural for us to develop a book together and to explore whether previous frustrations could be mixed with greater optimism. This book represents a curated selection of topics in implementation science that we view as central. Its primary aim is to take a critical but friendly approach to understanding what implementation science is, and isn't, specifically calling out areas where more evidence is needed.

In doing so, we are fundamentally encouraged by the progress of the discipline to date – it has without a doubt been impressive. However, we are also worried that, as we have often observed with the term "evidence-based practice," implementation science will become a term that people use for their own purposes – perhaps uncritically and without a clear understanding of what it is. Moreover, even with an understanding of what it is, we have often observed a lack of humility about how complicated implementation can be and what it takes to successfully bring evidence into widespread use within complex health and social care systems. It is no small task, and failure is frequent. In fact, much of what we have learned is a result of challenging experiences in our applied work. We hope that as implementation science moves from infancy to toddlerhood, this collection of work will inform its development. Indeed, we look forward to Implementation Science 3.0 even as we finish our take on Implementation Science 2.0 with this book.

Implementing evidence begins with an introductory chapter that reflects our take on how implementation science has emerged from the evidence-based movement and developed into a separate scientific discipline with its own distinct theoretical and conceptual thinking, methods, measures, and research designs as well as its own scientific challenges and discussions. As such, this chapter provides the lay of the land of implementation science and functions as a pathway into the field – especially for readers with an interest in a basic overview of the discipline. Following this introduction, Ariel Aloe and colleagues help us to focus on the "what" of implementation – the knowledge or intervention to be used and applied in practice. When identifying this knowledge, many – ourselves included – stress the need to first figure out what is already known about the phenomenon of interest, for example, in the form of systematic reviews, rather than just taking action without leaning on prior knowledge. However, when having sourced the necessary evidence, we often get hung up on interpreting what we find – because there is little in the literature that tells us how to interpret the findings within the context of the research at hand. Aloe and colleagues aim to fill this gap by introducing the CUTOS framework – a framework detailing how to take context into account when interpreting evidence while trying to decide which service or practice to implement. In doing so, the authors make the very interesting point that generalization is more than generalizing to a population – it is generalizing to a context.

Hereafter, two chapters focus on the role of the very popular implementation frameworks, models, and theories in implementation. While acknowledging the considerable overlap between different theories, models, and frameworks used in implementation science, Per Nilsen makes the case for the usability of all of them – if selected appropriately for aims and purposes to which they are relevant. Hence, rather than arguing for ending the substantial production of frameworks in the field, Nilsen recognizes their utility and argues for their informed, meaningful, and systematic use. This kind of framework use is then illustrated with the chapter by Melanie Barwick and colleagues who explore how the use of the Consolidated Framework for Implementation Research (CFIR) can help to build our understanding of the characteristics of successful implementation and those who implement. Based on three different case studies, they highlight the important role that an intervention's relative advantage, the tension for change within the organization, and a deep understanding of patient needs and resources have for successful implementation efforts. Using data collected in the USA, Norway, Mali, and Ethiopia, the authors illustrate that the CFIR has the potential to support the identification of crucial factors for each single case and, when used as a shared analytic frame across cases, to promote the comparison of results across contexts and studies over time. In this way, they argue, implementation frameworks can help to create a stronger foundation for planning the rollout of evidence-based interventions in practice by pointing to some of the key factors that appear to be necessary – or even sufficient – preconditions for successful implementation processes.

Chapters 5 and 6 then lead us toward the organizational context in implementation. Bryan Weiner and colleagues take a deep dive into our knowledge about organizational readiness – a concept attractive to many implementation scientists and practitioners because it resonates so well with our intuitive sense that success requires readiness from the beginning of an effort. However, what exactly is it – this organizational readiness – when drilling down into its details? Is it the sum of individual readiness, and, if so, what is that readiness of individual organizational members about? Also, could there be anything else that organizational readiness is a proxy for? For instance, are we observing a poorly functioning organization, or are we observing an organization that is not ready for this particular intervention because its key members are unmotivated (i.e., they could do it, but they do not want to)? Weiner and colleagues point to our need to be able to better differentiate between different understandings and versions of readiness and hence call for caution in preparing staff for implementation processes because the strategies used and/ or the readiness targeted may not be the appropriate choice. This, of course, creates a dilemma for implementation practice because implementation actions cannot be stopped just because reliable evidence is missing. Weiner and coauthors suggest some ways forward.

Nate Williams and Charles Glisson then open the discussion of yet another rather blurry and unclarified concept: the implementation context. It is probably one of the most referred to explanations of implementation results. However, as Williams and

Glisson highlight, we know next to nothing about what *context* implies in terms of implementation. How can it be adequately operationalized, theoretically described, and scientifically examined? What are the mechanisms of change, and how can they be effectively developed, tailored, and sustained? As was the case for organizational readiness, this gap has substantial consequences for implementation support practice, whose actors can rely only on limited evidence about how to help create enabling implementation contexts – leading the authors to call for a substantially increased research activity focused on defining and testing the effect of contextual factors in implementation.

In leaving the single and entering a cross-organizational perspective, the following two chapters are devoted to the role of implementation strategies. Unsurprisingly, these strategies have garnered considerable attention in recent years because they represent the "doing" of implementation. Understanding how they can be effectively designed, developed, and evaluated is therefore crucial for progressing the field toward a more consolidated evidence base. Luke Wolfenden and colleagues illustrate how this can occur through three Australian case studies exploring the implementation of interventions for chronic disease risk reduction in community settings. They show that the lack of clear evidence in the implementation strategy area – preventing the identification of particular strategies as effective under any circumstances – necessitates the use of a systematic and theoretically informed approach to the design, monitoring, and evaluation of strategies. This type of rigor applied in implementation practice will gradually create a stronger foundation of evidence for specific implementation strategies. Moving from multiple strategies to a description of a single strategy used in practice, Allison Metz and Leah Bartley detail their experience and further conceptualization of implementation teams. This strategy is increasingly used in research trials and practice and can be developed within or between agencies and systems. The aim of dedicated teams is to assign the responsibility for implementation to a group with the competencies necessary to shepherd an implementation through its different stages, including scaling up and sustainment. Metz and Bartley provide suggestions for what these competencies might entail and how they can be observed as part of expert implementation support practice.

From here, the focus of the book shifts toward implementation measurement – one of the hottest topics in implementation science. Cara C. Lewis and Caitlin Dorsey set the stage by both providing an overview of the state of the art of measurement in implementation and of needed developments to further progress their accuracy and applicability, which is so very central to enabling high-quality implementation research and practice. A persistent challenge to implementation measurement in recent years has been the lack of tools that are both pragmatic and have good psychometric properties (i.e., reliability and validity). While many instruments are available, most only apply to a particular setting or context and cannot be used across studies. In other words, the challenge is in the quality and not the quantity of measures – leading Lewis and Dorsey to call for establishing clear measurement reporting guidelines that can facilitate the reporting of data on each measure's reliability, face validity, and criterion validity.

From here, Tan, Parolini, and Jeffreys lead us into the world of big data – the power of which, they argue, can be anticipated and planned for rather than simply waiting for it to come. They describe what it will take to develop data systems, large and small, that can measure implementation and impact in real time. Such an approach, while in its infancy, has the potential to advance implementation quickly especially if data are collected in large systems or consistently across a number of systems. Fred Wulczyn and Sara Feldman then round off the topic of implementation measurement by providing an early example of the power of large-scale data to inform implementation and its influence on outcomes. They detail New York City's efforts to scale-up a linked, multilevel intervention for children receiving child welfare services – an intervention targeting multiple levels of the service system in order to take into account the interdependencies that exist in these systems but are often ignored.

With the final chapter of this book, Aaron Lyon and colleagues then raise the question, *where to from here*? As such, it takes a look into the future of implementation which has taken a somewhat ironic turn. Namely, Lyon and colleagues describe what amounts to a growing divide between the science and practice of implementation. While implementation science was originally conceptualized as being an applied discipline and its adherents committed to preventing the separation of those producing the science of implementation from those utilizing it, a gap has nevertheless emerged. Lyon and colleagues describe a lack of active and mutual exchange between research, practice, and policy, potentially putting the field at risk of these elements being trapped within their siloed professional identities, which would be a state of affairs familiar to other scientific disciplines. They therefore suggest a fundamental change in the training agenda, specifically gearing it to increase the production of more pragmatic research that involves practice, a greater use of team science, bringing researchers and practitioners together, and promoting comprehensive interprofessional education in order to facilitate shared learning experiences.

We hope that this collection of articles can be of inspiration and support for all those working in the field of implementation. A big thank you goes to all authors of the above chapters – both for their contribution and for the patience with which they have collaborated with us. We are looking forward to continuing our implementation discussions in the decade ahead and to follow the further development of the field of implementation science.

Copenhagen, Denmark   Bianca Albers
Clayton, Australia   Aron Shlonsky
Melbourne, Australia   Robyn Mildon

Contents

About the Editors

Bianca Albers, MSc & MA is a co-founder and the chair of the European Implementation Collaborative (EIC).

She is a seasoned organizational leader, investigator, and project manager with 15+ years' experience in promoting the use of evidence in policy and practice in child, youth, and family services in multiple Western countries. With a background in political science, she also has a great interest in the field of evidence-based policy and policy implementation. Ms Albers is also a member of the Editorial Board for *Implementation Research and Practice*.

In her work, she focuses on the development, implementation, and evaluation of evidence-informed programs, practices, and service models and on building the capacity within organizations and services to develop, implement, and sustain evidence-informed practices and policies. A key element in this work is the identification, selection, and translation of current best and relevant evidence.

Aron Shlonsky, PhD is Professor and Head of Department (Social Work) at Monash University's School of Primary and Allied Health Care and was formerly professor of Evidence Informed Practice (Social Work) and director of the Centre for Applied Research on Effective Services at the University of Melbourne School of Health Sciences.

He is an associate editor at *Children and Youth Services Review* and at the Campbell Collaboration Knowledge Translation and Implementation Coordinating Group.

After graduating from UC Berkeley with a doctorate in social welfare and a master's degree in public health, he was an assistant professor at Columbia University School of Social Work and was then Factor-Inwentash Chair in Child Welfare at the University of Toronto Faculty of Social Work. He is known internationally for his work in child welfare, particularly in the generation and implementation of evidence to inform practice and policy as well as longitudinal data analysis in the child and family services field.

Robyn Mildon, PhD is the founding executive director of the Centre for Evidence and Implementation (CEI). She is an internationally recognized leader with a long-standing career focused on the implementation, mainstreaming, and scaling-up of evidence to achieve social impact for children, families, and communities in a range of health and human service areas. She has led several national, ongoing initiatives aimed at improving the selection and use of evidence in real-world service and policy settings.

In addition to her Australian-based work, she has built a portfolio of projects collaborating with both government and nongovernment agencies in countries such as Singapore, Norway, Sweden, the USA, the UK, and New Zealand and has been a keynote speaker at multiple events around the globe.

She was the co-chair of the Global Evidence and Implementation Summit 2018, was the founding chair of the Scientific Program Committee for the first and second Australian Implementation Conference (AIC), and a co-chair for the third Biennial Australasian Implementation Conference. She is also the founding co-chair of the Knowledge Translation and Implementation Group with the Campbell Collaboration. She holds an honorary associate professorship with the University of Melbourne.

About the Contributors

Amir Alishahi-Tabriz is a physician-researcher and implementation scientist at the UNC Eshelman School of Pharmacy. He got his MPH in health policy and management and PhD in implementation science both from UNC Gillings School of Global Public Health. His research expertise stems from the multidisciplinary training and experiences he has gained through medical and graduate education and collaborations with diverse, global healthcare organizations and research settings such as WHO, Duke School of Medicine, and Durham VA Health Care System. His content expertise spans implementation science, emergency department operations, and cancer care delivery.

Ariel M. Aloe, PhD is an Associate Professor in Psychological and Quantitative Foundations at the University of Iowa, the Associate Director for Statistical Methods at the Iowa Reading Research Center, and the assistant director for Center for Advanced Studies in Measurement and Assessment (CASMA). He is interested in developing statistical techniques to study complex problems.

Leah Bartley, PhD, Master of Social Work (MSW) is an Implementation Specialist with the National Implementation Research Network (NIRN) at the Frank Porter Graham Child Development Institute at the University of North Carolina at Chapel Hill. In her current role, she is supporting implementation science application in child welfare and philanthropic initiatives. She was also the 2014–2016 Doris Duke Fellow for the Promotion of Child Well-Being through the University of Chicago Chapin Hall. Previously, she was a program manager for the Ruth Young Center for Children and Families where she provided technical assistance, data analysis, and implementation support to the replication of Family Connections, a child maltreatment prevention program. Furthermore, from 2008 to 2010, she was the Duke Endowment Fellow, following several years as a direct service social worker. Dr. Bartley's most recent publications include a review of variables that have impacted fidelity of child maltreatment prevention related interventions, and a coauthorship on cocreative conditions for sustaining research evidence in public child welfare.

Melanie Barwick, PhD, CPsych is a registered psychologist and senior scientist in the Research Institute at The Hospital for Sick Children (SickKids) in Toronto, Canada, with affiliations to the SickKids' Learning Institute and SickKids Centre for Global Child Health. She is a professor in the Department of Psychiatry, Faculty of Medicine, and in the Dalla Lana School of Public Health at the University of Toronto. She is a Governing Board Director for *Children's Mental Health Ontario* (CMHO), Associate Editor for the journal *Evidence & Policy*, and on the Editorial Board of *Implementation Research and Practice (IRaP)*. Dr. Barwick is an internationally recognized expert in implementation science and knowledge translation (KT), working in many areas of health, mental health, and global health. Her research aims to improve the implementation of evidence into practice and community and to broaden the reach of evidence more generally to support decision making, practice, policy, knowledge, and awareness. She developed and provides professional development in KT internationally through the *Specialist Knowledge Translation Training*™ and the *Knowledge Translation Professional Certificate*™ (http://tinyurl. com/p2p5du6). The KTPC is recognized as a Leading Practice by Accreditation Canada and has over 380 graduates worldwide. Since 2004, SKTT™ and its affiliated program SKTTAustralia™ have trained over 3000 learners internationally.

Alecia S. Clary, PhD, MSW is a Research Scientist with Avalere Health where she works in healthcare transformation and care delivery innovation. Specifically, Dr. Clary focuses on using real-world evidence to design and conduct high-quality studies to improve healthcare quality. In this role, she draws on her expertise in implementation science, program evaluation, and intervention design to assist clients in the execution of practice-based research studies.

Katherine A. Comtois, PhD, MPH is a professor of Psychiatry and Behavioral Sciences and an adjunct professor of Psychology at the University of Washington, USA. She also works as a clinical psychologist and is the director of the UW Center for Suicide Prevention and Recovery. She has been working in the area of health services, treatment development, and clinical trials research to prevent suicide for over 25 years. She is the director of Dissemination and Implementation for the Military Suicide Research Consortium and is founder and past president of the Society for Implementation Research Collaboration (SIRC). Dr. Comtois is a trainer and implementation consultant in large mental health systems working to reduce suicidal behavior in the United States, Britain, Canada, Germany, Norway, and Australia.

Laura Damschroder, MPH, MS is a research scientist in the Veterans Affairs (VA) Center for Clinical Management Research and project principle investigator in the Quality Enhancement Research Initiative (QUERI) in Ann Arbor, Michigan. She is a researcher embedded within the VA's healthcare system focusing on translating evidence-based practices into routine clinical care. Ms. Damschroder is an international leader in advancing the science of implementation and is lead author of the Consolidated Framework for Implementation Research (CFIR), one of the most widely cited papers in implementation science.

Caitlin Dorsey is a Research Specialist III at Kaiser Permanente Washington Health Research Institute. She earned her BAH from Indiana University and shortly thereafter was hired as a Project Coordinator in the Training Research and Implementation in Psychology (TRIP) Lab at Indiana University. Caitlin joined KPWHRI in August 2016, and her current work aims to investigate instrumentation issues within the field of implementation science.

Raluca Dubrowski, MA, PhD is a grants officer at Ontario Tech University and a research associate at the Hospital for Sick Children. Raluca's expertise is in knowledge translation and implementation science. Working in collaboration with Dr. Barwick, Raluca has conducted research focused on the implementation of evidence-based programs in various sectors, including mental health, health, public health, and education. The goal of these projects was to improve health and mental health outcomes by optimizing the quality and fidelity of implementation and examining the contextual factors that influence implementation outcomes. In addition, Raluca has worked on several global health projects examining the implementation of exclusive breastfeeding in Ethiopia and Mali in collaboration with Care and Save the Children, and the implementation of typhoid control interventions in nine countries in Africa, Asia, and South America. The focus of this work was to systematically examine the implementation context and its impact on outcomes.

Sara Feldman, PhD is a Senior Researcher at Chapin Hall. She studies the implementation and impact of child welfare reform efforts, with a focus on the at-scale adoption of both evidence-based and experimental models. Feldman has worked extensively with organizations around worker time use, workload, and worker/supervisor burden. In addition to her research activities, Feldman is an instructor for the Data Center's signature seminar, *Advanced Analytics for Child Welfare Administration*, as well as for the Data Center's principal course on evidence use, *Evidence Driven Growth and Excellence (EDGE)*. Feldman received her Ph.D. in Social Work from Columbia University.

Meghan Finch, MPH, PhD is an experienced program manager and researcher specializing in evidence-based program planning applying implementation science. She has extensive experience in large-scale practice-based evaluations and in evidence synthesis and translation. She holds a position with the University of Newcastle in the School of Medicine and Public Health and is Managing Editor for the Knowledge Translation and Implementation Group with the Campbell Collaboration.

Charles Glisson, PhD University of Tennessee Chancellor's Professor Emeritus, has directed interdisciplinary mental health services research projects for four decades supported by the National Institute of Mental Health, MacArthur Foundation, WT Grant Foundation, and other funders. His research focuses on organizational culture and climate, and their impact on client outcomes in child welfare and mental health services, including the development of the Availability, Responsiveness, and Continuity (ARC) organizational intervention strategy.

Colleen Jeffreys, Bsc has an extensive work history in designing and developing IT software and database systems spanning more than three decades. During her career, she has worked in various roles in developing database solutions for the community services sector, state and local government sector and the private sector, including applications in banking, insurance and publishing. Since undertaking postgraduate studies in Business Intelligence and Data Warehousing a decade ago, she has specialised in applying those skills to the area of social welfare. Colleen is currently a Data Architect with a research team at the Department of Social Work, University of Melbourne.

Suzanne E. U. Kerns, PhD is a licensed clinical psychologist, research associate professor, and the executive director of the Center for Effective Interventions at the University of Denver (USA) Graduate School of Social Work. Her clinical and research interests focus on enhancing the wellbeing of children and families through ensuring access to proven-effective treatment approaches, including examining the acquisition, implementation, adaptation, and sustainability of evidence-based practices. She is a member of the International Evidence-Based Practices Consortium and the Society for Implementation Research Collaboration (SIRC) and works with Abt Associates as the principal investigator for the Title IV-E Prevention Services Clearinghouse.

Melanie Kingsland, PhD is a research practitioner specialising in initiatives to support the implementation of policies and practices in community and clinical settings. She is a Program Manager with Hunter New England Population Health and a National Health and Medical Research Council Research Fellow at the University of Newcastle, Australia. She is also the Chair of the Knowledge Translation Working Group with Cochrane Public Health. Her interests include maternal health, healthy sports settings and population-level initiatives to reduced alcohol-related harm.

Stacey L. Klaman, PhD, MPH is a research fellow in the San Diego Family Health Center Laura Rodriquez Research Institute. Dr. Klaman focuses on research with underserved populations. She has studied hepatitis C virus related to injection substance use, integrating reproductive health care into treatment programs for pregnant and parenting women who live with an opioid use disorder, and the implementation of hospital-based doula programs. Her articles have been published in *Journal of Addiction Medicine* and *Journal of Obstetric, Gynecologic, & Neonatal Nursing,* among others.

Sara J. Landes, PhD is a psychologist and researcher at the Central Arkansas Veterans Healthcare System and an associate professor in the Department of Psychiatry at the University of Arkansas for Medical Sciences (UAMS). At UAMS, she is core faculty for the Center for Implementation Research. Sara's clinical expertise is in treating suicide and self-harm behaviors. Her research interests are in the dissemination and implementation of evidence-based mental health treatments, with a focus on suicide prevention and larger health care systems. She is a past president of the Society for Implementation Research Collaboration (SIRC).

Cara C. Lewis, PhD is a clinical psychologist, associate investigator at Kaiser Permanente Washington Health Research Institute and affiliate faculty in the Department of Psychiatry and Behavioral Sciences at the University of Washington. She is a Beck Scholar and Past President of the Society for Implementation Research Collaboration. Her research focuses on advancing pragmatic and rigorous measures and methods for implementation science and practice, and informing tailored implementation of evidence-based practices, notably Cognitive Behavior Therapy in community mental health settings.

Aaron R. Lyon, PhD is an Associate Professor at the Department of Psychiatry and Behavioral Sciences, University of Washington (UW). He is also the Director of the UW School Mental Health Assessment, Research, and Training (SMART) Center, an implementation research and technical assistance center focused on supporting the use of evidence-based practices that promote social, emotional, and behavioral well-being in the education sector. Dr. Lyon's research emphasizes methods of increasing the accessibility, effectiveness, equity, and efficiency of interventions for children, adolescents, and families; delivered within contexts (e.g., schools) that routinely provide care to chronically underserved populations.

Allison Metz, PhD is a developmental psychologist, Director of the National Implementation Research Network (NIRN), Senior Research Scientist at the Frank Porter Graham Child Development Institute, Research Professor at the School of Social Work, and Adjunct Professor at the School of Global Public Health at The University of North Carolina at Chapel Hill. Allison specializes in the implementation, mainstreaming, and scaling of evidence to achieve social impact for children and families in a range of human service and education areas, with an emphasis on child welfare and early childhood service contexts. Allison's work focuses on several key areas including the development of evidence-informed practice models; the use of effective implementation and scaling strategies to improve the application of evidence in service delivery systems; and the development of coaching, continuous quality improvement, and sustainability strategies.

Nicole K. Nathan, PhD is a health promotion research practitioner. She is a Program Manager and Research Fellow with Hunter New England Population Health and a Conjoint Senior Lecturer with the University of Newcastle, Australia. Dr Nathan's research aims to reduce the prevalence of chronic diseases by increasing the implementation and sustainability of evidence-based obesity prevention services in community settings, in particular within schools.

Per Nilsen, PhD is a Professor of Social Medicine and Public Linköping University, Sweden, where he was responsible for building a research program on implementation science. He leads several projects on implementation of changes in health and welfare. Nilsen has developed masteral- and doctoral-level implementation courses, which have run annually since 2011. The PhD course attracts students from the Nordic countries and beyond. Nilsen takes particular interest in issues concerning practice change and the use of theories, models and frameworks for improved understanding and explanation of implementation challenges.

Arno Parolini, PhD is a Senior Research Fellow at the Department of Social Work, University of Melbourne, where he specialises in quantitative analytical methods and development of information systems to improve policy and practice in health and human service systems. He holds a doctoral degree in economics and master degrees in economics and business administration and has gained extensive experience working in industry, government and academia. Driven by learnings from his professional career, he has a particular research interest in understanding and modelling causal links of implementation decisions throughout service systems and especially their impact on client outcomes.

Deborah K. Reed, PhD is the director of the Iowa Reading Research Center (IRRC) and an associate professor at the University of Iowa. Her evaluation and research interests include effective practices for reading instruction, intervention, and assessment as well as the use of data-based decision-making within reading programs.

Rachel L. Sutherland, PhD is an experienced Public Health Nutritionist and Health Service Manager with more than 15 years' experience leading research within an integrated research practice unit. She was awarded an NHMRC Translating Research in Practice (TRIP) Fellowship due to her leading influential translational research focusing on the development and evaluation of implementation research interventions to scale-up population health services. As Deputy Program Director, she led aspects of the Good for Kids and Good for Life program, Australia's largest population-wide child obesity prevention service and research trial in community settings. Her PhD was the first trial internationally to demonstrate an increase in physical activity, reduction in unhealthy weight gain and demonstrate cost effective amongst disadvantaged adolescents. She has continued her research focus on implementation science and scaling-up interventions, currently leading major service delivery innovations across multiple health districts in New South Wales, Australia.

Wei Wu Tan is a Social Work PhD student and researcher at the University of Melbourne, where he does research in child protection systems and social service programmes. He is also involved in teaching research methodology and implementation science. Wei has a PhD in physics and has conducted research in atmospheric science. Prior to pursuing his second PhD at Melbourne, he worked as a high school principal in Malaysia for 6 years. Wei also has extensive experience in Buddhist studies and translations. He is interested in exploring how the insights of Buddhism and Social Work can enrich each other.

Christopher G. Thompson, PhD is an assistant professor of Research, Measurement, and Statistics in the Department of Educational Psychology at Texas

A&M University. His research focuses on methodological issues and applications of meta-analysis.

Kea Turner, PhD, MPH, MA is an assistant professor at Moffitt Cancer Center and the University of South Florida Morsani College of Medicine. Dr. Turner's research aims to improve the quality of cancer care delivery by evaluating the implementation of evidence-based interventions and assessing whether effective implementation improves patient outcomes. Dr. Turner's research has focused on the implementation of health informatics interventions (e.g., using telemedicine to improve healthcare access for rural patients) and patient safety interventions (e.g., using pharmacist-physician collaboration to improve medication management).

Bryan J. Weiner, PhD is Professor in the Departments of Global Health and Health Services at the University of Washington.

Dr. Weiner's research focuses on the implementation of innovations and evidence-based practices in health care. Over the past 23 years, he has examined a wide range of innovations including quality improvement practices, care management practices, and patient safety practices, as well as evidence-based clinical practices in cancer and cardiovascular disease. His research has advanced implementation science by creating knowledge about the organizational determinants of effective implementation, developing new theories of implementation, and improving the state of measurement in the field.

John H. Wiggers, PhD is a population health practitioner and researcher. He is the Director of Health Research, Translation and Population Health Hunter New England Local Health District, Director of the University of Newcastle Priority Research Centre for Health Behaviour Sciences and Director, WHO Collaborating Centre in NCD Program Implementation. His research has a focus on reducing preventable health risk behaviours through changing the care delivery practices of clinical and community organisations.

Christopher M. Williams, PhD is a physiotherapist and NHMRC Early Career Research Fellow. He also holds a Clinical Research Fellowship with the Hunter New England Local Health District and is the programme lead of the Musculoskeletal Health Program, a programme conducted within a practice-research partnership at the Hunter New England Population Health Research Group. His work relates to the management of musculoskeletal conditions, and their interaction with chronic disease and associated health risk behaviours (such as weight gain, inactivity, poor diet, alcohol misuse and smoking). This involves pragmatic research designs, imbedded with routine health services, as well as testing setting-based implementation strategies, which aim to improve evidence-based health care.

Nathaniel J. Williams, PhD is a Licensed Clinical Social Worker and Assistant Professor in the School of Social Work at Boise State University in Boise, Idaho, USA. In addition, he serves as Co-leader of the Methods Core in the University of

Pennsylvania's National Institute of Mental Health (NIMH) ALACRITY Center for the transformation of behavioral health services. Dr. Williams' research focuses on strategies to improve the implementation of evidence-based practices in mental health service systems, the relationship between organizational culture and climate and implementation, and statistical methods for modeling data and testing mechanisms in multilevel implementation trials.

Luke Wolfenden, PhD is a behavioural and implementation scientist. He is a National Health and Medical Research Council (NMHRC) and Heart Foundation Future Leaders Fellow at the University of Newcastle, Australia. He is also the Director of an NHMRC Centre for Research Excellence in Implementation for Community Chronic Disease Prevention. His research seeks to reduce the burden of chronic disease through the development of effective public health interventions, and testing strategies to implement such interventions in community contexts.

Fred Wulczyn, PhD is a Senior Research Fellow at Chapin Hall at the University of Chicago. After helping to launch Chapin Hall in 1985, Wulczyn received a PhD from the School of Social Service Administration at the University of Chicago. He was elected to the American Academy of Social Work and Social Welfare in 2015.

Serene Yoong, PhD is a dietician and implementation scientist undertaking research to reduce the modifiable risk factors for chronic disease in the population. She seeks to advance the field of implementation science by undertaking large-scale, applied trials and bedding innovative studies to explore new concepts in the field. She was awarded an Australian Research Council Discovery Early Career Award to undertake this research.

Chapter 1
En Route to Implementation Science 3.0

Bianca Albers, Aron Shlonsky, and Robyn Mildon

In a highly referenced commentary published on Forbes.com[1] in 2004, Guy Kawasaki very briefly states "Ideas are easy. Implementation is hard. Keep thinking." Back then, this simple truth was used to remind aspiring entrepreneurs that it can be tough to get a business idea off the ground. In this book, we are reaching back to this motto to frame our exploration of the current state of implementation science and the shape of things to come. While the development of this discipline in the past 20 years has been truly impressive, we are still a long way from successfully "implementing implementation."

The interest in successful implementation is not new – within political science, it has existed since the early 1970s with a distinct focus on the barriers and enablers of fruitful policy implementation (Hupe, 2010; Hupe & Hill, 2015; Pressman & Wildavsky, 1974; Weatherley & Lipsky, 1977). The concept of implementation was pushed to new levels when it was linked with the evidence-based practice (EBP) movement. EBP first took hold in health as evidence-based medicine (Sackett, Rosenberg, Gray, Haynes, & Richardson, 1996) and then migrated to social welfare (Petrosino, Boruch, Soydan, Duggan, & Sanchez-Meca, 2001) and education (Simons, Kushner, Jones, & James, 2003). In our preferred model, optimal evidence-based decision-making – reflected in Fig. 1.1 below – is the intersection of what we currently know (current best evidence), what consumers prefer and are likely to

---

[1] Retrieved from https://www.forbes.com/2004/11/04/cx_gk_1104artofthestart.html#4af9fecd1efe on August 27, 2018.

B. Albers (✉)
European Implementation Collaborative, Copenhagen, Denmark
e-mail: balbers@implementation.eu

A. Shlonsky
Monash University, Clayton, Australia

R. Mildon
Centre for Evidence and Implementation, Melbourne, Australia

© Springer Nature Switzerland AG 2020
B. Albers et al. (eds.), *Implementation Science 3.0*,
https://doi.org/10.1007/978-3-030-03874-8_1

1

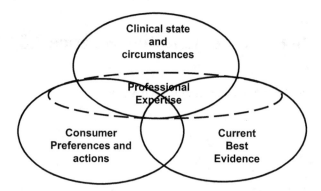

Fig. 1.1 Evidence-based model of professional decision-making. (This figure is an adapted version of thinking reflected in Fig. 2 in Haynes, Deveraux, and Gyatt (2002))

accept (consumer preferences and actions), and their individual circumstances as they relate to the issue at hand (clinical state and circumstances).

There have been continuing academic arguments about what evidence-based and evidence-informed practice entails (Chalmers, 2003, 2005; Gambrill, 2003; Mullen, Shlonsky, Bledsoe, & Bellamy, 2005; Mullen & Streiner, 2004; Shlonsky, Noonan, Littell, & Montgomery, 2010), but there is little doubt that the mere existence of evidence does not mean that such evidence can and will be used in practice. Even if a practitioner or provider is committed to finding and integrating current best evidence into assessment and treatment decisions, this evidence may not be available. In some cases, this may be because the research has not yet been conducted, which supports a push for more discovery research and evaluations of existing programs. In other cases, the data evidence may be patchy or poorly synthesized supporting the need for high-quality systematic reviews. Importantly, there is also every indication that even if evidence has been discovered and properly synthesized, the research to practice gap – in health terminology, the time it takes for evidence to make its way from the lab to the bedside – is substantial and may take as long as 17 years (Balas & Boren, 2000; Grant, Green, & Mason, 2003). Moreover, even though knowledge exists, the capacity of a service provider to find and use this knowledge effectively is contingent on the context in which services are delivered. Often illustrated through a "funnel of attrition" (Glasziou, 2005; White, 2018), the multiple steps required to achieve outcomes in real-world practice through the use of evidence potentially lead to a loss of impact – because a broad range of barriers hamper or prevent this use at each stage (Fig. 1.2). The number of people who actually receive and benefit from a known, effective intervention is far smaller than the number of people who could use it.

In other words, the economic, political, professional, and sociohistorical context in which service delivery organizations operate cannot be ignored and will impede or facilitate the use of evidence in practice (Raghavan, Bright, & Shadoin, 2008; Regehr, Stern, & Shlonsky, 2007; Schoenwald, Hoagwood, Atkins, Evans, &

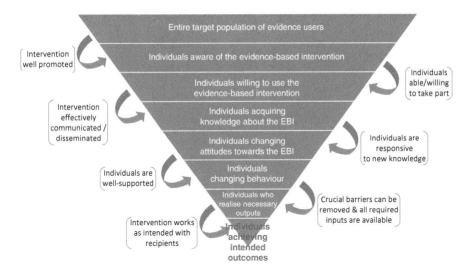

Fig. 1.2 The funnel of attrition. (Developed based on (Glasziou, 2005; White, 2018))

Ringeisen, 2010). The realization that consumers[2] only benefit from services they actually receive, and that delivery is at least as complicated as development, has driven the emergence of implementation science as a field of practice and scholarship.

Implementation 1.0: Conceptualizing Implementation

Implementation science is "the scientific study of methods to promote the systematic uptake of research findings and other evidence-based practices into routine practice, and hence, to improve the quality and effectiveness of health services and care" (Eccles & Mittman, 2006).

The emergence of implementation science as a discipline can be observed in many ways, but perhaps the most visually compelling representation can be made using the published academic literature. We conducted a simple search of academic publications using the terms "implementation" and "evidence-based" and their derivations over 20 years of publications between 1998 and 2017 (Fig. 1.3).[3,4,5,6]

---

[2] The use of "consumers" here refers to patients, clients, students, or other intended beneficiaries of services and implies that decisions about services are made with their input.

[3] Databases used: Ovid Medline, Embase, Psycinfo, Cochrane Collaboration Registry of Controlled Trials, Cochrane Database of Systematic Reviews.

[4] Search terms used for evidence-based: Evidence-based OR evidence based OR evidence-informed OR evidence informed.

[5] Search terms used for implementation: Implementation OR knowledge translation OR knowledge exchange OR knowledge mobilization OR knowledge transfer.

[6] Inclusive indexing including any use of the terms in titles, abstracts, and subject headings.

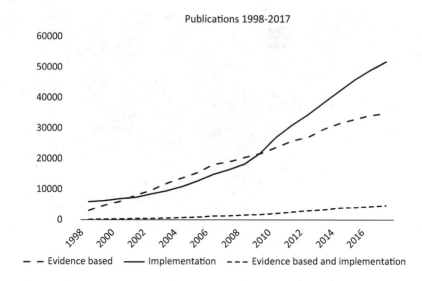

Fig. 1.3 Publications including the terms "implementation" and/or "evidence-based" and their derivations

The use of "evidence-based" and related terms rose from just 3076 in 1998 to 31,848 in 2017, representing an order of magnitude increase. The use of implementation and related terms saw a similar explosion beginning in 1998 with only 5937 articles and ending with 51,581 in 2017, an 870% increase. Although both sets of terms had massive increases, they have increased in different ways. Evidence-based terms have increased steadily and uniformly while implementation terms began a marked increase in volume in 2009. The number of implementation articles more than doubled between 2009 and 2017 (rate ratio = 2.35). When evidence and implementation terms are combined,[7] the overall numbers are smaller (as expected), but the overall percent increase over time is even more dramatic. In 1998, there were a mere 141 articles using both of these terms. By 2017, we found 4676 articles using both terms – a more than 3000 percent increase. While there are substantial limitations to this search,[8] these findings nevertheless tell a story of an emerging

---

[7] Evidence-based OR evidence based OR evidence-informed OR evidence informed AND implementation OR knowledge translation OR knowledge exchange OR knowledge mobilization OR knowledge transfer.

[8] Limitations include the fact that these data are correlational only, the overall number of published studies has increased, duplicates across databases (while controlled for) may still exist in substantial numbers, authors in the field may be referencing themselves in large numbers, all disciplines are not uniquely represented (e.g., education), indexing may be inaccurate or has changed over time, and terms may not be defined the same way by individual authors. Complete search available upon request.

discipline that is strongly linked with the evidence-based movement that began in the 1990s.

Scholars operating in this field were driven by an interest in closing the research-practice gap through the identification and examination of activities and processes that effectively support the dissemination, uptake, and implementation of evidence in real-world practice and policy settings. As such, the field of implementation science has – from the beginning – been interdisciplinary and aimed at enabling better service delivery in health and human services. This big tent includes traditional and allied health, social welfare, and education – the three main areas we draw from in this book – and hence embraces service sectors such as primary care, behavioral health, education, criminal justice, or child welfare.

The first decade of scientific inquiry – taking place between 2000 and 2010 – was clearly exploratory and resulted in the development of a large number of implementation constructs that were conceptual in nature and aimed at capturing the essence of implementation processes at the organizational and individual levels. Factors influencing implementation (e.g., the implementer and the setting in which he or she operates (Parahoo, 1999)) as well as activities aimed at supporting implementation (e.g., the monitoring of fidelity (Schoenwald, Henggeler, Brondino, & Rowland, 2000) or facilitation (Harvey et al., 2002)) gained increasing attention.

Many of these constructs were rolled up into implementation frameworks that attempted to capture both the elements and a process describing how they might be used together to understand and facilitate successful implementation. Multiple highly-cited articles from this time present implementation frameworks (Damschroder et al., 2009; Fixsen, Naoom, Blase, Friedman, & Wallace, 2005; Greenhalgh, Robert, Macfarlane, Bate, & Kyriakidou, 2004; Rycroft-Malone, 2004) and theories (May & Finch, 2009) and reflect a strong interest in identifying overarching determinants of implementation success or failure. While the purpose and structures of these frameworks differ, they have contributed to a shared understanding of key factors crucial to implementation. These are probably best reflected in the QIF – the Quality Implementation Framework (Meyers, Wandersman, & Durlak, 2012) – which integrates the content of 25 other implementation frameworks, 23 of which were developed in the first decade of implementation science. It echoes the common acknowledgment in the field that implementation

- Occurs in stages – with the QIF suggesting four
- Requires an assessment of needs prior to the selection of an intervention to implement
- Depends on the readiness of individuals and organizations
- Necessitates considering how an intervention may need to be adapted
- Implies to build capacities among all stakeholders involved – internal as well as external
- Entails developing an infrastructure to support the implementation – e.g., in the form of proper planning, team building, or system alignment
- Demands continuous monitoring of and support to practice, preferably embedded within continuous feedback mechanisms

Unsurprisingly, following the wave of framework development, many implementation studies focused on identifying and describing barriers and facilitators of the uptake of evidence in practice or policy – an interest that has been maintained over time (Addington, Kyle, Desai, & Wang, 2010; Brunette et al., 2008; Forman, Olin, Hoagwood, Crowe, & Saka, 2008; Kadu, 2015; Khanassov, Vedel, & Pluye, 2014; Morgan et al., 2016).

Simultaneously, others began examining and operationalizing key implementation concepts in greater detail, for example, organizational readiness (Holt, Armenakis, Feild, & Harris, 2007; Holt, Armenakis, Harris, & Feild, 2007; Weiner, 2009), the implementation context (Aarons, 2004; Aarons, McDonald, Sheehan, & Walrath-Greene, 2007; McCormack et al., 2002; Stetler, 2003; Stetler, McQueen, Demakis, & Mittman, 2008; Weiner, Lewis, & Linnan, 2008; Woltmann et al., 2008), implementation leadership (Dopson & Fitzgerald, 2006; Gifford, Edwards, Griffin, & Lybanon, 2007; Hodson & Cooke, 2004; Øvretveit, 2009; Proctor et al., 2007), and fidelity (Kendall & Beidas, 2007; Perepletchikova & Kazdin, 2005; Perepletchikova, Treat, & Kazdin, 2007), to name just a few. The primary aim of these publications was to synthesize current best knowledge; propose foundational definitions; or point to ambiguities, gaps, and pertinent questions that would have to be addressed by implementation scientists in the future. Empirical studies examining the relationship between implementation indicators on the one hand and clinical outcomes on the other were relatively rare with a few but highly prominent exceptions (Durlak & DuPre, 2008; Lipsey, 2009).

The growing production of implementation publications in this decade accelerated further from 2005 with the establishment of two scientific, peer-reviewed journals focused on implementation. First came "Evidence and Policy", describing itself as "dedicated to the comprehensive and critical assessment of the relationship between research evidence and the concerns of policymakers and practitioners, as well as researchers." A year later, "Implementation Science" (IS) followed, which aimed at encompassing "all aspects of research relevant to the scientific study of methods to promote the uptake of research findings into routine settings in clinical, community and policy contexts" (Eccles & Mittman, 2006).

Moreover, organizations dedicated to building implementation science capacities began to emerge, with the US-based Implementation Research Institute, IRI (Proctor et al., 2013), and a research program focused on Implementation and Learning (I&L) established at Linköping University in Sweden (Carlfjord, Roback, & Nilsen, 2017) being among the first to be founded in 2009. They have since been followed by multiple other capacity-building initiatives (Chambers, Proctor, Brownson, & Straus, 2017; Proctor & Chambers, 2017) such as the Training Institute for Dissemination and Implementation Research in Health (TIDIHR; Meissner et al., 2013) in 2011, King's College London's Centre for Implementation

Science[9] in 2013, and Australia's National Health and Medical Research Council's Translating Research into Practice (TRIP) Fellowships[10] in 2013.

In experiencing this substantial growth in productivity, IS scholars increasingly acknowledged and discussed challenges linked to the highly diverse terminology used in the field. "Implementation science" was used next to "knowledge translation and exchange" (Mitton, Adair, McKenzie, Patten, & Perry, 2007; Straus, Tetroe, & Graham, 2009), "knowledge mobilization" (Ward, 2017), and "knowledge brokering" (Ward, House, & Hamer, 2009) – leading some to call for a clearer conceptualization and mapping of terms (Graham et al., 2006) and others to develop suggestions for shared definitions (Rabin, Brownson, Haire-Joshu, Kreuter, & Weaver, 2008). While this has not resulted in a fully streamlined terminology without any overlaps, there now exists greater agreement on "knowledge translation and exchange"–related terminology describing processes of spreading and disseminating research findings and "implementation" denoting active efforts to effectively apply these findings in practice (Green, Ottoson, García, & Hiatt, 2009).

Based on a steadily increasing productivity and high numbers of outputs reflected in the many concepts developed, implementation science scholars entered into the next decade with a growing sense of being part of an "emerging science" (Proctor, Landsverk, Aarons, Chambers, & Mittman, 2008) that, despite its conceptual and methodological diversities and challenges, offered prospects and new pathways toward a better understanding of how to effectively integrate research findings into the daily routines of individual practitioners, their teams and organizations, and the wider service systems they are part of.

Implementation 2.0: Laying the Foundations of Implementation Research

The second decade of the implementation science movement, beginning around 2010, has been characterized by the emergence of rigorous research testing concepts, models, and theories in an effort to build on the *science* part of implementation science. This has not curbed the interest in and associated work to develop implementation concepts, models, and theories. However, there has clearly been a recognition that development and use of proper methods for measuring and testing the effectiveness of implementation elements, processes, theories, and concepts are needed to meaningfully advance the field. A core interest within this work stream is the enhancement of designs and tools used to evaluate implementation processes as part of dedicated implementation studies.

Extending the searches for evidence and implementation, we conducted an additional search to measure the extent to which the experimentation and knowl-

---

[9] http://www.clahrc-southlondon.nihr.ac.uk/centre-implementation-science

[10] https://www.nhmrc.gov.au/funding/find-funding/translating-research-practice-trip-fellowships

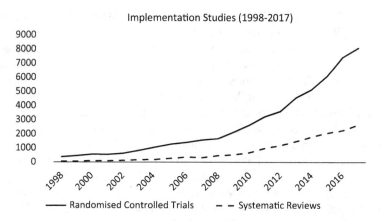

Fig. 1.4 Randomized controlled trials and systematic reviews with a focus on implementation

edge building required to successfully develop a new discipline is being conducted. One way to measure whether there is high-quality experimentation occurring in a discipline is to measure the extent to which randomized controlled trials are being used to test the effectiveness of interventions. Knowledge building requires evidence synthesis, and systematic reviews of the literature are the most exhaustive and rigorous method for synthesizing research questions within and between disciplines. As such, we searched for all randomized controlled trials (RCTs) and systematic reviews (SRs) within the implementation science discipline over 20 years of publications between 1998 and 2017 (Fig. 1.4).[11,12,13,14,15] Similar to the earlier analysis, RCTs and SRs involving implementation have increased considerably. RCTs in the discipline increased from a low of 371 in 1998 to 8091 in 2017, a 22-fold increase. SRs also saw a considerable rise from a low of 58 in 1998 to a high of 2642 in 2017, a 45-fold increase. Also similar to the earlier analysis, the yearly output of rigorous implementation studies (as measured by the use of RCTs) increased steadily from 1998 to 2008 and then increased dramatically between 2009 (1674 studies) and 2017 (8091 studies), representing an almost 300 percent increase. SRs had a lagged but similar increase beginning in 2010 (669 studies) and ending in 2017 (2642 studies), representing just over a 200 percent increase. These findings overwhelmingly suggest that implementation science is well on its way to becoming a major discipline in the health and social sciences.

---

[11] Databases used: Ovid Medline, Embase, Psycinfo, Cochrane Collaboration Registry of Controlled Trials, Cochrane Database of Systematic Reviews.

[12] Search terms used for RCTs: RCT or randomi* or (random* adj3 (assign* or allocat*)) or blinded or double blind* or doubleblind*.

[13] Search terms used for SRs: ((metaanal* or meta anal* or (systematic adj2 review*) or systematic synthesis).mp. or (meta analysis or metasynthesis or "systematic review").

[14] Search terms used for implementation: Implementation OR knowledge translation OR knowledge exchange OR knowledge mobilization OR knowledge transfer.

[15] Inclusive indexing including any use of the terms in titles, abstracts, and subject headings.

One key debate therefore has centered on identifying the study designs that are available to scientists to evaluate implementation. This has generated a strong interest in the potential of hybrid trials to assess the quality and effectiveness of implementation activities while simultaneously evaluating the effectiveness of an intervention (Brown et al., 2017; Curran, Bauer, Mittman, Pyne, & Stetler, 2012; Peters, Adam, Alonge, Agyepong, & Tran, 2013). These can take a number of forms, but most can be classified into the following three distinct approaches (Curran et al., 2012):

- Hybrid Type 1: Testing a clinical intervention while gathering information on its delivery during an effectiveness trial and/or on its potential for implementation in a real-world situation
- Hybrid Type 2: Simultaneous testing of a clinical intervention and an implementation intervention/strategy
- Hybrid Type 3: Testing an implementation intervention/strategy while observing/gathering information on the clinical intervention and related outcomes

These designs can be seen as an acknowledgment that measuring clinical outcomes without also measuring implementation outcomes is insufficient. In particular, if implementation is not measured, observed clinical outcomes may be in error or, at best, not well understood. If a trial does not measure implementation outcomes (i.e., whether the intervention was implemented to a high standard) and finds no difference between the treatment and control groups, it is unclear whether the lack of difference was a result of poor implementation or whether the intervention was not effective. If the result of the trial is negative, it is unclear whether poor implementation was to blame or the intervention itself is harmful. If the trial is positive, it cannot be assumed that the intervention was implemented as well as it could have been (which might have resulted in an even larger effect size). An increasing number of such hybrid trials have begun to generate findings (Damschroder et al., 2017; Galaviz et al., 2017; Santesteban-Echarri et al., 2018) and – given the large number of study protocols currently entered into registries – will generate further results in the coming years (Brunkert, Ruppen, Simon, & Zúñiga, 2018; Engell, Follestad, Andersen, & Hagen, 2018; Grazioli et al., 2019; Smith et al., 2018).

There are a few specific designs within the hybrid framework that warrant mention given their power to generate evidence about implementation outcomes during trials or using observational data. The Stepped-Wedge design is a cluster randomized, wait-list control trial that is extended to include the randomization of start

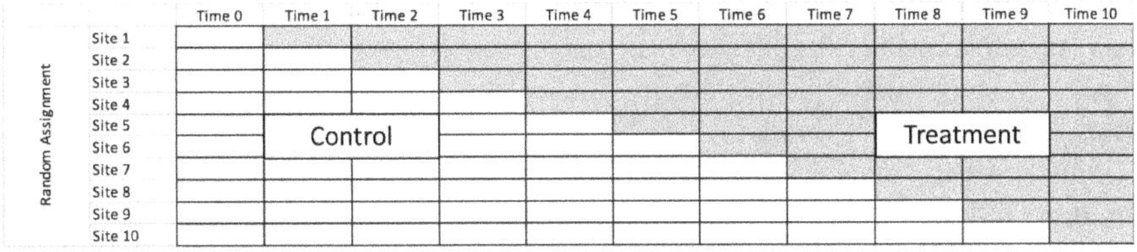

Fig. 1.5 Stepped-Wedge hybrid design

times for each trial site. The researcher randomly assigns both the time and place at which an intervention is delivered (Fig. 1.5). All sites in Fig. 1.5 will eventually enter the trial, but they are assigned (randomly) to begin the trial at different times. As the trial rolls out over time, implementation outcomes can be assessed as part of a Hybrid I design. Given the time series nature of the trial, different implementation strategies that are learned along the way can be deployed as new sites begin implementing. Conversely, an implementation strategy can be tested, and its corresponding effect on clinical outcomes can be observed (Hybrid Type 3). In both instances, the timed beginning of the intervention being tested allows for measurement between sites and within sites – with each site (except the first one) serving as both a treatment and control. Randomization of individuals at each site can also be used to strengthen the design.

Two other methodical innovations for knowledge development in implementation science have been named by Powell et al. (2019). In citing the work of colleagues (Collins, Murphy, & Strecher, 2007), they highlight Multiphase Optimization Strategy (MOST) and Sequential Multiple Assignment Randomized Trial (SMART) as novel approaches to study design. These two designs, while originally conceptualized for testing interventions, can also be used to test implementation strategies. MOST is a framework for improving interventions prior to testing with an RCT. The idea is, essentially, to optimize treatment effects through the better selection of individual intervention components, their mix, ordering, and/or their dose through a series of experiments prior to formal testing of the intervention. These individual experiments can involve simple or more complex factorial designs or even SMART designs, making them somewhat more efficient than standard RCTs. SMART designs are specifically geared to test two or more interventions administered to individuals, based on their progress with the first intervention in a chain of possible treatments (e.g., a different intervention is given to someone who responds poorly to the initial intervention as opposed to someone who responds well). This approach better reflects a real-world setting where interventions, even those that are well evidenced, do not produce hoped-for results and something else needs to be tried. The difference is that each stage has a randomization component, establishing a viable causal chain that can be rigorously evaluated for its effectiveness. Another approach that has promise for testing multiple intervention strategies within the same trial is a counterbalanced design (Sarkies et al., 2019). This design takes advantage of settings that have different contexts (e.g., hospitals with inpatients, outpatients, medical, or surgical units) but model the same outcome (e.g., mortality) in order to test a number of implementation strategies simultaneously without compromising internal validity through contamination (control group receives all or part of the benefit of the intervention) or ordering (order in which strategies are delivered). The approach can be used to concurrently test the impact of a number of different strategies within the same cluster of an RCT (2–4 strategies illustrated in Fig. 1.6), providing evidence of effectiveness that is strengthened by its testing across multiple contexts.

The establishment of causality in implementation science is becoming increasingly complex. Rigorous experimental designs can be expensive even using SMART

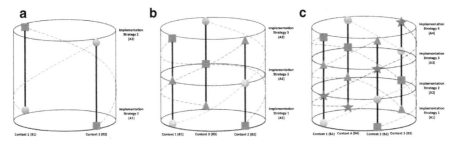

Fig. 1.6 The counterbalanced implementation study model. (Source: Sarkies et al. (2019). This figure is unadapted from its original version and licensed under a Creative Commons Generic License (CC BY 4.0 OA). It is attributed to Sarkies et al. (2019))

designs, and traditional RCTs are limited in terms of what they can reasonably test (i.e., they only test one or, at best, a few interventions at a time). There are now movements in implementation science to take advantage of the information age and its vast capacity to generate and store potentially meaningful data. Innovative observational study designs and statistical approaches can harness these data to model the effect of different implementation strategies within complex health and social interventions. In particular, the combination of Bayesian and artificial intelligence (AI) approaches – the probabilistic expert systems also called Knowledge Engineering with Bayesian Networks (Korb & Nicholson, 2011) – offers a way to model the likelihood of outcomes and even to create system maps that can be used to simulate the effect of clinical and implementation interventions carried out at known decision points (Parolini, Tan, & Shlonsky, 2018).

The prospective design of information systems and the ongoing content they collect also have a great deal of promise, especially as systems become more flexible in their capacity to add meaningful data such as reliable and valid measures of client progress and implementation outcomes (Tan, Jeffreys, and Parolini – this book, Chap. 10). The advantages of this approach are that knowledge can be generated in real time under both experimental and nonexperimental conditions using existing data; the information can be used to simulate (predict) how implementation strategies, delivered as individual units or in combination with others and in varying order, are likely to play out when introduced at key decision points; and the predictions can then be tested for accuracy and fed back into the models in a never-ending quality assurance process. The danger of such approaches is that they rely on high-quality data (which are often not present) and can be way off the mark either through the inclusion of information that is not normally available to decision-makers (e.g., using predictors that are only known after the decision is made), information that is predictive but at a level that is non-informative (e.g., young teen mothers are at higher risk for interaction with the child protection system – this is already well known), or black box solutions to problems that make no sense in the practice context. The way to contend with these challenges is to meaningfully bring theory into the picture – specifically defining strategies and actively testing them (Lewis et al., 2018; Parolini et al., 2018) rather than simply leaving it to the machine. Also essential is involving content experts (those at the coal face of service provision, consumers, line managers) in the identification of key decision points, the interpretation of findings, and the response to what is found. Bayesian approaches are well suited to such inclusive building of models since they rely on, and can actively solicit, the input of stakeholders to generate initial probabilities for simulated models (Korb & Nicholson, 2011).

Simultaneously, the field has begun to critically examine both the opportunities and limitations of traditional randomized, controlled study designs for implementation science and to search for alternatives that can help to balance rigor with relevance and enable meaningful methodological innovation (Brown et al., 2017; Hill, Cooper, & Parker, 2019; Landsverk, Brown, Rolls-Reutz, Palinkas, & Horwitz, 2010; Mazzucca et al., 2018; Palinkas et al., 2010; Schliep, Alonzo, & Morris, 2018).

As a logical consequence of this desire to enhance the methods for conducting implementation research, scholars have paid greater attention to the design elements of this research, namely, implementation outcomes and measures. One of the major advancements has been the development of a framework that outlines eight distinct implementation outcomes and separates these from service and clinical outcomes (Proctor et al., 2010). Closely linked to the development of these implementation outcomes are questions about how to best measure these and the processes aimed at generating them. In the past five years, there have therefore been multiple initiatives to map available measurement tools and resources (Lewis, 2015; Lewis et al., 2015, 2018), to discuss these critically (Clinton-McHarg et al., 2016; Martinez, Lewis, & Weiner, 2014), and to develop new implementation measures tailored to specific aspects of implementation such as implementation climate (Ehrhart, Torres, Wright, Martinez, & Aarons, 2016); leadership (Aarons, Ehrhart, & Farahnak, 2014); acceptability, feasibility, and appropriateness (Weiner et al., 2017); or quality and speed (Chamberlain, Brown, & Saldana, 2011). As part of these efforts, scholars have increasingly called for pragmatic tools designed with strong psychometric properties but also with a high degree of utility for stakeholders who adopt them within real-world settings as part of routine service delivery (Glasgow & Riley, 2013; Halko, Stanick, Powell, & Lewis, 2017; Powell et al., 2017; Stanick et al., 2018). While this is a work in progress, a selection of results from these efforts is presented in Table 1.1 below, listing pragmatic implementation measures aimed at supporting implementation practice in operational ways for which validation studies have been conducted or are in progress.

These scientific enhancements have helped pave the way to a deeper conceptualization of the activities that form implementation, namely, implementation strategies and implementation mechanisms.

As part of this work, "implementation strategies" have become a commonly shared umbrella term for "methods or techniques used to enhance the adoption, implementation and sustainability" (Proctor, Powell, & McMillen, 2013, p. 2) of research-informed programs. Their recognition as the "how-to" practices that help to enable change in practice or policy has led to suggestions for how to categorize (Mazza et al., 2013; Michie et al., 2013; Pantoja et al., 2017; Powell et al., 2015; Waltz et al. 2014, 2015), report (Leeman, Birken, Powell, Rohweder, & Shea, 2017;

Table 1.1 A selection of pragmatic implementation tools

Tool name	Tool purpose	Tool references
The Evidence-Based Practice Attitude Scale (*EBPAS*)	To measure the attitudes of service providers toward adopting an EBP	Aarons (2004), Aarons, Cafri, Lugo, and Sawitzky (2010), Cook et al. (2018), Egeland, Ruud, Ogden, Lindstrøm, and Heiervang (2016), Rye, Torres, Friborg, Skre, and Aarons (2017), and van Sonsbeek et al. (2015)
The Implementation Leadership Scale (*ILS*)	To assess the presence of characteristics of leadership conducive of implementation	Aarons et al. (2014), Aarons, Ehrhart, Torres, Finn, and Roesch (2016), Finn, Torres, Ehrhart, Roesch, and Aarons (2016), Lyon et al. (2018), and Torres et al. (2018)
The Implementation Climate Scale (*ICS*)	To assess the presence of critical factors of implementation climate	Ehrhart et al. (2016), Ehrhart, Aarons, and Farahnak (2014), and Lyon et al. (2018)
The Organizational Readiness for Implementing Change (*ORIC*) Questionnaire	To measure the organizational implementation readiness within health-care settings	Ruest, Léonard, Thomas, Desrosiers, and Guay (2019), Shea, Jacobs, Esserman, Bruce, and Weiner (2014), and Storkholm, Mazzocato, Tessma, and Savage (2018)
NoMad: Implementation measure based on Normalization Process Theory	To assess, monitor, and measure factors that affect the implementation of complex intervention within routine practice (i.e., "normalization")	Elf et al. (2018), Finch et al. (2013, 2018), Rapley et al. (2018), and Vis et al. (2019)
The Stages of Implementation Completion (SIC) tool	To track the time required to achieve key milestones for the implementation of an EBP	Chamberlain et al. (2011), Saldana (2014); Saldana et al. (2019), and Saldana, Chamberlain, Wang, and Brown (2011)

Pinnock, 2015; Proctor, Powell, & McMillen, 2013), and evaluate their use (Boyd, Powell, Endicott, & Lewis, 2018; Bunger et al., 2017). Furthermore, the field has paid growing attention to ways in which targeted implementation strategies can be selected and designed for either research or practice purposes (Ageberg, Bunke, Lucander, Nilsen, & Donaldson, 2018; Lewis, Scott, & Marriott, 2018; Powell et al., 2015).

Following this focus on strategies, the field has recently taken a logical next step by also exploring the mechanisms through which these strategies may help generate positive implementation outcomes (Dalkin, Greenhalgh, Jones, Cunningham, & Lhussier, 2015; Lewis, Klasnja, et al., 2018; Parolini et al., 2018; Williams, Glisson, Hemmelgarn, & Green, 2016), thereby working toward a greater understanding of which strategies to choose for which purposes.

While this exploration is in its infancy, it has recently been integrated into a research agenda aiming to capture some of the key issues implementation science ought to address in the decade ahead (Powell et al., 2019). The focus is on further strengthening the field's abilities to describe, develop, refine, and test key implementation components, including linking implementation determinants with strategies, mechanisms, and outcomes to thereby generate the empirical data needed to understand "when, where, why and how implementation strategies exert their effects" (Powell et al., 2019, p. 506). This argument builds on the fact that, to date, effect sizes for the use of particular implementation strategies have been small – both for "single component," "multifaceted," or "tailored" strategies. Moreover, the overall evidence on their effectiveness remains ambiguous, and limited guidance is available on how to systematically identify key implementation determinants and match these with appropriate implementation strategies able to address determinants (Dalkin et al., 2015). The authors therefore call for setting multiple key priorities in order to enhance the impact of implementation strategies:

- Enhancing the methods for designing and tailoring implementation strategies, including ways to prioritize and evaluate determinants and linking these to strategies
- Specifying and testing the mechanisms of change that link strategies to determinants, involving a stronger use of theory and the development and use of more sophisticated mediation models
- Conducting more effectiveness and economic studies of implementation strategies conducive to identifying ways to, for example, optimize, tailor, or sequence implementation strategies
- Improving the structured tracking and reporting of implementation strategies to enhance the transparency and replicability of implementation studies and to promote a more consistent use of strategy terminology

This debate about implementation strategies has also garnered increased attention for those enacting the strategies – implementation actors or implementers (Leeman et al., 2017; Proctor, Powell, & McMillen, 2013). This attention is focused on finding ways to consider the knowledge, skills, and attitudes of the implementer and the quality with which this person enables implementation – for example, by assessing barriers and facilitators, designing or selecting strategies, providing implementation support, and addressing determinants. At the risk of creating a cult of personality, it appears crucial for the field to walk the talk on capacity building, that is, to not just "teach" key concepts and tools but to actively build implementation practice capacities. This requires training and supporting frontline workers and managers to "do implementation" using effective methods that can enable learning, practice change, and effective feedback and coaching. It also requires the incorporation of failure into the learning process. Allowing room for failure – and encouraging yet another attempt – is an essential component of capacity building for implementation competence among practitioners, supervisors, managers, and senior leaders and is core to an implementation-informed culture of service delivery.

But is this all there is to it? Surely not. The field faces a diverse range of challenges that are both empirical and theoretical in nature (Papoutsi, Ruth, Foy, Grimshaw, & Rycroft-Malone, 2016; Williams & Beidas, 2018). Scholars, therefore, have continued to show a strong interest in conceptual and theoretical implementation science aimed at describing, defining, and modelling key constructs that – thus far – have eluded detailed investigation. One example is the role of context – specifically its complexity and impact on implementation processes (May, Johnson, & Finch, 2016; Waltz, Powell, Fernandez, Abadie, & Damschroder, 2019). A number of studies have attempted to capture its key determinants (Pfadenhauer et al., 2015; Squires, 2015; Watson et al., 2018), develop approaches to specifying it as part of research (Booth et al., 2019), and provide guidance about how to assess (Pfadenhauer et al., 2017) and measure it in practice (Bergström et al., 2015; Hølge Hazelton et al., 2019; Squires et al., 2015). Similar attention has been paid to key constructs such as:

- *De-implementation* – that is, the process of abandoning low-value health-care practices shown to be ineffective, unnecessary, or harmful (Hasson, Nilsen, Augustsson, & von Thiele Schwarz, 2018). Introducing an evidence- and implementation-informed culture implicitly calls for ending the use of unproven and ineffective interventions. However, only recently have scientists begun to consider how, under what conditions, and with which implications such abandonment can and should occur, leading to primarily conceptual publications (Greenhalgh et al., 2017; McKay, Morshed, Brownson, Proctor, & Prusaczyk, 2018; Niven et al., 2015; Prasad & Ioannidis, 2014) with few empirical studies in the making (Hasson et al., 2018; McKay, Dolcini, & Hoffer, 2017).
- *Adaptation* – that is, the "process of thoughtful and deliberate alteration to the design or delivery of an intervention, with the goal of improving its fit or effectiveness in a given context" (Stirman, Baumann, & Miller, 2019). There are now specific frameworks available to guide an adaptation (Escoffery et al., 2018; Stirman et al., 2019; Stirman, Miller, Toder, & Calloway, 2013), also helping to increase an awareness of the importance of taking a planned approach to such a process (Baumann et al., 2015). Furthermore, particular methods have been suggested for use in adaptation (Highfield et al., 2015; Tabak et al., 2018).
- *Sustainment* – describing a situation in which the delivery of an intervention and the behavior change implied can be maintained over time, with intended benefits being achieved continuously and adaptations conducted as relevant (Moore, Mascarenhas, Bain, & Straus, 2017). Scholars have worked to conceptualize sustainment (Chambers, Glasgow, & Stange, 2013; Moore et al., 2017; Schell et al., 2013), examine its determinants (Aarons et al., 2016; Cooper, Bumbarger, & Moore, 2013; Noel, 2017; Whelan, Love, Millar, Allender, & Bell, 2018; Willging, Green, Gunderson, Chaffin, & Aarons, 2015), and measure it (Ehrhart et al., 2018; Ford, Stumbo, & Robinson, 2018; Huang et al., 2017). However, the evidence base explaining how sustainment can be achieved and interventions developed with sustainability in mind remains scarce.
- *Scaling* – that is, "deliberate efforts to increase the impact of health service innovations successfully tested in pilot or experimental projects so as to benefit more people and to foster policy and program development on a lasting basis" (World Health Organization, 2009, p. 1). This concept was still defined as "emerging" at the beginning of the second decade of implementation science (Milat, King, Bauman, & Redman, 2013) and has since been explored through both systematic reviews

(Ben Charif et al., 2017; Willis et al., 2016) – with further reviews in the making (Power et al., 2019; Wolfenden, Albers, & Shlonsky, 2018) – and theoretical and empirical studies. The latter of which conceptualize and examine particular facets of scaling, such as "scaling out" (Aarons, Sklar, Mustanski, Benbow, & Brown, 2017) or "scaling penalties" (McCrabb et al., 2019; Tommeraas & Ogden, 2015).

Compared to other constructs, scaling in particular has become a key agenda item within implementation science, due to its potential to satisfy aspirations to enhance the reach of effective human services and improve population outcomes at a global level (Indig, Lee, Grunseit, Milat, & Bauman, 2018; Kruk et al., 2016; Richter et al., 2017). There is a growing recognition of a hitherto ethnocentric – Western – bias in implementation science reflected in, for example, key implementation concepts being developed primarily within settings of Western service and governance systems and a limited number of studies conducted in low and middle countries (Ridde, 2016). This has inhibited both the development of the discipline and the meaningful application of models and concepts in under-resourced settings experiencing substantial health, welfare, and education disparities (Alonge et al., 2019; McNulty et al., 2019). Simultaneously, scholars have called for a more intentional use of implementation science to address disparities present in Western countries due to social, economic, or environmental factors – mirrored in, for example, substantial health disadvantages present in indigenous populations, racial minorities, or other groups in society in need of support (Chinman, Woodward, Curran, & Hausmann, 2017). In recent years, this has led to a stronger focus on considering and conceptualizing equity – the fair and equal treatment of everyone – within implementation. This focus informs the design of new concepts and models, involving the development of frameworks suggested to be used by researchers during the design (Jull et al., 2017; Mbuagbaw et al., 2017), execution (Woodward, Matthieu, Uchendu, Rogal, & Kirchner, 2019), and reporting of trials (Welch et al., 2015, 2017) in order to integrate an equity perspective in their research. Within service settings, models are available to decision-makers supporting the consideration of equity-related questions during program planning, design, implementation, and evaluation (Eslava-Schmalbach et al., 2019; Harding & Oetzel, 2019; Nápoles & Stewart, 2018). Furthermore, equity-focused implementation trials are in progress, aimed at harnessing implementation science to, for example, decrease high rates of stillbirths and neonatal deaths in low- and middle-income countries (Gurung et al., 2019; Jernigan, D'Amico, & Kaholokula, 2018), improve child maternal health in rural Nepal using community health workers as implementers of evidence-based interventions (Maru et al., 2018), or improve opioid risk management among agencies serving veterans in the US (Chinman et al., 2019). However, multiple issues emerging from an equity perspective on implementation remain to be discussed and systematically examined, including, for example, appropriate research designs (Chinman et al., 2017; Wallerstein & Duran, 2010), strategies matching the substantial resource constraints characterizing disadvantaged countries and communities, ways to build the implementation capacity of frontline workers, approaches to ensure sustainment, and the transfer of knowledge from resource-poor to resource-rich contexts (Alonge et al., 2019; Wallerstein & Duran, 2010; Yapa & Bärnighausen, 2018).

Stakeholders to implementation have also been a center point of scholarly interest in recent years. One aspect of this interest are the ways in which organizational leaders support implementation processes, both at the top- and the middle-manager level (Bäck, von Thiele Schwarz, Hasson, & Richter, 2019; Birken et al., 2015; Hodson & Cooke, 2004). While this has generated a broad understanding of the behaviors supportive of evidence adoption and implementation (Gifford et al., 2018; Guerrero, Padwa, Fenwick, Harris, & Aarons, 2016; Reichenpfader, Carlfjord, & Nilsen, 2015), less is known about the determinants of implementation leadership (Birken et al., 2018; Mosson, von Thiele Schwarz, Richter, & Hasson, 2018), a gap that has and will feed studies aiming to build our understanding of how optimal implementation leadership can be fostered. The still few existing interventions in this area currently being tested are, for example, the Leadership and Organizational Change for Implementation (LOCI) program (Aarons, 2015; Aarons, Ehrhart, Moullin, Torres, & Green, 2017; Egeland et al., 2019) developed in the US or the Swedish iLEAD program (Mosson, von Thiele Schwarz, Hasson, Lundmark, & Richter, 2018; Richter et al., 2016). Both reflect a strong interest in utilizing some of the techniques that have shown to be of benefit in supporting practitioners' use of evidence-based interventions with leaders and managers. They combine elements of dynamic training with the provision of ongoing support and continuous feedback while also targeting leaders at multiple levels of an organization or system to create an implementation-minded leadership culture. While first data point to the feasibility and acceptability of such an approach (Aarons, 2015), further research is required to assess its impact on not only individual leadership behavior but also its impact on organizations and their implementation work.

A second central aspect of implementation stakeholder research is the dependency of implementation success on the active and constructive engagement of individuals and organizations who oftentimes have divergent preferences and interests. This raises questions about, for example, how to select relevant stakeholders across different implementation stages, how to facilitate fruitful coordination, collaboration and problem-solving among them, or how to utilize the resources they have at their disposal. Among the more prominent concepts developed in response to these and other questions have been

- "Co-creation," that is, "collaborative knowledge generation by academics working alongside other stakeholders" (Greenhalgh, Jackson, Shaw, & Janamian, 2016; p. 393)
- Different types of "change agents" (Alagoz, Chih, Hitchcock, Brown, & Quanbeck, 2018; Bornbaum, Kornas, Peirson, & Rosella, 2015; Long, Cunningham, & Braithwaite, 2013)
- A range of partnership models particularly focused on creating community engagement in implementation (Drahota et al., 2016; Haldane et al., 2019; Hearld, Bleser, Alexander, & Wolf, 2016)

These trends have been further strengthened through requirements for the involvement of consumers in conducting clinical trials (Montgomery et al., 2013) and systematic reviews (Pollock et al., 2018) as well as training programs aimed at strengthening researchers' ability to involve consumers and communities in their work (McKenzie, Alpers, Heyworth, Phuong, & Hanley, 2016).

In synthesizing the results of promoting broad stakeholder engagement in implementation, systematic reviews often present positive findings (McKenzie et al., 2016) but also highlight that this engagement builds on a "complex process influenced by an array of social and cultural factors" (Haldane et al., 2019; p. 21). The field is far from having understood these factors – be they determinants of, or strategies for, engagement – especially when it comes to patient, client, and other stakeholders who are the recipients of the evidence-based interventions to be implemented (Greenhalgh et al., 2019; Olasoji et al., 2019).

Another current debate within implementation science centers on questions about how it is differentiated from other fields of science. From its early beginnings, implementation science had a natural affiliation with behavioral science. This has been reflected in a strong engagement of behavioral scientists in scholarly discussions about implementation (Atkins & Michie, 2013; Eccles et al., 2009; Michie, Fixsen, Grimshaw, & Eccles, 2009) and the development and extensive use of behavioral frameworks in the field (Atkins et al., 2017; Birken et al., 2017; Cane, O'Connor, & Michie, 2012; Michie, van Stralen, & West, 2011). Certainly, implementation science uses behavioral science to understand the ways in which people interact with the programs, practices, and services they are asked to deliver, and techniques from this discipline have guided the selection of strategies designed to improve implementation outcomes.

Not quite so natural has been its affiliation with improvement science, which in the first decade was considered a separate discipline. This view has changed in recent years, leading to a growing agreement between both disciplines that improvement and implementation science are compatible (Churruca et al., 2019; Granger, 2018; Koczwara et al., 2018; Øvretveit, Mittman, Rubenstein, & Ganz, 2017). The affinity between the two disciplines has become evident by the growing number of studies utilizing concepts of quality improvement to answer implementation research questions and vice versa (Boaz et al., 2016; Robinson et al., 2017; Williams, Sevdalis, & Gaughran, 2019). Even at the institutional level, there are indicators of a growing "rapprochement" between the disciplines, as mirrored in the recently established *Healthcare Improvement Studies Institute* (THIS),[16] based in the UK, which counts multiple centers for implementation science among its partners, enhancing opportunities for joint research projects and publications.

Less examined and agreed upon is the role that complexity science – representing efforts to describe and understand the behavior of complex systems, understood as being more than the sum of their individual components and parts – can play in implementation science. While there is an acknowledgment of the need to move

---

[16] https://www.thisinstitute.cam.ac.uk/

away from the simplistic and often linear models of thinking that have dominated the first decade of implementation science (Hawe, 2015; Northridge & Metcalf, 2016), concrete suggestions for how to integrate systems and complexity thinking into models, methods, and designs of implementation studies have – thus far – primarily been made at a programmatic level at which they remain under debate (Braithwaite, Churruca, Long, Ellis, & Herkes, 2018; Bucknall & Hitch, 2018; Greenhalgh & Papoutsi, 2018; Kitson et al., 2018; Kitson et al., 2018). This has also broadened the range of methods suggested to be of value in examining complexity, including, for example, social network analysis (Oliver & Faul, 2018; Shelton et al., 2018; Valente, Palinkas, Czaja, Chu, & Brown, 2015), agent-based modelling (McKay, Hoffer, Combs, & Dolcini, 2018), ethnographic approaches (Palinkas, Mendon, & Hamilton, 2019), and the use of large-scale observational data to model implementation pathways within systems (Lewis et al., 2018; Parolini et al., 2018).

A fourth area of science suggested to be of relevance for implementation scientists to consider is that of policy implementation. A key publication pointing to its potential value was published early in the most recent decade (Nilsen, Ståhl, Roback, & Cairney, 2013) – but without leading to a visibly closer dialogue between implementation scholars on the one hand and political scientists on the other. There is a certain mutual recognition on both sides, both theoretically (DeSisto et al., 2019; Moulton & Sandfort, 2017; Purtle, Brownson, & Proctor, 2016; Roll, Moulton, & Sandfort, 2017) and empirically (Powell et al., 2016; Purtle, Brownson, & Proctor, 2016). However, evidence-based policy research appears to be located within a separate network of scholars who keep a strong focus on whether aspirations to infuse politics and policies with evidence are realistic (Cairney, Oliver, & Wellstead, 2016; Liverani, Hawkins, & Parkhurst, 2013; Newman, Cherney, & Head, 2015; Oliver, Innvar, Lorenc, Woodman, & Thomas, 2014). An active cross-disciplinary debate involving both these networks, together with other sociologists, political and implementation scientists, and focusing on, for example, how to categorize, understand, and measure policy dynamics at play in implementation processes has yet to fully emerge.

Finally, organizational science – "an interdisciplinary domain focusing on behavior, in, around and of organizations" (Rousseau, 2007; p. 50) – has also gathered increasing interest among implementation scholars. With organizational behavior being a key determinant in implementation, it is only natural to consider how theories aiming to explain this behavior may be utilized to support implementation research and practice (Birken et al., 2017; Dadich & Doloswala, 2018). However, this work is in early beginnings. Organization science provides an abundance of theories centered around key discussions on whether to understand organizations as closed or open systems; their ability to learn, create shared meanings, tackle diverting stakeholder interests and influences, and manage unpredictability; and their exertion of power, control, and dominance (Astley & Van de Ven, 1983; Örtenblad, Putnam, & Trehan, 2016). In addition, the differences between public organizations serving citizens and the public interest and corporate companies focused on shareholder revenue and preferences have been a long-standing point of interest in this field (Bozeman & Bretschneider, 1994; Denhardt & Baker, 2007; Torfing, Sørensen,

& Røiseland, 2018) informing the thinking about organizations. In order to take advantage of this knowledge base in relevant and appropriate ways within implementation science, further mining of the evidence, deeper analysis of its utility in implementation, and stronger multidisciplinary collaboration involving organizational as well as implementation scientists will be required.

Despite these gaps, needs, and deficiencies, implementation science today – at the end of its second decade of forming – appears to be more developed and more diverse. The field has refined its understanding of many concepts resulting in greater sophistication. The production of empirical data is growing (Norton, Lungeanu, Chambers, & Contractor, 2017). Funding streams and other investments in the research infrastructure have been made to build capacity into the future (Norton, Kennedy, & Chambers, 2017; Purtle, Peters, & Brownson, 2016). Multiple international networks exist working to bring implementation scientists and practitioners together on a regular basis, be it for webinars, master classes, conferences, or other activities (Darnell et al., 2017). Moreover, with the recent launch of "Implementation Science Communications," a sister journal to "Implementation Science," the Society for Implementation Research Collaboration (SIRC)[17] launching "Implementation Research and Practice", a new journal dedicated to implementation science – and further publications in the making elsewhere – the conditions are conducive for growing and diversifying the discipline.

Of course, greater diversity has also created a larger number of questions to be addressed by implementation scientists – with some of these outlined above. While progress has been made in multiple areas of the field, further advancements are needed. Toward the end of the second decade, a compelling commentary (Wensing & Grol, 2019) has been introduced, disparaging the slow accumulation of knowledge in the field and a lack of substantial research programs with sufficient capacity to enable implementation and improvement science to make society-wide differences for the health and well-being of people and communities. The authors criticize that there remains a mismatch between scientific problems and the ways in which these are solved because implementation researchers and other relevant stakeholders lack sufficient training; they also highlight the proliferation of conceptual models insufficiently tested and validated, point to the need for developing systematic approaches for stakeholder involvement, and emphasize the importance of further advancing rigorous implementation evaluations and measures. As such, they echo points made both in this introduction and to be outlined further in this book. This brings us back to our starting point: Ideas are easy. Implementation is hard. Keep thinking.

---

[17] https://societyforimplementationresearchcollaboration.org/

References

Aarons, G. A. (2004). Mental health provider attitudes toward adoption of evidence-based practice: The evidence-based practice attitude scale (EBPAS). *Mental Health Services Research, 6*(2), 61–74.

Aarons, G. A. (2015). Leadership and organizational change for implementation (LOCI): A randomized mixed method pilot study of a leadership and organization development intervention for evidence-based practice implementation. *Implementation Science, 10*(1), 1–12. https://doi.org/10.1186/s13012-014-0192-y

Aarons, G. A., Cafri, G., Lugo, L., & Sawitzky, A. C. (2010). Expanding the domains of attitudes towards evidence-based practice: The evidence based practice attitude scale-50. *Administration and Policy in Mental Health and Mental Health Services Research, 39*(5), 331–340. https://doi.org/10.1007/s10488-010-0302-3

Aarons, G. A., Ehrhart, M. G., & Farahnak, L. R. (2014). The implementation leadership scale (ILS): Development of a brief measure of unit level implementation leadership. *Implementation Science, 9*(1), 1–10. https://doi.org/10.1186/1748-5908-9-45

Aarons, G. A., Ehrhart, M. G., Moullin, J. C., Torres, E. M., & Green, A. E. (2017). Testing the leadership and organizational change for implementation (LOCI) intervention in substance abuse treatment: A cluster randomized trial study protocol. *Implementation Science, 12*(29), 1–11. https://doi.org/10.1186/s13012-017-0562-3

Aarons, G. A., Ehrhart, M. G., Torres, E. M., Finn, N. K., & Roesch, S. C. (2016). Validation of the implementation leadership scale (ILS) in substance use disorder treatment organizations. *Journal of Substance Abuse Treatment, 68*(C), 31–35. https://doi.org/10.1016/j.jsat.2016.05.004

Aarons, G. A., Green, A. E., Trott, E., Willging, C. E., Torres, E. M., Ehrhart, M. G., & Roesch, S. C. (2016). The roles of system and organizational leadership in system- wide evidence-based intervention sustainment: A mixed- method study. *Administration and Policy in Mental Health and Mental Health Services Research*, 1–18. https://doi.org/10.1007/s10488-016-0751-4.

Aarons, G. A., McDonald, E. J., Sheehan, A. K., & Walrath-Greene, C. M. (2007). Confirmatory factor analysis of the evidence-based practice attitude scale (EBPAS) in a geographically diverse sample of community mental health providers. *Administration and Policy in Mental Health and Mental Health Services Research, 34*(5), 465–469. https://doi.org/10.1007/s10488-007-0127-x

Aarons, G. A., Sklar, M., Mustanski, B., Benbow, N., & Brown, C. H. (2017). "Scaling-out" evidence-based interventions to new populations or new health care delivery systems. *Implementation Science, 12*(1), 1–13. https://doi.org/10.1186/s13012-017-0640-6

Addington, D., Kyle, T., Desai, S., & Wang, J. L. (2010). Facilitators and barriers in implementing quality measurements in primary mental health care. *Canadian Family Physician, 56*, 1322–1331.

Ageberg, E., Bunke, S., Lucander, K., Nilsen, P., & Donaldson, A. (2018). Facilitators to support the implementation of injury prevention training in youth handball: A concept mapping approach. *Scandinavian Journal of Medicine & Science in Sports, 29*(2), 275–285. https://doi.org/10.1111/sms.13323

Alagoz, E., Chih, M.-Y., Hitchcock, M., Brown, R., & Quanbeck, A. (2018). The use of external change agents to promote quality improvement and organizational change in healthcare organizations: A systematic review. *BMC Health Services Research, 18*(42), 1–13. https://doi.org/10.1186/s12913-018-2856-9

Alonge, O., Rodriguez, D. C., Brandes, N., Geng, E., Reveiz, L., & Peters, D. H. (2019). How is implementation research applied to advance health in low-income and middle-income countries? *BMJ Global Health, 4*(2), e001257–e001210. https://doi.org/10.1136/bmjgh-2018-001257

Astley, G., & Van de Ven, A. H. (1983). Central perspectives and debates in organization theory. *Administrative Science Quarterly, 28*(2), 245–273.

Atkins, L., & Michie, S. (2013). Changing eating behaviour: What can we learn from behavioural science? *Nutrition Bulletin, 38*(1), 30–35. https://doi.org/10.1111/nbu.12004

Atkins, L., Francis, J. J., Islam, R., O'Connor, D., Patey, A., Ivers, N., ... Michie, S. (2017). A guide to using the Theoretical Domains Framework of behaviour change to investigate implementation problems. *Implementation Science, 12*(1), 1–18. https://doi.org/10.1186/s13012-017-0605-9

Bäck, A., von Thiele Schwarz, U., Hasson, H., & Richter, A. (2019). Aligning perspectives?— Comparison of top and middle-level managers' views on how organization influences implementation of evidence-based practice. *British Journal of Social Work, 35*(1), 255–220. https://doi.org/10.1093/bjsw/bcz085

Balas, E. A., & Boren, S. A. (2000). Managing clinical knowledge for health care improvement. *Yearbook of Medical Informatics*, 65–70.

Baumann, A. A., Powell, B. J., Kohl, P. L., Tabak, R. G., Penalba, V., Proctor, E. K., ... Cabassa, L. J. (2015). Cultural adaptation and implementation of evidence-based parent-training: A systematic review and critique of guiding evidence. *Children and Youth Services Review, 53*, 113–120. https://doi.org/10.1016/j.childyouth.2015.03.025

Ben Charif, A., Zomahoun, H. T. V., LeBlanc, A., Langlois, L., Wolfenden, L., Yoong, S. L., ... Légaré, F. (2017). Effective strategies for scaling up evidence- based practices in primary care: A systematic review. *Implementation Science, 12*(139), 1–13. https://doi.org/10.1186/s13012-017-0672-y

Bergström, A., Skeen, S., Duc, D. M., Blandon, E. Z., Estabrooks, C. A., Gustavsson, P., ... Wallin, L. (2015). Health system context and implementation of evidence-based practices— Development and validation of the Context Assessment for Community Health (COACH) tool for low- and middle-income settings. *Implementation Science, 10*(1), 1–15. https://doi.org/10.1186/s13012-015-0305-2

Birken, S. A., Bunger, A. C., Powell, B. J., Turner, K., Clary, A. S., Klaman, S. L., ... Weiner, B. J. (2017). Organizational theory for dissemination and implementation research. *Implementation Science, 12*(1), 1–15. https://doi.org/10.1186/s13012-017-0592-x

Birken, S. A., Clary, A., Tabriz, A. A., Turner, K., Meza, R., Zizzi, A., ... Charns, M. (2018). Middle managers' role in implementing evidence-based practices in healthcare: A systematic review. *Implementation Science, 13*(149), 1–14. https://doi.org/10.1186/s13012-018-0843-5

Birken, S. A., Lee, S.-Y. D., Weiner, B. J., Chin, M. H., Chiu, M., & Schaefer, C. T. (2015). From strategy to action. *Health Care Management Review, 40*(2), 159–168. https://doi.org/10.1097/HMR.0000000000000018

Birken, S. A., Powell, B. J., Presseau, J., Kirk, M. A., Lorencatto, F., Gould, N. J., ... Damschroder, L. J. (2017). Combined use of the consolidated framework for implementation research (CFIR) and the theoretical domains framework (TDF): A systematic review. *Implementation Science, 12*(2), 1–14. https://doi.org/10.1186/s13012-016-0534-z

Boaz, A., Robert, G., Locock, L., Sturmey, G., Gager, M., Vougioukalou, S., ... Fielden, J. (2016). What patients do and their impact on implementation. *Journal of Health Organization and Management, 30*(2), 258–278. https://doi.org/10.1108/JHOM-02-2015-0027

Booth, A., Moore, G., Flemming, K., Garside, R., Rollins, N., Tunçalp, Ö., & Noyes, J. (2019). Taking account of context in systematic reviews and guidelines considering a complexity perspective. *BMJ Global Health, 4*(Suppl 1), e000840–e000815. https://doi.org/10.1136/bmjgh-2018-000840

Bornbaum, C. C., Kornas, K., Peirson, L., & Rosella, L. C. (2015). Exploring the function and effectiveness of knowledge brokers as facilitators of knowledge translation in health-related settings: A systematic review and thematic analysis. *Implementation Science, 10*(162), 1–12. https://doi.org/10.1186/s13012-015-0351-9

Boyd, M. R., Powell, B. J., Endicott, D., & Lewis, C. C. (2018). A method for tracking implementation strategies: An exemplar implementing measurement-based care in community behavioral health clinics. *Behavior Therapy, 49*(4), 525–537. https://doi.org/10.1016/j.beth.2017.11.012

Bozeman, B., & Bretschneider, S. (1994). The "Publicness Puzzle" in organization theory: A test of alternative explanations of differences between public and private organizations*. *J-Part, 4*(2), 197–223.

Braithwaite, J., Churruca, K., Long, J. C., Ellis, L. A., & Herkes, J. (2018). When complexity science meets implementation science: A theoretical and empirical analysis of systems change. *BMC Medicine, 16*(1), 1–14. https://doi.org/10.1186/s12916-018-1057-z

Brown, C. H., Curran, G., Palinkas, L. A., Aarons, G. A., Wells, K. B., Jones, L., … Cruden, G. (2017). An overview of research and evaluation designs for dissemination and implementation. *Annual Review of Public Health, 38*(1), 1–22. https://doi.org/10.1146/annurev-publhealth-031816-044215

Brunette, M. F., Asher, D., Whitley, R., Lutz, W. J., Wieder, B. L., Jones, A. M., & McHugo, G. J. (2008). Implementation of integrated dual disorders treatment: A qualitative analysis of facilitators and barriers. *Psychiatric Services, 69*(9), 989–995.

Brunkert, T., Ruppen, W., Simon, M., & Zúñiga, F. (2018). A theory-based hybrid II implementation intervention to improve pain management in Swiss nursing homes: A mixed-methods study protocol. *Journal of Advanced Nursing, 75*(2), 432–442. https://doi.org/10.1111/jan.13817

Bucknall, T. K., & Hitch, D. (2018). Connections, communication and collaboration in healthcare's complex adaptive systems comment on "using complexity and network concepts to inform healthcare knowledge translation". *Kerman University of Medical Sciences, 7*(6), 556–559. https://doi.org/10.15171/ijhpm.2017.138

Bunger, A. C., Powell, B. J., Robertson, H. A., MacDowell, H., Birken, S. A., & Shea, C. M. (2017). Tracking implementation strategies: A description of a practical approach and early findings. *Health Research Policy and Systems, 15*(1), 1–12. https://doi.org/10.1186/s12961-017-0175-y

Cairney, P., Oliver, K., & Wellstead, A. (2016). To bridge the divide between evidence and policy: Reduce ambiguity as much as uncertainty. *Public Administration Review, 76*(3), 399–402. https://doi.org/10.1111/puar.12555

Cane, J., O'Connor, D., & Michie, S. (2012). Validation of the theoretical domains framework for use in behaviour change and implementation research. *Implementation Science, 7*(37), 1–17.

Carlfjord, S., Roback, K., & Nilsen, P. (2017). Five years' experience of an annual course on implementation science: An evaluation among course participants. *Implementation Science, 12*(1), 1–8. https://doi.org/10.1186/s13012-017-0618-4

Chalmers, I. (2003). Trying to do more good than harm in policy and practice: The role of rigorous, transparent, up-to-date evaluations. *The Annals of the American Academy of Political and Social Science, 589*(1), 22–40. https://doi.org/10.1177/0002716203254762

Chalmers, I. (2005). If evidence-informed policy works in practice, does it matter if it doesn't work in theory? *Evidence & Policy: a Journal of Research, Debate and Practice, 1*(2), 227–242.

Chamberlain, P., Brown, C. H., & Saldana, L. (2011). Observational measure of implementation progress in community based settings: The stages of implementation completion (SIC). *Implementation Science, 6*(1), 116. https://doi.org/10.1186/1748-5908-6-116

Chambers, D. A., Glasgow, R. E., & Stange, K. C. (2013). The dynamic sustainability framework: Addressing the paradox of sustainment amid ongoing change. *Implementation Science, 8*(117), 1–11. https://doi.org/10.1186/1748-5908-8-117

Chambers, D. A., Proctor, E. K., Brownson, R. C., & Straus, S. E. (2017). Mapping training needs for dissemination and implementation research: Lessons from a synthesis of existing D&I research training programs. *Translational Behavioral Medicine*, 1–9. https://doi.org/10.1007/s13142-016-0399-3

Chinman, M. J., Gellad, W. F., McCarthy, S., Gordon, A. J., Rogal, S., Mor, M. K., & Hausmann, L. R. M. (2019). Protocol for evaluating the nationwide implementation of the VA Stratification Tool for Opioid Risk Management (STORM). *Implementation Science, 14*(5), 1–11. https://doi.org/10.1186/s13012-019-0852-z

Chinman, M. J., Woodward, E. N., Curran, G. M., & Hausmann, L. R. M. (2017). Harnessing implementation science to increase the impact of health equity research. *Medical Care, 55*(9), S16–S23.

Churruca, K., Ludlow, K., Taylor, N., Long, J. C., Best, S., & Braithwaite, J. (2019). The time has come: Embedded implementation research for health care improvement. *Journal of Evaluation in Clinical Practice, 297*(4), 403–408. https://doi.org/10.1111/jep.13100

Clinton-McHarg, T., Yoong, S. L., Tzelepis, F., Regan, T., Fielding, A., Skelton, E., … Wolfenden, L. (2016). Psychometric properties of implementation measures for public health and community settings and mapping of constructs against the Consolidated Framework for Implementation Research: A systematic review. *Implementation Science, 11*(148), 1–22. https://doi.org/10.1186/s13012-016-0512-5

Collins, L. M., Murphy, S. A., & Strecher, V. (2007). The multiphase optimization strategy (MOST) and the sequential multiple assignment randomized trial (SMART): New methods for more potent eHealth interventions. *American Journal of Preventive Medicine, 32*(5 Suppl), S112–S118.

Cook, C. R., Davis, C., Brown, E. C., Locke, J., Ehrhart, M. G., Aarons, G. A., … Lyon, A. R. (2018). Confirmatory factor analysis of the evidence-based practice attitudes scale with school-based behavioral health consultants. *Implementation Science, 13*(1), 1–8. https://doi.org/10.1186/s13012-018-0804-z

Cooper, B. R., Bumbarger, B. K., & Moore, J. E. (2013). Sustaining evidence-based prevention programs: Correlates in a large-scale dissemination initiative. *Prevention Science, 16*(1), 145–157. https://doi.org/10.1007/s11121-013-0427-1

Curran, G., Bauer, M. S., Mittman, B. S., Pyne, J. M., & Stetler, C. B. (2012). Effectiveness-implementation hybrid designs. *Medical Care, 50*, 217–226.

Dadich, A., & Doloswala, N. (2018). What can organisational theory offer knowledge translation in healthcare? A thematic and lexical analysis. *BMC Health Services Research, 18*(351), 1–20. https://doi.org/10.1186/s12913-018-3121-y

Dalkin, S. M., Greenhalgh, J., Jones, D., Cunningham, B., & Lhussier, M. (2015). What's in a mechanism? Development of a key concept in realist evaluation. *Implementation Science, 10*(49), 1–7. https://doi.org/10.1186/s13012-015-0237-x

Damschroder, L. J., Aron, D. C., Keith, R. E., Kirsh, S. R., Alexander, J. A., & Lowery, J. C. (2009). Fostering implementation of health services research findings into practice: A consolidated framework for advancing implementation science. *Implementation Science, 4*(1), 50. https://doi.org/10.1186/1748-5908-4-50

Damschroder, L. J., Reardon, C. M., AuYoung, M., Moin, T., Datta, S. K., Sparks, J. B., … Richardson, C. R. (2017). Implementation findings from a hybrid III implementation-effectiveness trial of the Diabetes Prevention Program (DPP) in the Veterans Health Administration (VHA). *Implementation Science, 12*(94), 1–14. https://doi.org/10.1186/s13012-017-0619-3

Darnell, D., Dorsey, C. N., Melvin, A., Chi, J., Lyon, A. R., & Lewis, C. C. (2017). A content analysis of dissemination and implementation science resource initiatives: What types of resources do they offer to advance the field? *Implementation Science, 12*(137), 1–15. https://doi.org/10.1186/s13012-017-0673-x

Denhardt, R. B., & Baker, D. L. (2007). Five great issues in organization theory. In *Handbook of public administration* (pp. 121–147). Boca Raton, FL: Taylor & Francis.

DeSisto, C. L., Kroelinger, C. D., Estrich, C., Velonis, A., Uesugi, K., Goodman, D. A., … Rankin, K. M. (2019). Application of an implementation science framework to policies on immediate postpartum long-acting reversible contraception. *Public Health Reports, 134*(2), 189–196. https://doi.org/10.1177/0033354918824329

Dopson, S., & Fitzgerald, L. (2006). The role of the middle manager in the implementation of evidence-based health care. *Journal of Nursing Management, 14*, 43–51.

Drahota, A., Meza, R. D., Brikho, B., Naaf, M., Estabillo, J. A., Gomez, E. D., … Aarons, G. A. (2016). Community-academic partnerships: A systematic review of the state of the literature and recommendations for future research. *The Milbank Quarterly, 94*(1), 163–214.

Durlak, J. A., & DuPre, E. P. (2008). Implementation matters: A review of research on the influence of implementation on program outcomes and the factors affecting implementation. *American Journal of Community Psychology, 41*(3–4), 327–350. https://doi.org/10.1007/s10464-008-9165-0

Eccles, M. P., Armstrong, D., Baker, R., Cleary, K., Davies, H. T. O., Davies, S., … Sibbald, B. (2009). An implementation research agenda. *Implementation Science, 4*(18), 1–7. https://doi.org/10.1186/1748-5908-4-18

Eccles, M. P., & Mittman, B. S. (2006). Welcome to implementation science. *Implementation Science, 1*(1), 89–83. https://doi.org/10.1186/1748-5908-1-1

Egeland, K. M., Ruud, T., Ogden, T., Lindstrøm, J. C., & Heiervang, K. S. (2016). Psychometric properties of the Norwegian version of the Evidence-Based Practice Attitude Scale (EBPAS): To measure implementation readiness. *Health Research Policy and Systems, 14*(1), 1–10. https://doi.org/10.1186/s12961-016-0114-3

Egeland, K. M., Skar, A.-M. S., Endsjø, M., Laukvik, E. H., Bækkelund, H., Babaii, A., … Aarons, G. A. (2019). Testing the leadership and organizational change for implementation (LOCI) intervention in Norwegian mental health clinics: A stepped-wedge cluster randomized design study protocol, 1–12. https://doi.org/10.1186/s13012-019-0873-7.

Ehrhart, M. G., Aarons, G. A., & Farahnak, L. R. (2014). Assessing the organizational context for EBP implementation: The development and validity testing of the Implementation Climate Scale (ICS). *Implementation Science, 9*(157), 1–11. https://doi.org/10.1186/s13012-014-0157-1

Ehrhart, M. G., Torres, E. M., Green, A. E., Trott, E. M., Willging, C. E., Moullin, J. C., & Aarons, G. A. (2018). Leading for the long haul: A mixed-method evaluation of the Sustainment Leadership Scale (SLS). *Implementation Science, 13*(17), 1–11. https://doi.org/10.1186/s13012-018-0710-4

Ehrhart, M. G., Torres, E. M., Wright, L. A., Martinez, S. Y., & Aarons, G. A. (2016). Validating the implementation climate scale (ICS) in child welfare organizations. *Child Abuse & Neglect, 53*, 17–26. https://doi.org/10.1016/j.chiabu.2015.10.017

Elf, M., Nordmark, S., Lyhagen, J., Lindberg, I., Finch, T. L., & Åberg, A. C. (2018). The Swedish version of the Normalization Process Theory Measure S-NoMAD: Translation, adaptation, and pilot testing. *Implementation Science, 13*(1), 1–12. https://doi.org/10.1186/s13012-018-0835-5

Engell, T., Follestad, I. B., Andersen, A., & Hagen, K. A. (2018). Knowledge translation in child welfare – Improving educational outcomes for children at risk: Study protocol for a hybrid randomized controlled pragmatic trial. *Trials, 19*(714), 1–17. https://doi.org/10.1186/s13063-018-3079-4

Escoffery, C. T., Lebow-Skelley, E., Haardoerfer, R., Boing, E., Udelson, H., Wood, R., … Mullen, P. D. (2018). A systematic review of adaptations of evidence-based public health interventions globally. *Implementation Science, 13*(125), 1–21. https://doi.org/10.1186/s13012-018-0815-9

Eslava-Schmalbach, J., Garzón-Orjuela, N., Elias, V., Reveiz, L., Tran, N., & Langlois, E. V. (2019). Conceptual framework of equity-focused implementation research for health programs (EquIR). *International Journal for Equity in Health, 18*(80), 1–11. https://doi.org/10.1186/s12939-019-0984-4

Finch, T. L., Girling, M., May, C. R., Mair, F. S., Murray, E., Treweek, S., … Rapley, T. (2018). Improving the normalization of complex interventions: Part 2 – Validation of the NoMAD instrument for assessing implementation work based on normalization process theory (NPT). *BMC Medical Research Methodology, 18*(135), 1–13. https://doi.org/10.1186/s12874-018-0591-x

Finch, T. L., Rapley, T., Girling, M., Mair, F. S., Murray, E., Treweek, S., … May, C. R. (2013). Improving the normalization of complex interventions: Measure development based on normalization process theory (NoMAD): Study protocol. *Implementation Science, 8*(43), 1–8.

Finn, N. K., Torres, E. M., Ehrhart, M. G., Roesch, S. C., & Aarons, G. A. (2016). Cross-validation of the implementation leadership scale (ILS) in child welfare service organizations. *Child Maltreatment, 21*(3), 250–255. https://doi.org/10.1177/1077559516638768

Fixsen, D., Naoom, S. F., Blase, K. A., Friedman, R. M., & Wallace, F. (2005). *Implementation research: A synthesis of the literature* (pp. 1–125). Tampa, FL: University of South Florida, Louis de la Parte Florida Mental Health Institute, The National Implementation Research Network.

Ford, J. H., Stumbo, S. P., & Robinson, J. M. (2018). Assessing long-term sustainment of clinic participation in NIATx200_ Results and a new methodological approach. *Journal of Substance Abuse Treatment, 92*, 51–63. https://doi.org/10.1016/j.jsat.2018.06.012

Forman, S. G., Olin, S.-C. S., Hoagwood, K. E., Crowe, M., & Saka, N. (2008). Evidence-based interventions in schools: Developers' views of implementation barriers and facilitators. *School Mental Health, 1*(1), 26–36. https://doi.org/10.1007/s12310-008-9002-5

Galaviz, K. I., Estabrooks, P. A., Ulloa, E. J., Lee, R. E., Janssen, I., Taylor, J. L. Y., … Lévesque, L. (2017). Evaluating the effectiveness of physician counseling to promote physical activity in Mexico: An effectiveness-implementation hybrid study. *Translational Behavioral Medicine, 7*, 731–740. https://doi.org/10.1007/s13142-017-0524-y

Gambrill, E. D. (2003). Evidence-based practice: Sea change or the emperor's new clothes? *Journal of Social Work Education, 39*(1), 3–23.

Gifford, W. A., Edwards, N., Griffin, P., & Lybanon, V. (2007). Managerial leadership for nurses' use of research evidence: An integrative review of the literature. *Worldviews on Evidence-Based Nursing, 4*(3), 126–145.

Gifford, W. A., Squires, J. E., Angus, D. E., Ashley, L. A., Brosseau, L., Craik, J. M., … Graham, I. D. (2018). Managerial leadership for research use in nursing and allied health care professions: A systematic review. *Implementation Science, 13*(127), 1–23. https://doi.org/10.1186/s13012-018-0817-7

Glasgow, R. E., & Riley, W. T. (2013). Pragmatic measures. *American Journal of Preventive Medicine, 45*(2), 237–243. https://doi.org/10.1016/j.amepre.2013.03.010

Glasziou, P. (2005). The paths from research to improved health outcomes. *Evidence Based Medicine, 10*(1), 4–7. https://doi.org/10.1136/ebm.10.1.4-a

Graham, I. D., Logan, J., Harrison, M. B., Straus, S. E., Tetroe, J. M., Caswell, W., & Robinson, N. (2006). Lost in knowledge translation: Time for a map? *Journal of Continuing Education in the Health Professions, 26*(1), 13–24. https://doi.org/10.1002/chp.47

Granger, B. B. (2018). Science of improvement versus science of implementation: Integrating both into clinical inquiry. *AACN Advanced Critical Care, 29*(2), 208–212. https://doi.org/10.4037/aacnacc2018757

Grant, J., Green, L., & Mason, B. (2003). Basic research and health: A reassessment of the scientific basis for the support of biomedical science. *Research Evaluation, 12*(3), 217–224.

Grazioli, V. S., Moullin, J. C., Kasztura, M., Canepa-Allen, M., Hugli, O., Griffin, J., … Bodenmann, P. (2019). Implementing a case management intervention for frequent users of the emergency department (I-CaM): An effectiveness-implementation hybrid trial study protocol. *BMC Health Services Research, 19*(28), 1–11. https://doi.org/10.1186/s12913-018-3852-9

Green, L. W., Ottoson, J. M., García, C., & Hiatt, R. A. (2009). Diffusion theory and knowledge dissemination, utilization, and integration in public health. *Annual Review of Public Health, 30*(1), 151–174. https://doi.org/10.1146/annurev.publhealth.031308.100049

Greenhalgh, T., Hinton, L., Finlay, T., Macfarlane, A., Fahy, N., Clyde, B., & Chant, A. (2019). Frameworks for supporting patient and public involvement in research: Systematic review and co-design pilot. *Health Expectations, 362*(1), k3193–k3117. https://doi.org/10.1111/hex.12888

Greenhalgh, T., Jackson, C., Shaw, S., & Janamian, T. (2016). Achieving research impact through co-creation in community-based health services: Literature review and case study. *The Milbank Quarterly, 94*(2), 392–429.

Greenhalgh, T., & Papoutsi, C. (2018). Studying complexity in health services research: Desperately seeking an overdue paradigm shift, 1–6. https://doi.org/10.1186/s12916-018-1089-4.

Greenhalgh, T., Robert, G., Macfarlane, F., Bate, P., & Kyriakidou, O. (2004). Diffusion of innovations in service organizations: Systematic review and recommendations. *The Milbank Quarterly, 82*(4), 581–629.

Greenhalgh, T., Wherton, J., Papoutsi, C., Lynch, J., Hughes, G., A'Court, C., … Shaw, S. (2017). Beyond adoption: A new framework for theorizing and evaluating nonadoption, abandonment, and challenges to the scale-up, spread, and sustainability of health and care technologies. *Journal of Medical Internet Research, 19*(11), e367–e330. https://doi.org/10.2196/jmir.8775

Guerrero, E. G., Padwa, H., Fenwick, K., Harris, L. M., & Aarons, G. A. (2016). Identifying and ranking implicit leadership strategies to promote evidence-based practice implementation in addiction health services. *Implementation Science, 11*(1), 1–13. https://doi.org/10.1186/s13012-016-0438-y

Gurung, R., Jha, A. K., Pyakurel, S., Gurung, A., Litorp, H., Wrammert, J., … Kc, A. (2019). Scaling up safer birth bundle through quality improvement in Nepal (SUSTAIN)—A stepped wedge cluster randomized controlled trial in public hospitals. *Implementation Science, 14*(65), 1–9. https://doi.org/10.1186/s13012-019-0917-z

Haldane, V., Chuah, F. L. H., Srivastava, A., Singh, S. R., Koh, G. C. H., Seng, C. K., & Legido-Quigley, H. (2019). Community participation in health services development, implementation, and evaluation: A systematic review of empowerment, health, community, and process outcomes. *PLoS One, 14*(5), e0216112–e0216125. https://doi.org/10.1371/journal.pone.0216112

Halko, H., Stanick, C., Powell, B. J., & Lewis, C. C. (2017). Defining the "pragmatic" measures construct: A stakeholder-driven approach. *The Behavior Therapist, 40*(7), 248–251.

Harding, T., & Oetzel, J. (2019). Implementation effectiveness of health interventions for indigenous communities: A systematic review. *Implementation Science, 14*(76), 1–18. https://doi.org/10.1186/s13012-019-0920-4

Harvey, G., Loftus-Hills, A., Rycroft-Malone, J., Titchen, A., Kitson, A. L., McCormack, B. G., & Seers, K. (2002). Getting evidence into practice: The role and function of facilitation. *Journal of Advanced Nursing, 37*(6), 577–588.

Hasson, H., Nilsen, P., Augustsson, H., & von Thiele Schwarz, U. (2018). Empirical and conceptual investigation of de-implementation of low-value care from professional and health care system perspectives: A study protocol. *Implementation Science, 13*(67), 1–8. https://doi.org/10.1186/s13012-018-0760-7

Hawe, P. (2015). Lessons from complex interventions to improve health. *Annual Review of Public Health, 36*(1), 307–323. https://doi.org/10.1146/annurev-publhealth-031912-114421

Haynes, B. R., Devereaux, P. J., & Guyatt, G. H. (2002). Clinical expertise in the era of evidence-based medicine and patient choice. *Evidence Based Medicine, 7*(March/April), 1–3.

Hearld, L. R., Bleser, W. K., Alexander, J. A., & Wolf, L. J. (2016). A systematic review of the literature on the sustainability of community health collaboratives. *Medical Care Research and Review, 73*(2), 127–181. https://doi.org/10.1177/1077558715607162

Highfield, L., Hartman, M. A., Mullen, P. D., Rodriguez, S. A., Fernandez, M. E., & Bartholomew, L. K. (2015). Intervention mapping to adapt evidence-based interventions for use in practice: Increasing mammography among African American women. *BioMed Research International, 2015*(1), 1–11. https://doi.org/10.1155/2015/160103

Hill, L. G., Cooper, B. R., & Parker, L. A. (2019). Qualitative comparative analysis: A mixed-method tool for complex implementation questions. *The Journal of Primary Prevention, 40*(1), 69–87. https://doi.org/10.1007/s10935-019-00536-5

Hodson, R., & Cooke, E. (2004). Leading the drive for evidence-informed practice. *Journal of Integrated Care, 12*(1), 12–18.

Hølge Hazelton, B., Bruun, L. Z., Slater, P., McCormack, B. G., Thomsen, T. G., Klausen, S. H., & Bucknall, T. K. (2019). Danish translation and adaptation of the context assessment index with implications for evidence-based practice. *Worldviews on Evidence-Based Nursing, 16*(3), 221–229. https://doi.org/10.1111/wvn.12347

Holt, D. T., Armenakis, A. A., Feild, H. S., & Harris, S. G. (2007). Readiness for organizational change: The systematic development of a scale. *The Journal of Applied Behavioral Science, 43*(2), 232–255. https://doi.org/10.1177/0021886306295295

Holt, D. T., Armenakis, A. A., Harris, S. G., & Feild, H. S. (2007). Toward a comprehensive definition of readiness for change: A review of research and instrumentation. *Research in Organizational Change and Development, 16*, 289–336. https://doi.org/10.1016/S0897-3016(06)16009-7

Huang, W., Hunter, S. B., Ayer, L., Han, B., Slaughter, M. E., Garner, B. R., & Godley, S. H. (2017). Measuring sustainment of an evidence based treatment for adolescent substance use. *Journal of Substance Abuse Treatment, 83*, 55–61. https://doi.org/10.1016/j.jsat.2017.10.005

Hupe, P. (2010). The thesis of incongruent implementation: Revisiting Pressman and Wildavsky. *Public Policy and Administration, 26*(1), 63–80. https://doi.org/10.1177/0952076710367717

Hupe, P. L., & Hill, M. J. (2015). "And the rest is implementation." Comparing approaches to what happens in policy processes beyond great expectations. *Public Policy and Administration, 31*(2), 103–121. https://doi.org/10.1177/0952076715598828

Indig, D., Lee, K., Grunseit, A., Milat, A. J., & Bauman, A. (2018). Pathways for scaling up public health interventions. *BMC Public Health, 18*(68), 1–11. https://doi.org/10.1186/s12889-017-4572-5

Jernigan, V. B. B., D'Amico, E. J., & Kaholokula, J. K. (2018). Prevention research with indigenous communities to expedite dissemination and implementation efforts, 1–9. https://doi.org/10.1007/s11121-018-0951-0.

Jull, J., Whitehead, M., Petticrew, M., Kristjansson, E., Gough, D., Petkovic, J., … Welch, V. (2017). When is a randomised controlled trial health equity relevant? Development and validation of a conceptual framework. *BMJ Open, 7*(9), e015815–e015818. https://doi.org/10.1136/bmjopen-2016-015815

Kadu, M. K. (2015). Facilitators and barriers of implementing the chronic care model in primary care: A systematic review. *BMC Family Practice, 16*(1), 1–14. https://doi.org/10.1186/s12875-014-0219-0

Kendall, P. C., & Beidas, R. S. (2007). Smoothing the trail for dissemination of evidence-based practices for youth: Flexibility within fidelity. *Professional Psychology Research and Practice, 38*(1), 13–20. https://doi.org/10.1037/0735-7028.38.1.13

Khanassov, V., Vedel, I., & Pluye, P. (2014). Barriers to implementation of case management for patients with dementia: A systematic mixed studies review. *The Annals of Family Medicine, 12*(5), 456–465. https://doi.org/10.1370/afm.1677

Kitson, A. L., Brook, A., Harvey, G., Jordan, Z., Marshall, R., O'Shea, R., & Wilson, D. (2018). Using complexity and network concepts to inform healthcare knowledge translation. *Kerman University of Medical Sciences, 7*(3), 231–243. https://doi.org/10.15171/ijhpm.2017.79

Kitson, A. L., O'Shea, R., Brook, A., Harvey, G., Jordan, Z., Marshall, R., & Wilson, D. (2018). The knowledge translation complexity network (KTCN) model: The whole is greater than the sum of the parts – A response to recent commentaries. *Kerman University of Medical Sciences, 7*(8), 768–770. https://doi.org/10.15171/ijhpm.2018.49

Koczwara, B., Stover, A. M., Davies, L., Davis, M. M., Fleisher, L., Ramanadhan, S., … Proctor, E. (2018). Harnessing the synergy between improvement science and implementation science in cancer: A call to action. *Journal of Oncology Practice, 14*(6), 335–340. https://doi.org/10.1200/JOP.17.00083

Korb, K. B., & Nicholson, A. E. (2011). *Bayesian artificial intelligence* (2nd ed.). Boca Raton, FL: CRC Press.

Kruk, M. E., Yamey, G., Angell, S. Y., Beith, A., Cotlear, D., Guanais, F., … Goosby, E. (2016). Transforming global health by improving the science of scale-up. *PLoS Biology, 14*(3), e1002360–e1002316. https://doi.org/10.1371/journal.pbio.1002360

Landsverk, J., Brown, C. H., Rolls-Reutz, J., Palinkas, L. A., & Horwitz, S. M. (2010). Design elements in implementation research: A structured review of child welfare and child mental health studies. *Administration and Policy in Mental Health and Mental Health Services Research, 38*(1), 54–63. https://doi.org/10.1007/s10488-010-0315-y

Leeman, J., Birken, S. A., Powell, B. J., Rohweder, C., & Shea, C. M. (2017). Beyond "implementation strategies": Classifying the full range of strategies used in implementation science and practice. *Implementation Science, 12*(1), 1–9. https://doi.org/10.1186/s13012-017-0657-x

Lewis, C. C. (2015). The society for implementation research collaboration instrument review project: A methodology to promote rigorous evaluation. *Implementation Science, 10*(1), 1–18. https://doi.org/10.1186/s13012-014-0193-x

Lewis, C. C., Fischer, S., Weiner, B. J., Stanick, C., Kim, M., & Martinez, R. G. (2015). Outcomes for implementation science: An enhanced systematic review of instruments using evidence-based rating criteria. *Implementation Science, 10*(1), 1–17. https://doi.org/10.1186/s13012-015-0342-x

Lewis, C. C., Klasnja, P., Powell, B. J., Lyon, A. R., Tuzzio, L., Jones, S., ... Weiner, B. (2018). From classification to causality: Advancing understanding of mechanisms of change in implementation science. *Frontiers in Public Health, 6*, 65–66. https://doi.org/10.3389/fpubh.2018.00136

Lewis, C. C., Mettert, K. D., Dorsey, C. N., Martinez, R. G., Weiner, B. J., Nolen, E., ... Powell, B. J. (2018). An updated protocol for a systematic review of implementation-related measures. *Systematic Reviews, 7*(66), 1–8. https://doi.org/10.1186/s13643-018-0728-3

Lewis, C. C., Puspitasari, A., Boyd, M. R., Scott, K., Marriott, B. R., Hoffman, M., ... Kassab, H. (2018). Implementing measurement based care in community mental health: A description of tailored and standardized methods. *BMC Research Notes, 11*(1), 606–607. https://doi.org/10.1186/s13104-018-3193-0

Lewis, C. C., Scott, K., & Marriott, B. R. (2018). A methodology for generating a tailored implementation blueprint: An exemplar from a youth residential setting. *Implementation Science, 13*(68), 1–13. https://doi.org/10.1186/s13012-018-0761-6

Lipsey, M. W. (2009). The primary factors that characterize effective interventions with juvenile offenders: A meta-analytic overview. *Victims & Offenders, 4*(2), 124–147. https://doi.org/10.1080/15564880802612573

Liverani, M., Hawkins, B., & Parkhurst, J. O. (2013). Political and institutional influences on the use of evidence in public health policy. A systematic review. *PLoS One, 8*(10), e77404. https://doi.org/10.1371/journal.pone.0077404.s004

Long, J. C., Cunningham, F. C., & Braithwaite, J. (2013). Bridges, brokers and boundary spanners in collaborative networks: A systematic review. *BMC Health Services Research, 13*(158), 1–13.

Lyon, A. R., Cook, C. R., Brown, E. C., Locke, J., Davis, C., Ehrhart, M. G., & Aarons, G. A. (2018). Assessing organizational implementation context in the education sector: Confirmatory factor analysis of measures of implementation leadership, climate, and citizenship. *Implementation Science, 13*(5), 1–14. https://doi.org/10.1186/s13012-017-0705-6

Martinez, R. G., Lewis, C. C., & Weiner, B. J. (2014). Instrumentation issues in implementation science. *Implementation Science, 9*(118), 1–9. https://doi.org/10.1186/s13012-014-0118-8

Maru, S., Nirola, I., Thapa, A., Thapa, P., Kunwar, L., Wu, W.-J., ... Maru, D. (2018). An integrated community health worker intervention in rural Nepal: A type 2 hybrid effectiveness-implementation study protocol. *Implementation Science, 13*(53), 1–11. https://doi.org/10.1186/s13012-018-0741-x

May, C. R., & Finch, T. L. (2009). Implementing, embedding, and integrating practices: An outline of normalization process theory. *Sociology, 43*(3), 535–554. https://doi.org/10.1177/0038038509103208

May, C. R., Johnson, M., & Finch, T. L. (2016). Implementation, context and complexity. *Implementation Science, 11*(1), 1–12. https://doi.org/10.1186/s13012-016-0506-3

Mazza, D., Bairstow, P., Buchan, H., Chakraborty, S. P., van Hecke, O., Grech, C., & Kunnamo, I. (2013). Refining a taxonomy for guideline implementation: Results of an exercise in abstract classification. *Implementation Science, 8*(32), 1–10. https://doi.org/10.1186/1748-5908-8-32

Mazzucca, S., Tabak, R. G., Pilar, M., Ramsey, A. T., Baumann, A. A., Kryzer, E., ... Brownson, R. C. (2018). Variation in research designs used to test the effectiveness of dissemination and implementation strategies: A review. *Frontiers in Public Health, 6*, 1–10. https://doi.org/10.3389/fpubh.2018.00032

Mbuagbaw, L., Aves, T., Shea, B., Jull, J., Welch, V., Taljaard, M., ... Tugwell, P. (2017). Considerations and guidance in designing equity-relevant clinical trials. *International Journal for Equity in Health, 16*(93), 1–9. https://doi.org/10.1186/s12939-017-0591-1

McCormack, B. G., Kitson, A. L., Harvey, G., Rycroft-Malone, J., Titchen, A., & Seers, K. (2002). Getting evidence into practice: The meaning of 'context'. *Journal of Advanced Nursing, 38*(1), 94–104.

McCrabb, S., Lane, C., Hall, A., Milat, A. J., Bauman, A., Sutherland, R., ... Wolfenden, L. (2019). Scaling-up evidence-based obesity interventions: A systematic review assessing intervention adaptations and effectiveness and quantifying the scale-up penalty. *Obesity Reviews, 20*(7), 964–982. https://doi.org/10.1111/obr.12845

McKay, V. R., Dolcini, M. M., & Hoffer, L. D. (2017). The dynamics of de-adoption: A case study of policy change, de-adoption, and replacement of an evidence-based HIV intervention. *Translational Behavioral Medicine, 7*(4), 1–11. https://doi.org/10.1007/s13142-017-0493-1

McKay, V. R., Hoffer, L. D., Combs, T. B., & Dolcini, M. M. (2018). The dynamic influence of human resources on evidence-based intervention sustainability and population outcomes: An agent-based modeling approach, 1–10. https://doi.org/10.1186/s13012-018-0767-0.

McKay, V. R., Morshed, A. B., Brownson, R. C., Proctor, E. K., & Prusaczyk, B. (2018). Letting go: Conceptualizing intervention de-implementation in public health and social service settings. *American Journal of Community Psychology, 38*(Suppl 4), 4–14. https://doi.org/10.1002/ajcp.12258

McKenzie, A., Alpers, K., Heyworth, J., Phuong, C., & Hanley, B. (2016). Consumer and community involvement in health and medical research: Evaluation by online survey of Australian training workshops for researchers. *Research Involvement and Engagement, 2*(16), 1–15. https://doi.org/10.1186/s40900-016-0030-2

McNulty, M., Smith, J. D., Villamar, J., Burnett-Ziegler, I., Vermeer, W., Benbow, N., … Hendricks Brown, C. (2019). Implementation research methodologies for achieving scientific equity and health equity. *Ethnicity & Disease, 29*(Suppl 1), 83–92.

Meissner, H. I., Glasgow, R. E., Vinson, C. A., Chambers, D. A., Brownson, R. C., Green, L. W., … Mittman, B. (2013). The U.S. training institute for dissemination and implementation research in health. *Implementation Science, 8*(12), 1–9.

Meyers, D. C., Wandersman, A., & Durlak, J. A. (2012). The quality implementation framework: A synthesis of critical steps in the implementation process. *American Journal of Community Psychology, 50*(3–4), 462–480. https://doi.org/10.1007/s10464-012-9522-x

Michie, S., Fixsen, D., Grimshaw, J., & Eccles, M. P. (2009). Specifying and reporting complex behaviour change interventions: The need for a scientific method. *Implementation Science, 4*(1), 1238–1236. https://doi.org/10.1186/1748-5908-4-40

Michie, S., Richardson, M., Johnston, M., Abraham, C., Francis, J. J., Hardeman, W., … Wood, C. E. (2013). The behavior change technique taxonomy (v1) of 93 hierarchically clustered techniques: Building an international consensus for the reporting of behavior change interventions. *Annals of Behavioral Medicine, 46*(1), 81–95. https://doi.org/10.1007/s12160-013-9486-6

Michie, S., van Stralen, M. M., & West, R. (2011). The behaviour change wheel: A new method for characterising and designing behaviour change interventions. *Implementation Science, 6*(1), 42. https://doi.org/10.1186/1748-5908-6-42

Milat, A. J., King, L., Bauman, A., & Redman, S. (2013). The concept of scalability: Increasing the scale and potential adoption of health promotion interventions into policy and practice. *Health Promotion International, 28*(3), 285–298. https://doi.org/10.1093/heapro/dar097

Mitton, C., Adair, C. E., McKenzie, E., Patten, S. B., & Perry, B. W. (2007). Knowledge transfer and exchange: Review and synthesis of the literature. *The Milbank Quarterly, 85*(4), 729–768.

Montgomery, P., Grant, S., Hopewell, S., Macdonald, G., Moher, D., Michie, S., & Mayo-Wilson, E. (2013). Protocol for CONSORT-SPI: An extension for social and psychological interventions. *Implementation Science, 8*(1), 1–7. https://doi.org/10.1186/1748-5908-8-99

Moore, J. E., Mascarenhas, A., Bain, J., & Straus, S. E. (2017). Developing a comprehensive definition of sustainability. *Implementation Science, 12*(1), 1–8. https://doi.org/10.1186/s13012-017-0637-1

Morgan, F., Battersby, A., Weightman, A. L., Searchfield, L., Turley, R., Morgan, H., … Ellis, S. (2016). Adherence to exercise referral schemes by participants – What do providers and commissioners need to know? A systematic review of barriers and facilitators. *BMC Public Health, 16*(227), 1–11. https://doi.org/10.1186/s12889-016-2882-7

Mosson, R., von Thiele Schwarz, U., Hasson, H., Lundmark, R., & Richter, A. (2018). How do iLead? Validation of a scale measuring active and passive implementation leadership in Swedish healthcare. *BMJ Open, 8*(6), e021992–e021911. https://doi.org/10.1136/bmjopen-2018-021992

Mosson, R., von Thiele Schwarz, U., Richter, A., & Hasson, H. (2018). The impact of inner and outer context on line managers' implementation leadership. *British Journal of Social Work, 48*(5), 1447–1468. https://doi.org/10.1093/bjsw/bcx077

Moulton, S., & Sandfort, J. (2017). The strategic action field framework for policy implementation research. *Policy Studies Journal, 45*(1), 144–169.

Mullen, E. J., Shlonsky, A., Bledsoe, S. E., & Bellamy, J. L. (2005). From concept to implementation: Challenges facing evidence-based social work. *Evidence & Policy: a Journal of Research, Debate and Practice, 1*(1), 61–84.

Mullen, E. J., & Streiner, D. L. (2004). The evidence for and against evidence-based practice. *Brief Treatment and Crisis Intervention, 4*(2), 111–121. https://doi.org/10.1093/brief-treatment/mhh009

Nápoles, A. M., & Stewart, A. L. (2018). Transcreation: An implementation science framework for community-engaged behavioral interventions to reduce health disparities. *BMC Health Services Research*, 1–15. https://doi.org/10.1186/s12913-018-3521-z.

Newman, J., Cherney, A., & Head, B. W. (2015). Do policy makers use academic research? Reexamining the "two communities" theory of research utilization. *Public Administration Review, 76*(1), 24–32. https://doi.org/10.1111/puar.12464

Nilsen, P., Ståhl, C., Roback, K., & Cairney, P. (2013). Never the twain shall meet? – A comparison of implementation science and policy implementation research. *Implementation Science, 8*(63), 1–12. https://doi.org/10.1186/1748-5908-8-63

Niven, D. J., Mrklas, K. J., Holodinsky, J. K., Straus, S. E., Hemmelgarn, B. R., Jeffs, L. P., & Stelfox, H. T. (2015). Towards understanding the de-adoption of low-value clinical practices: A scoping review. *BMC Medicine, 13*(1), 1–21. https://doi.org/10.1186/s12916-015-0488-z

Noel, V. A. (2017). Barriers and facilitators to sustainment of an evidence-based supported employment program. *Administration and Policy in Mental Health and Mental Health Services Research, 44*(3), 331–338. https://doi.org/10.1007/s10488-016-0778-6

Northridge, M. E., & Metcalf, S. S. (2016). Enhancing implementation science by applying best principles of systems science. *Health Research Policy and Systems, 14*(74), 1–8. https://doi.org/10.1186/s12961-016-0146-8

Norton, W. E., Kennedy, A. E., & Chambers, D. A. (2017). Studying de-implementation in health: An analysis of funded research grants. *Implementation Science, 12*(144), 1–13. https://doi.org/10.1186/s13012-017-0655-z

Norton, W. E., Lungeanu, A., Chambers, D. A., & Contractor, N. (2017). Mapping the growing discipline of dissemination and implementation science in health. *Scientometrics, 286*, 1–24. https://doi.org/10.1007/s11192-017-2455-2

Olasoji, M., Cross, W., Reed, F., Wang, W., Jacob, S., & Plummer, V. (2019). Mental health nurses' attitudes towards consumer involvement in nursing handover pre and post an educational implementation. *International Journal of Mental Health Nursing, 30*(2), 12–11. https://doi.org/10.1111/inm.12631

Oliver, K., & Faul, M. V. (2018). Networks and network analysis in evidence, policy and practice. *Evidence & Policy: a Journal of Research, Debate and Practice, 14*(3), 369–379. https://doi.org/10.1332/174426418X15314037224597

Oliver, K., Innvar, S., Lorenc, T., Woodman, J., & Thomas, J. (2014). A systematic review of barriers to and facilitators of the use of evidence by policymakers. *BMC Health Services Research, 14*(1), 1–12. https://doi.org/10.1186/1472-6963-14-2

Örtenblad, A., Putnam, L. L., & Trehan, K. (2016). Beyond Morgan's eight metaphors: Adding to and developing organization theory. *Human Relations, 69*(4), 875–889. https://doi.org/10.1177/0018726715623999

Øvretveit, J. (2009). *Leading improvement effectively* (pp. 1–105). London, UK: The Health Foundation.

Øvretveit, J., Mittman, B. S., Rubenstein, L., & Ganz, D. A. (2017). Using implementation tools to design and conduct quality improvement projects for faster and more effective improvement. *International Journal of Health Care Quality Assurance, 30*(8), 755–768. https://doi.org/10.1108/IJHCQA-01-2017-0019

Palinkas, L. A., Aarons, G. A., Horwitz, S. M., Chamberlain, P., Hurlburt, M., & Landsverk, J. (2010). Mixed method designs in implementation research. *Administration and Policy in Mental Health and Mental Health Services Research, 38*(1), 44–53. https://doi.org/10.1007/s10488-010-0314-z

Palinkas, L. A., Mendon, S. J., & Hamilton, A. B. (2019). Innovations in mixed methods evaluations. *Annual Review of Public Health, 40*(1), 423–442. https://doi.org/10.1146/annurev-publhealth-040218-044215

Pantoja, T., Opiyo, N., Lewin, S., Paulsen, E., Ciapponi, A., Wiysonge, C. S., ... Oxman, A. D. (2017). Implementation strategies for health systems in low-income countries: An overview of systematic reviews. (Cochrane Effective Practice and Organisation of Care Group, Ed.) *Cochrane Database of Systematic Reviews, 10*, 63–135.

Papoutsi, C., Ruth, B., Foy, R., Grimshaw, J., & Rycroft-Malone, J. (2016). Challenges for Implementation Science. In *Challenges, solutions and future directions in the evaluation of service innovations in health care and public health* (pp. 121–132). National Institute for Health Research: Southhampton (U.K.).

Parahoo, K. (1999). Barriers to, and facilitators of, research utilization among nurses in Northern Ireland. *Journal of Advanced Nursing, 31*(1), 89–98.

Parolini, A., Tan, W. W., & Shlonsky, A. (2018). A blueprint for causal inference in implementation systems. *Social Science Research Network*, 1–38.

Perepletchikova, F., & Kazdin, A. E. (2005). Treatment integrity and therapeutic change: Issues and research recommendations. *Clinical Psychology: Science and Practice, 12*(4), 365–383. https://doi.org/10.1093/clipsy/bpi045

Perepletchikova, F., Treat, T. A., & Kazdin, A. E. (2007). Treatment integrity in psychotherapy research: Analysis of the studies and examination of the associated factors. *Journal of Consulting and Clinical Psychology, 75*(6), 829–841. https://doi.org/10.1037/0022-006X.75.6.829

Peters, D. H., Adam, T., Alonge, O., Agyepong, I. A., & Tran, N. (2013). Implementation research: What it is and how to do it. *British Medical Journal, 347*(nov20 1), f6753. https://doi.org/10.1136/bmj.f6753.

Petrosino, A., Boruch, R. F., Soydan, H., Duggan, L., & Sanchez-Meca, J. (2001). Meeting the challenges of evidence-based policy: The Campbell Collaboration. *The Annals of the American Academy of Political and Social Science, 578*(1), 14–34.

Pfadenhauer, L. M., Gerhardus, A., Mozygemba, K., Lysdahl, K. B., Booth, A., Hofmann, B., ... Rehfuess, E. (2017). Making sense of complexity in context and implementation: The Context and Implementation of Complex Interventions (CICI) framework. *Implementation Science, 12*(1), 1–17. https://doi.org/10.1186/s13012-017-0552-5

Pfadenhauer, L. M., Mozygemba, K., Gerhardus, A., Hofmann, B., Booth, A., Lysdahl, K. B., ... Rehfuess, E. A. (2015). Context and implementation: A concept analysis towards conceptual maturity. *Theriogenology, 109*(2), 103–114. https://doi.org/10.1016/j.zefq.2015.01.004

Pinnock, H. (2015). Developing standards for reporting implementation studies of complex interventions (StaRI): A systematic review and e-Delphi. *Implementation Science, 10*(1), 1–10. https://doi.org/10.1186/s13012-015-0235-z

Pollock, A., Campbell, P., Struthers, C., Synnot, A., Nunn, J., Hill, S., ... Morley, R. (2018). Stakeholder involvement in systematic reviews: A scoping review. *Systematic Reviews*, 1–26. https://doi.org/10.1186/s13643-018-0852-0.

Powell, B. J., Beidas, R. S., Lewis, C. C., Aarons, G. A., McMillen, J. C., Proctor, E. K., & Mandell, D. S. (2015). Methods to improve the selection and tailoring of implementation strategies. *Journal of Behavioral Health Services Research, 44*(2), 177–194. https://doi.org/10.1007/s11414-015-9475-6

Powell, B. J., Beidas, R. S., Rubin, R. M., Stewart, R. E., Wolk, C. B., Matlin, S. L., ... Mandell, D. S. (2016). Applying the policy ecology framework to Philadelphia's behavioral health transformation efforts. *Administration and Policy in Mental Health and Mental Health Services Research,* 1–18. https://doi.org/10.1007/s10488-016-0733-6.

Powell, B. J., Fernandez, M. E., Williams, N. J., Aarons, G. A., Beidas, R. S., Lewis, C. C., … Weiner, B. J. (2019). Enhancing the impact of implementation strategies in healthcare: A research agenda. *Frontiers in Public Health, 7,* 503–509. https://doi.org/10.3389/fpubh.2019.00003

Powell, B. J., Stanick, C. F., Halko, H. M., Dorsey, C. N., Weiner, B. J., Barwick, M. A., … Lewis, C. C. (2017). Toward criteria for pragmatic measurement in implementation research and practice: A stakeholder-driven approach using concept mapping. *Implementation Science, 12*(118), 1–7. https://doi.org/10.1186/s13012-017-0649-x

Powell, B. J., Waltz, T. J., Chinman, M. J., Damschroder, L. J., Smith, J. L., Matthieu, M. M., … Kirchner, J. E. (2015). A refined compilation of implementation strategies: Results from the Expert Recommendations for Implementing Change (ERIC) project. *Implementation Science, 10*(1), 1–14. https://doi.org/10.1186/s13012-015-0209-1

Power, J., Gilmore, B., Vallières, F., Toomey, E., Mannan, H., & McAuliffe, E. (2019). Adapting health interventions for local fit when scaling-up: A realist review protocol. *BMJ Open, 9*(1), e022084–e022011. https://doi.org/10.1136/bmjopen-2018-022084

Prasad, V., & Ioannidis, J. P. A. (2014). Evidence-based de-implementation for contradicted, unproven, and aspiring healthcare practices. *Implementation Science, 9*(1), 1–5.

Pressman, J. L., & Wildavsky, A. B. (1974). Implementation. ICON Group International.

Proctor, E. K., & Chambers, D. A. (2017). Training in dissemination and implementation research: A field-wide perspective. *Translational Behavioral Medicine,* 1–12. https://doi.org/10.1007/s13142-016-0406-8.

Proctor, E. K., Knudsen, K. J., Fedoravicius, N., Hovmand, P., Rosen, A., & Perron, B. (2007). Implementation of evidence-based practice in community behavioral health: Agency director perspectives. *Administration and Policy in Mental Health and Mental Health Services Research, 34*(5), 479–488. https://doi.org/10.1007/s10488-007-0129-8

Proctor, E. K., Landsverk, J., Aarons, G. A., Chambers, D. A., & Mittman, B. S. (2008). Implementation research in mental health services: An emerging science with conceptual, methodological, and training challenges. *Administration and Policy in Mental Health and Mental Health Services Research, 36*(1), 24–34. https://doi.org/10.1007/s10488-008-0197-4

Proctor, E. K., Landsverk, J., Baumann, A. A., Mittman, B. S., Brownson, R. C., Glisson, C., & Chambers, D. A. (2013). The implementation research institute: Training mental health implementation researchers in the United States. *Implementation Science, 8*(105), 1–12. https://doi.org/10.1186/1748-5908-8-105

Proctor, E. K., Powell, B. J., & McMillen, J. C. (2013). Implementation strategies: Recommendations for specifying and reporting. *Implementation Science, 8*(139), 1–11.

Proctor, E. K., Silmere, H., Raghavan, R., Hovmand, P., Aarons, G. A., Bunger, A. C., … Hensley, M. (2010). Outcomes for implementation research: Conceptual distinctions, measurement challenges, and research agenda. *Administration and Policy in Mental Health and Mental Health Services Research, 38*(2), 65–76. https://doi.org/10.1007/s10488-010-0319-7

Purtle, J., Brownson, R. C., & Proctor, E. K. (2016). Infusing science into politics and policy: The importance of legislators as an audience in mental health policy dissemination research. *Administration and Policy in Mental Health and Mental Health Services Research, 44*(2), 160–163. https://doi.org/10.1007/s10488-016-0752-3

Purtle, J., Peters, R., & Brownson, R. C. (2016). A review of policy dissemination and implementation research funded by the National Institutes of Health, 2007–2014. *Implementation Science, 11*(1), 1–8. https://doi.org/10.1186/s13012-015-0367-1

Rabin, B. A., Brownson, R. C., Haire-Joshu, D., Kreuter, M. W., & Weaver, N. L. (2008). A glossary for dissemination and implementation research in health. *Journal of Public Health Management and Practice, 14*(2), 117–123. https://doi.org/10.1097/01.PHH.0000311888.06252.bb

Raghavan, R., Bright, C., & Shadoin, A. L. (2008). Toward a policy ecology of implementation of evidence-based practices in public mental health settings. *Implementation Science, 3*(1), 26–29. https://doi.org/10.1186/1748-5908-3-26

Rapley, T., Girling, M., Mair, F. S., Murray, E., Treweek, S., McColl, E., … Finch, T. L. (2018). Improving the normalization of complex interventions: Part 1 – Development of the NoMAD instrument for assessing implementation work based on normalization process theory (NPT). *BMC Medical Research Methodology, 18*(133), 1–17. https://doi.org/10.1186/s12874-018-0590-y

Regehr, C., Stern, S., & Shlonsky, A. (2007). Operationalizing evidence-based practice: The development of an institute for evidence-based social work. *Research on Social Work Practice, 17*(3), 408–416. https://doi.org/10.1177/1049731506293561

Reichenpfader, U., Carlfjord, S., & Nilsen, P. (2015). Leadership in evidence-based practice: A systematic review. *Leadership in Health Services, 28*(4), 298–316. https://doi.org/10.1108/LHS-08-2014-0061

Richter, A., von Thiele Schwarz, U., Lornudd, C., Lundmark, R., Mosson, R., & Hasson, H. (2016). iLead—A transformational leadership intervention to train healthcare managers' implementation leadership. *Implementation Science, 11*(1), 1–13. https://doi.org/10.1186/s13012-016-0475-6

Richter, L. M., Daelmans, B., Lombardi, J., Heymann, J., Boo, F. L., Behrman, J. R., … Paper 3 Working Group and the Lancet Early Childhood Development Series Steering Committee. (2017). Investing in the foundation of sustainable development: Pathways to scale up for early childhood development. *The Lancet, 389*(10064), 103–118. https://doi.org/10.1016/S0140-6736(16)31698-1.

Ridde, V. (2016). Need for more and better implementation science in global health. *BMJ Global Health, 1*(2), e000115–e000113. https://doi.org/10.1136/bmjgh-2016-000115

Robinson, T. E., Janssen, A., Harnett, P., Museth, K. E., Provan, P. J., Hills, D. J., & Shaw, T. (2017). Embedding continuous quality improvement processes in multidisciplinary teams in cancer care: Exploring the boundaries between quality and implementation science. *Australian Health Review, 41*(3), 291–296. https://doi.org/10.1071/AH16052

Roll, S., Moulton, S., & Sandfort, J. (2017). A comparative analysis of two streams of implementation research. *Journal of Public and Nonprofit Affairs, 3*(1), 3–20. https://doi.org/10.20899/jpna.3.1.3-22

Rousseau, D. M. (2007). Standing out in the fields of organization science. *Journal of Organizational Behavior, 28*(7), 849–857. https://doi.org/10.1002/job.457

Ruest, M., Léonard, G., Thomas, A., Desrosiers, J., & Guay, M. (2019). French cross-cultural adaptation of the Organizational Readiness for Implementing Change (ORIC). *BMC Health Services Research, 19*(535), 1–14. https://doi.org/10.1186/s12913-019-4361-1

Rycroft-Malone, J. (2004). The PARIHS framework – A framework for guiding the implementation of evidence-based practice. *Journal of Nursing Care Quality, 19*(4), 297–304.

Rye, M., Torres, E. M., Friborg, O., Skre, I., & Aarons, G. A. (2017). The evidence-based practice attitude scale- 36 (EBPAS-36): A brief and pragmatic measure of attitudes to evidence-based practice validated in US and Norwegian samples. *Implementation Science, 12*(44), 1–11. https://doi.org/10.1186/s13012-017-0573-0

Sackett, D. L., Rosenberg, W. C., Gray, J. A. M., Haynes, B. R., & Richardson, W. S. (1996). Evidence based medicine: What it is and what it isn't. *British Medical Journal, 312*, 71–73.

Saldana, L. (2014). The stages of implementation completion for evidence-based practice: Protocol for a mixed methods study. *Implementation Science, 9*(43), 1–11. https://doi.org/10.1186/1748-5908-9-43

Saldana, L., Bennett, I., Powers, D., Vredevoogd, M., Grover, T., Schaper, H., & Campbell, M. (2019). Scaling implementation of collaborative care for depression: Adaptation of the stages of implementation completion (SIC). *Administration and Policy in Mental Health and Mental Health Services Research*, 1–9. https://doi.org/10.1007/s10488-019-00944-z.

Saldana, L., Chamberlain, P., Wang, W., & Brown, C. H. (2011). Predicting program start-up using the stages of implementation measure. *Administration and Policy in Mental Health and Mental Health Services Research, 39*(6), 419–425. https://doi.org/10.1007/s10488-011-0363-y

Santesteban-Echarri, O., Hernández-Arroyo, L., Rice, S. M., Güerre-Lobera, M. J., Serrano-Villar, M., Espín-Jaime, J. C., & Jiménez-Arriero, M. Á. (2018). Adapting the brief coping cat for children with anxiety to a group setting in the Spanish public mental health system: A hybrid effectiveness-implementation pilot study. *Journal of Child and Family Studies, 27*, 3300–3315. https://doi.org/10.1007/s10826-018-1154-9

Sarkies, M. N., Skinner, E. H., Bowles, K.-A., Morris, M. E., Williams, C., O'Brien, L., … Haines, T. P. (2019). A novel counterbalanced implementation study design: Methodological description and application to implementation research. *Implementation Science, 14*(45), 1–11. https://doi.org/10.1186/s13012-019-0896-0

Schell, S. F., Luke, D. A., Schooley, M. W., Elliott, M. B., Herbers, S. H., Mueller, N. B., & Bunger, A. C. (2013). Public health program capacity for sustainability: A new framework. *Implementation Science, 8*(15), 1–9. https://doi.org/10.1186/1748-5908-8-15

Schliep, M. E., Alonzo, C. N., & Morris, M. A. (2018). Beyond RCTs: Innovations in research design and methods to advance implementation science. *Evidence-Based Communication Assessment and Intervention*, 1–17. https://doi.org/10.1080/17489539.2017.1394807.

Schoenwald, S. K., Henggeler, S. W., Brondino, M. J., & Rowland, M. D. (2000). Multisystemic therapy: Monitoring treatment fidelity. *Family Process, 39*, 83–103.

Schoenwald, S. K., Hoagwood, K. E., Atkins, M. S., Evans, M. E., & Ringeisen, H. (2010). Workforce development and the organization of work: The science we need. *Administration and Policy in Mental Health and Mental Health Services Research, 37*(1–2), 71–80. https://doi.org/10.1007/s10488-010-0278-z

Shea, C. M., Jacobs, S. R., Esserman, D. A., Bruce, K., & Weiner, B. J. (2014). Organizational readiness for implementing change: A psychometric assessment of a new measure. *Implementation Science, 9*(7), 1–15.

Shelton, R. C., Lee, M., Brotzman, L. E., Crookes, D. M., Jandorf, L., Erwin, D., & Gage-Bouchard, E. A. (2018). Use of social network analysis in the development, dissemination, implementation, and sustainability of health behavior interventions for adults: A systematic review. *Social Science & Medicine, 220*, 81–101. https://doi.org/10.1016/j.socscimed.2018.10.013

Shlonsky, A., Noonan, E., Littell, J. H., & Montgomery, P. (2010). The role of systematic reviews and the Campbell collaboration in the realization of evidence-informed practice. *Clinical Social Work Journal, 39*(4), 362–368. https://doi.org/10.1007/s10615-010-0307-0

Simons, H., Kushner, S., Jones, K., & James, D. (2003). From evidence-based practice to practice-based evidence: The idea of situated generalisation. *Research Papers in Education, 18*(4), 347–364. https://doi.org/10.1080/0267152032000176855

Smith, J. D., Berkel, C., Rudo-Stern, J., Montaño, Z., St George, S. M., Prado, G., … Dishion, T. J. (2018). The family check-up 4 health (FCU4Health): Applying implementation science frameworks to the process of adapting an evidence-based parenting program for prevention of pediatric obesity and excess weight gain in primary care. *Frontiers in Public Health, 6*, 243–217. https://doi.org/10.3389/fpubh.2018.00293

Squires, J. E. (2015). Identifying the domains of context important to implementation science: A study protocol. *Implementation Science, 10*(135), 1–9. https://doi.org/10.1186/s13012-015-0325-y

Squires, J. E., Hayduk, L., Hutchinson, A. M., Mallick, R., Norton, P. G., Cummings, G. G., & Estabrooks, C. A. (2015). Reliability and validity of the Alberta context tool (ACT) with professional nurses: Findings from a multi-study analysis. *PLoS One, 10*(6), e0127405–e0127417. https://doi.org/10.1371/journal.pone.0127405

Stanick, C. F., Halko, H. M., Dorsey, C. N., Weiner, B. J., Powell, B. J., Palinkas, L. A., & Lewis, C. C. (2018). Operationalizing the "pragmatic" measures construct using a stakeholder feedback and a multi-method approach. *BMC Health Services Research, 18*(882), 1–12. https://doi.org/10.1186/s12913-018-3709-2

Stetler, C. B. (2003). Role of the organization in translating research into evidence-based practice. *Outcomes Management, 7*(3), 97–103.

Stetler, C. B., McQueen, L., Demakis, J., & Mittman, B. S. (2008). An organizational framework and strategic implementation for system-level change to enhance research-based practice: QUERI series. *Implementation Science, 3*(1), 30. https://doi.org/10.1186/1748-5908-3-30

Stirman, S. W., Baumann, A. A., & Miller, C. J. (2019). The FRAME: An expanded framework for reporting adaptations and modifications to evidence-based interventions, 1–10. https://doi.org/10.1186/s13012-019-0898-y.

Stirman, S. W., Miller, C. J., Toder, K., & Calloway, A. (2013). Development of a framework and coding system for modifications and adaptations of evidence-based interventions. *Implementation Science, 8*(65), 1–12. https://doi.org/10.1186/1748-5908-8-65

Storkholm, M. H., Mazzocato, P., Tessma, M. K., & Savage, C. (2018). Assessing the reliability and validity of the Danish version of Organizational Readiness for Implementing Change (ORIC). *Implementation Science, 13*(1), 1–7. https://doi.org/10.1186/s13012-018-0769-y

Straus, S. E., Tetroe, J., & Graham, I. D. (2009). Defining knowledge translation. *Canadian Medical Association Journal, 181*(3–4), 165–168. https://doi.org/10.1503/cmaj.081229

Tabak, R. G., Strickland, J. R., Stein, R. I., Dart, H., Colditz, G. A., Kirk, B., … Evanoff, B. A. (2018). Development of a scalable weight loss intervention for low-income workers through adaptation of interactive obesity treatment approach (iOTA). *BMC Public Health, 18*(1), 1–11. https://doi.org/10.1186/s12889-018-6176-0

Tommeraas, T., & Ogden, T. (2015). Is there a scale-up penalty? Testing behavioral change in the scaling up of parent management training in Norway. *Administration and Policy in Mental Health and Mental Health Services Research*, 1–14. https://doi.org/10.1007/s10488-015-0712-3.

Torfing, J., Sørensen, E., & Røiseland, A. (2018). Transforming the public sector into an arena for co-creation: Barriers, drivers, benefits, and ways forward. *Administration & Society, 51*(5), 795–825. https://doi.org/10.1177/0095399716680057

Torres, E. M., Ehrhart, M. G., Beidas, R. S., Farahnak, L. R., Finn, N. K., & Aarons, G. A. (2018). Validation of the implementation leadership scale (ILS) with supervisors' self-ratings. *Community Mental Health Journal, 54*(1), 49–53. https://doi.org/10.1007/s10597-017-0114-y

Valente, T. W., Palinkas, L. A., Czaja, S., Chu, K.-H., & Brown, C. H. (2015). Social network analysis for program implementation. *PLoS One, 10*(6), e0131712–e0131718. https://doi.org/10.1371/journal.pone.0131712

van Sonsbeek, M. A. M. S., Hutschemaekers, G. J. M., Veerman, J. W., Kleinjan, M., Aarons, G. A., & Tiemens, B. G. (2015). Psychometric properties of the Dutch version of the evidence-based practice attitude scale (EBPAS). *Health Research Policy and Systems, 13*(69), 1–12. https://doi.org/10.1186/s12961-015-0058-z

Vis, C., Ruwaard, J., Finch, T. L., Rapley, T., de Beurs, D., van Stel, H., … Smit, J. (2019). Toward an objective assessment of implementation processes for innovations in health care: Psychometric evaluation of the normalization measure development (NoMAD) questionnaire among mental health care professionals. *Journal of Medical Internet Research, 21*(2), e12376–e12316. https://doi.org/10.2196/12376

Wallerstein, N., & Duran, B. (2010). Community-based participatory research contributions to intervention research: The intersection of science and practice to improve health equity. *American Journal of Public Health, 100*(S1), S40–S47. https://doi.org/10.2105/AJPH.2009

Waltz, T. J., Powell, B. J., Chinman, M. J., Smith, J. L., Matthieu, M. M., Proctor, E. K., … Kirchner, J. E. (2014). Expert recommendations for implementing change (ERIC): Protocol for a mixed methods study. *Implementation Science, 9*(39), 1–12.

Waltz, T. J., Powell, B. J., Fernandez, M. E., Abadie, B., & Damschroder, L. J. (2019). Choosing implementation strategies to address contextual barriers: Diversity in recommendations and future directions. *Implementation Science, 14*(1), 1–15. https://doi.org/10.1186/s13012-019-0892-4

Waltz, T. J., Powell, B. J., Matthieu, M. M., Damschroder, L. J., Chinman, M. J., Smith, J. L., … Kirchner, J. E. (2015). Use of concept mapping to characterize relationships among implementation strategies and assess their feasibility and importance: Results from the Expert Recommendations for Implementing Change (ERIC) study. *Implementation Science, 10*(1), 1–8. https://doi.org/10.1186/s13012-015-0295-0

Ward, V. (2017). Why, whose, what and how? A framework for knowledge mobilisers. *Evidence & Policy: a Journal of Research, Debate and Practice, 13*(3), 477–497. https://doi.org/10.133 2/174426416X14634763278725

Ward, V., House, A., & Hamer, S. (2009). Knowledge brokering: The missing link in the evidence to action chain? *Evidence & Policy: a Journal of Research, Debate and Practice, 5*(3), 267–279. https://doi.org/10.1332/174426409X463811

Watson, D. P., Adams, E. L., Shue, S., Coates, H., McGuire, A., Chesher, J., ... Omenka, O. I. (2018). Defining the external implementation context: An integrative systematic literature review. *BMC Health Services Research, 18*(1), 1–14. https://doi.org/10.1186/s12913-018-3046-5

Weatherley, R., & Lipsky, M. (1977). Street-level bureaucrats and institutional innovation: Implementing special-education reform. *Harvard Educational Review, 17*(2), 171–197.

Weiner, B. J. (2009). A theory of organizational readiness for change. *Implementation Science, 4*(1), 67. https://doi.org/10.1186/1748-5908-4-67

Weiner, B. J., Lewis, C. C., Stanick, C., Powell, B. J., Dorsey, C. N., Clary, A. S., ... Halko, H. (2017). Psychometric assessment of three newly developed implementation outcome measures. *Implementation Science, 12*(1), 65–13. https://doi.org/10.1186/s13012-017-0635-3

Weiner, B. J., Lewis, M. A., & Linnan, L. A. (2008). Using organization theory to understand the determinants of effective implementation of worksite health promotion programs. *Health Education Research, 24*(2), 292–305. https://doi.org/10.1093/her/cyn019

Welch, V., Jull, J., Petkovic, J., Armstrong, R., Boyer, Y., Cuervo, L. G., ... Tugwell. (2015). Protocol for the development of a CONSORT-equity guideline to improve reporting of health equity in randomized trials. *Implementation Science, 10*(146), 1–11. https://doi.org/10.1186/ s13012-015-0332-z

Welch, V. A., Norheim, O. F., Jull, J., Cookson, R., Sommerfelt, H., Tugwell, P., & CONSORT-Equity and Boston Equity Symposium. (2017). CONSORT-Equity 2017 extension and elaboration for better reporting of health equity in randomised trials. *British Medical Journal, 359*, j5085–j5014. https://doi.org/10.1136/bmj.j5085

Wensing, M., & Grol, R. (2019). Knowledge translation in health: How implementation science could contribute more. *Implementation Science, 17*(88), 1–6. https://doi.org/10.1186/ s12916-019-1322-9

Whelan, J., Love, P., Millar, L., Allender, S., & Bell, C. (2018). Sustaining obesity prevention in communities: A systematic narrative synthesis review. *Obesity Reviews, 19*(6), 839–851. https://doi.org/10.1111/obr.12675

White, H. (2018). Theory-based systematic reviews. *Journal of Development Effectiveness, 10*(1), 17–38. https://doi.org/10.1080/19439342.2018.1439078

Willging, C. E., Green, A. E., Gunderson, L. M., Chaffin, M. J., & Aarons, G. A. (2015). From a "Perfect Storm" to "Smooth Sailing": Policymaker perspectives on implementation and sustainment of an evidence-based practice in two states. *Child Maltreatment, 20*(1), 24–36. https:// doi.org/10.1177/1077559514547384

Williams, J., Sevdalis, N., & Gaughran, F. (2019). Evaluation of a Physical health plan for people with psychosis: a protocol for a quality improvement study, 1–9. https://doi.org/10.1186/ s40814-019-0396-7.

Williams, N. J., & Beidas, R. S. (2018). Annual research review: The state of implementation science in child psychology and psychiatry: A review and suggestions to advance the field. *Journal of Child Psychology and Psychiatry, 60*(4), 430–450. https://doi.org/10.1111/jcpp.12960

Williams, N. J., Glisson, C., Hemmelgarn, A., & Green, P. (2016). Mechanisms of change in the ARC organizational strategy: Increasing mental health clinicians' EBP adoption through improved organizational culture and capacity. *Administration and Policy in Mental Health and Mental Health Services Research*, 1–15. https://doi.org/10.1007/s10488-016-0742-5.

Willis, C. D., Riley, B. L., Stockton, L., Abramowicz, A., Zummach, D., Wong, G., ... Best, A. (2016). Scaling up complex interventions: Insights from a realist synthesis. *Health Research Policy and Systems, 14*(88), 1–16. https://doi.org/10.1186/s12961-016-0158-4

Wolfenden, L., Albers, B., & Shlonsky, A. (2018). Strategies for scaling up the implementation of interventions in social welfare: Protocol for a systematic review. *Campbell Systematic Reviews, 14*(1), 1–33.

Woltmann, E. M., Whitley, R., McHugo, G. J., Brunette, M., Torrey, W. C., Coots, L., ... Drake, R. E. (2008). The role of staff turnover in the implementation of evidence-based practices in mental health care. *Psychiatric Services, 59,* 732–737.

Woodward, E. N., Matthieu, M. M., Uchendu, U. S., Rogal, S., & Kirchner, J. E. (2019). The health equity implementation framework: Proposal and preliminary study of hepatitis C virus treatment. *Implementation Science, 14*(26), 1–18. https://doi.org/10.1186/s13012-019-0861-y

World Health Organization. (2009). *Practical guidance for scaling up health service innovations* (pp. 1–64). Geneva, Switzerland: World Health Organization.

Yapa, H. M., & Bärnighausen, T. (2018). Implementation science in resource-poor countries and communities. *Implementation Science, 13*(154), 1–13. https://doi.org/10.1186/s13012-018-0847-1

Chapter 2
CUTOS: A Framework for Contextualizing Evidence

Ariel M. Aloe, Christopher G. Thompson, and Deborah K. Reed

We always stress the need to first find evidence to figure out what we already know about a given problem rather than starting from scratch. This is one of the foundations of evidence-based practice. In education, as in many other fields, systematic reviews are being touted as the ultimate source for what the evidence says. Yet consumers of research often find it difficult to interpret and apply results from systematic reviews, even if they are of high quality. Unfortunately, there is little in the literature that tells us how to interpret the findings in the context of the research at hand, despite stressing the importance of doing so.

The CUTOS framework presented in this chapter provides a set of tools for disentangling what is known (and unknown) and a space to contemplate whether, which, and how findings are applicable. As such, it has the potential to support key steps identified as crucial to high-quality implementation, including determining what is known (i.e., what the evidence is) and how this knowledge applies to a specific context (population, organization, resources, etc.). Furthermore, the framework can be used as part of collaborative decision-making among multiple stakeholders involved in implementation processes.

A. M. Aloe (✉)
The University of Iowa, Iowa City, IA, USA
e-mail: ariel-aloe@uiowa.edu

C. G. Thompson
Texas A&M University, College Station, TX, USA

D. K. Reed
Iowa Reading Research Center, Iowa City, IA, USA

© Springer Nature Switzerland AG 2020
B. Albers et al. (eds.), *Implementation Science 3.0*,
https://doi.org/10.1007/978-3-030-03874-8_2

Introduction

When attempting to solve problems of practice, decision makers often are required to rely on previous studies that investigated the problem at hand and/or alternative solutions to the problem. Depending on the specific problem of practice, studies may have reported the effect of an intervention or program with a unique set of participants. Much has been written about issues of generalizing studies' findings in the social and health sciences, but little has been done to improve the applicability of primary studies' findings to related but different contexts or practices (Ercikan & Roth, 2014; Slavin, 2008). In this chapter, we propose a novel, systematic approach to contextualizing and appraising the results of previous studies. Although we rely on Cronbach's (1982) generalization framework, we apply this framework to establish the validity of research findings in a particular problem of practice.

School systems may struggle with a number of questions about how to help students be successful. *Is adopting a new curricular program beneficial to increasing student achievement? Is reducing class size beneficial to increasing students' academic achievement? Is the amount of homework assigned beneficial to increasing students' academic achievement? Is modifying the school calendar beneficial to increasing students' academic achievement?* These questions have one common theme: they attempt to inform decisions about the effectiveness of a program, intervention, or treatment. Previous research about these and other questions may exist, but assessing the quality and relevance of that evidence is usually a complex task. Many times, findings across different studies are contradictory, or those of individual studies might lack internal validity. Thus, in many disciplines, researchers rely on meta-analysis as a tool to synthesize empirical findings from multiple studies.

The term meta-analysis was coined by Glass (1976) to describe a statistical technique that combines the results of a series of studies addressing a common question. Results are typically transformed to the same metric and represented as effect sizes. Some use the term meta-analysis to signify the quantitative summaries used in a systematic review (also referred to as a research synthesis, research review, or quantitative review). A full discussion of systematic reviews and meta-analyses is outside of the scope of this manuscript, but other sources describe these in more detail (c.f., Cooper, Hedges, & Valentine, 2009; Higgins & Green, 2011). Although the framework and appraisal tool presented here can be used to contextualize evidence from primary studies, we recommended the use of them for evidence produced from meta-analytic studies.

This chapter is structured as follows. First, we distinguish between quality and relevance of the available evidence. Then, we briefly review the original UTOS framework before we introduce the CUTOS framework. Next, we discuss issues about relevant and irrelevant difference and then provide suggestions for how to use the framework and a corresponding tool to appraise evidence, including a heuristic application of the framework. We finalize our chapter with an illustration that applies the framework.

Quality vs Relevance of the Available Evidence

In many social sciences, it is common for researchers to be attuned to establishing internal and external validity (Campbell & Stanley, 1963; Cook & Campbell, 1979; Shadish, Cook, & Campbell, 2002). There is a long tradition of addressing threats to internal (e.g., selection bias, maturation, ambiguous temporal precedence of the intervention, attrition) and external validity (e.g., experimenter expectancy, compensatory rivalry, treatment diffusion) in primary studies. The basic idea is that if studies have high risk for threats to internal validity, there may be other reasons outside of the treatment responsible for producing the improvement of the measured outcome. If there are high risks for external validity, the findings of the given study may not be applicable to other subjects or settings outside of those in the study. In short, internal validity has to do with causality, and external validity has to do with generalization.

It is more common for the scientific community to focus on the quality of primary studies than their relevance. One example is apparent in the Cochrane Collaboration risk of bias tools for experimental and nonexperimental studies: the Grading of Recommendations Assessment, Development and Evaluation (GRADE working group, n.d.; Guyatt et al., 2011) and Methodological Expectations of Cochrane Intervention Reviews (MECIR; Chandler, Churchill, Higgins, Lasserson, & Tovey, 2013). There also are reporting statements such as Consolidated Standards of Reporting Trials (CONSORT; Schulz, Altman, and Moher, for the CONSORT Group, 2010), Transparent Reporting of Evaluations with Nonexperimental Design (TREND; Des Jarlais, Lyles, Crepaz, and the TREND Group, 2004), Preferred Reporting Items for Systematic Reviews and Meta-Analyses (PRISMA; Moher, Liberati, Tetzlaff, Altman, and the PRISMA Group, 2009), or Meta-analysis of Observational Studies in Epidemiology (MOOSE; Stroup et al., 2000). These tools are intended to ensure the rigor of the research. However, the fact that studies may be very well designed, analyzed, and reported does not guarantee that the evidence produced will be relevant for another context. Decision makers appear to be more concerned with the relevance of findings for their particular context (Innvaer, Vist, Trommald, & Oxman, 2002; Oliver, Innvar, Lorenc, Woodman, & Thomas, 2014).

Cronbach's UTOS

Generalization concerns whether and how findings from a particular population in a particular context can be extrapolated to different sets of participants and contexts (Campbell, 1986). Within program evaluation, Cronbach (1982) described a framework for the design and evaluation of studies, which has been proven useful for conceptualizing a wide variety of research studies (e.g., Becker, 1996). His original framework includes four elements: units, treatments, observing operations, and setting (UTOS).

Table 2.1 Relationship between UTOS and PICO frameworks

UTOS elements		PICO elements
U – unit	←——————————→	P – patient
T – treatment	←——————————→	I – intervention
O – observations	←	C – comparison
S – settings	—————————→	O – outcomes

Within this framework, units "U" refer to "the population of persons, sites, and so on about which a conclusion is sought" (1982, p. 78). "U" defines who the members of this population are. For studies of treatments, "T" defines what admissible treatment or intervention plans are. The curriculum implemented in a school setting is a form of treatment. Cronbach uses the example of curricular materials, workbooks, and lessons that may be implemented in different ways by the teachers using them.

"O" represents the plan for data collection or how data will be observed. Here, the researcher or evaluator would list the scales or instruments to be used or the interview questions that would be asked of participants. The theoretical definitions for constructs of interest, along with the operationalization of these, would constitute the "O." Finally, the setting "S" includes "the prevailing social attitudes, political divisions, economic context and so on" (1982, p. 79). These four elements are comparable to the elements of the Patient, Intervention, Comparison, and Outcomes framework (PICO) typically used in health science (e.g., Richardson, Wilson, Nishikawa, & Hayward, 1995), but some differences exist between UTOS and PICO (see Table 2.1). For instance, UTOS makes explicit the setting in which the evaluation takes place, and the setting arguably is implicitly considered in the PICO framework. Similarly, UTOS makes implicit the comparison intervention when this is stated explicitly in PICO.

The CUTOS Framework

When reporting and interpreting the results of their studies, it is common practice for researchers to make statements about probable implications for future research, practice, and policy. Typically, researchers' probable implications for practice and policy are suggestions, and no decision or action is immediately taken from them. Making suggestions is much easier and carries fewer consequences than making decisions. It is the practitioners and policymakers who must make decisions—decisions which hopefully are influenced by the accumulated evidence about the topic of interest. Even when a practitioner or a policymaker decides that there is not enough evidence to support a particular action and more evidence needs to be gathered before making a decision, the inaction is itself a form of decision. We argue for a truly synergistic collaboration between researcher and decision makers. Both researchers and decision makers bring skills and expertise that, when used properly, complement each other and should produce a better outcome. The framework and appraisal tool proposed here are intended to be used collaboratively by both researchers and decision makers for a specific context.

Distinguishing between external validity (can the results be generalized?), applicability (can this intervention be implemented elsewhere?), and transferability (can the results be replicated?) is a crucial step in assessing the relevance of empirical evidence (Burchett, Umoquit, & Dobrow, 2011). For some, transferability is synonymous with generalizability (e.g., Wang, Moss, & Hiller, 2005). But among other things, we argue that researchers are more concerned with generalizability while decision makers are more concerned with applicability and transferability.

In our framework, the same four elements (units, treatments, observing operations, and setting) of Cronbach's original framework are used but with exactly the reverse goal. We argue that, when solving problems of practice, the evidence used to support a decision must be systematically evaluated using the CUTOS framework, which adds a consideration of the research context (the "C") and sources of evidence. This new application of Cronbach's original framework attempts to answer a vital question of decision makers: "*Are the results of this study useful for me (within my practice)?*"

As depicted in Fig. 2.1, the CUTOS framework is positioned in the center to represent how it is affected by the different components.

We argue that the usefulness of evidence is anchored on the alignment between the specific context in which the intervention is going to be implemented and the context in which the evidence has been generated. Researchers and decision makers (stakeholders) play a crucial role in deciding the alignment between the specific representation of the elements (units, treatments, observing operations, and setting) represented in the evidence and in their particular context. Because researchers are typically more familiar with the evidence and stakeholders are typically more familiar with the context in which the program (or intervention) is going to be implemented, the goal of the framework is to build a synergistic cooperation between researchers and decision makers in assessing the alignment among the CUTOS elements. When deciding to implement a new program, explicit knowledge of how the characteristics of the new context align with the characteristics of the evidence is believed (at least in our framework) to aid in achieving the desired outcome.

Relevant and Irrelevant Differences

Interventions or implemented programs, as well as questions posed by researchers, typically represent values within a society because they target perceived concerns or areas that researchers believe need to be improved. The interventions occur in a particular context, and this may differ in many aspects, including but not limited to political and sociocultural characteristics. The intervention may be valued by some members of the society but present a conflict to the values of other members. For these and other reasons, it is important to carefully assess the relevancy among scenarios in which evidence and contexts differ. Moreover, differences in contexts may impact one or more of the UTOS elements (units, treatments, observations, and setting), as well as one or more of the features within a single element.

For example, consider the potential unit (U) characteristics that need to be assessed when determining whether to implement a new program for improving phonemic awareness or the ability to identify and manipulate the individual sounds in a word. The evidence for that intervention may have been gathered from a sample at the same grade level in which a school intends to implement the program, but perhaps the original program's effectiveness was studied with a group of children who have visual impairments. The school is planning to implement the intervention with children who may or may not have visual impairments. Because phonemic awareness relies solely on the ability to hear and produce sound, this specific difference between units is likely irrelevant in this case. However, the school still needs to determine whether there are other differences among the remaining unit features as well as the other elements of the UTOS framework (i.e., treatments, observations, and setting).

In many situations, distinguishing between relevant and irrelevant differences may not be a simple task (Cook, 1991). Ideally, one could rely on a variety of empirical evidence to conclude which characteristics of UTOS elements are relevant and irrelevant to a proposed context or application. Moderator and mediation analyses included in efficacy and effectiveness studies might be helpful in this

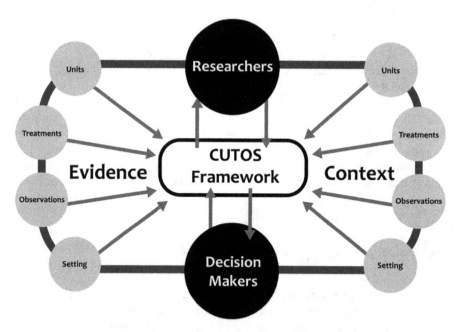

Fig. 2.1 The CUTOS framework. (Published with kind permission of © Ariel M. Aloe 2017. All Rights Reserved)

regard, but such analyses typically are exploratory and do not support making a casual inference. Thus, the interaction between researchers and decision makers is vital when deciding on evaluation components.

Applying the Framework

To aid the collaboration between researchers and decision makers when implementing this framework, we have developed an appraisal tool that contains the four UTOS framework elements (i.e., units, treatments, observations, and settings). Our intention is not only to acknowledge the potential diversity of the elements of UTOS but also to ensure the tool is accessible to a diverse group of researchers and decision makers. Researchers and decision makers can input specific characteristics of the UTOS elements and, then, score the individual items. By taking into account the different scores, users can make an overall decision about whether the research evidence is aligned to their intended application well enough to warrant implementing the intervention.

We developed an algorithm of recommended steps for researchers and decision makers to follow when applying this appraisal tool.

The steps are as follows (see Fig. 2.2):

1. *Locate empirical evidence.* We recommend that a literature search be conducted to identify the evidence of effectiveness for the specific intervention or program of interest. When multiple forms of empirical evidence are located, we suggest searching for a systematic review of the existing literature. If one is not located and time is not a major factor in the decision process, we suggest conducting a systematic review. In the example provided in the next section, we identified a meta-analysis on phonemic awareness (Ehri et al., 2001) as empirical evidence.

2. *Decide the sources of evidence relevant for each element of the CUTOS framework.* This step of the framework is designed to be truly a joint effort between researchers and decision makers. Both research and practical expertise can aid in determining what sources of evidence are relevant and irrelevant to a given application. For example, the gender of units may be relevant in one intervention but not another.

3. *Make a judgment about the alignment between the sources of evidence and the specific context in which the intervention or program is intended to be implemented.* In this step, both researchers and decision makers work collaboratively to score each one of the sources of evidence. The iteration of the appraisal tool provided here uses numerical values. However, in another version of the tool, we used color-coding schemes to avoid making unwarranted claims based on quantities given to a specific source of evidence. Thus, the example of the tool we provide in the section employs the number 3 for *mostly agree*, 2 for *somewhat agree*, 1 for *mostly disagree*, and NI for *no information*. The NI score is an important one. When the empirical evidence does not provide information about

a relevant element of UTOS, one cannot assume that there is or is not alignment. Also, bear in mind that scoring these elements is a somewhat subjective task in which judgment may play an important role. This is another reason (in addition to the different types of expertise) why we encourage the collaboration of researchers and decision makers in the scoring step.

4. *Give a rationale (i.e., a reason) for the score assigned to a particular source of evidence.* This step is arguably a part of the previous step, but because of its importance, we distinguish it as its own step. Using the comment section of the appraisal tool, justify scores given to each element of the framework. This information is particularly relevant when weighting the different elements of UTOS in the final step.

5. *Make a decision informed by the alignment of the sources of evidence.* Information in the appraisal tool should guide the decision-making process. Even in cases in which the appraisal tool is completed with more NI values than other scores, the tool remains valuable to making decisions based on the available and relevant evidence.

The appraisal tool might be better understood when anchored to a sample application of its use. We present such a scenario in the following section.

Example of CUTOS Appraisal Tool

In this section, we provide an example of the CUTOS appraisal tool using data from a study on phonemic awareness. Specifically, we used a beta version of the CUTOS appraisal tool, an open-source application designed to facilitate the use of this framework, to evaluate one of two meta-analyses (Ehri et al., 2001) to come from the alphabetics subgroup of the National Reading Panel (NICHD, 2000). The overall purpose of the meta-analysis was to examine the impact of phonemic awareness instruction on phonemic awareness, overall reading ability, and spelling outcomes. For the example in this chapter, we focus exclusively on the reading outcome, which combined measures of word reading, pseudo word reading, reading comprehension, oral text reading, reading speed, time to reach a criterion of learning, and miscues or errors made while reading aloud. Along with effect sizes, Ehri and colleagues coded five sets of moderator variables: outcome measures, characteristics of participants, properties of phonemic awareness instruction, features of the design, and

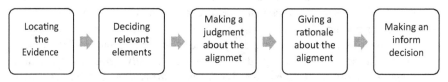

Fig. 2.2 Steps when appraising the alignment

characteristics of the study. Within each set are multiple characteristics, some continuous and others categorical. We incorporate several of these characteristics into the CUTOS appraisal tool.

In Ehri et al. (2001), a total of 96 standardized mean differences[1] were extracted from 52 experimental and quasi-experimental studies. The standardized mean difference was an appropriate effect size metric as tasks and outcomes used to assess children's phonemic awareness were heterogeneous. Effect sizes compared the difference of a treatment group receiving some sort of phonemic awareness instruction to a nonphonemic awareness or non-special instruction control group on the reading outcome. The statistically significant overall effect of $d = 0.53$ from the meta-analysis favored the phonemic awareness instruction treatment group. Although a significant overall effect was found, caution must be taken when linking policy decisions pertaining to specific school districts.

Data and moderators from Ehri et al. (2001) were compared to data from a large district in the state of Iowa, which we will refer to as District X, from the 2014 to 2015 school year.[2] This district was attempting to make decisions about the format and delivery of phonemic awareness instruction they should implement to improve students' reading abilities, so this example will highlight the applicability of the meta-analysis to this specific context. District X reading data were available for grades 3, 4, 5, 6, 7, 8, and 11, whereas studies in the meta-analysis included preschool, kindergarten, and grades 1–6. The primary interest in the implementation of the phonemic awareness instruction in District X was for students in grades 3, 4, 5, and 6 with reading disabilities. Moderators selected as sources of evidence and context as well as the judgment and the rationale are input in the CUTOS appraisal tool beta version in the respective panels for units, treatments, observations, and settings (see Table 2.2). The first step is entering the number of elements that will be needed to appraise the units (i.e., top of the panel). This will open as many spaces to input the labels of the elements (U elements, in this case), judgments, and the rationale for each judgment. In the next sections, we further discuss each of the rating score decisions.

Units Reading proficiency evidence from the Ehri et al. (2001) meta-analysis was classified as the number of effect sizes associated with students falling into the categories "At Risk," "Disabled," or "Normal Progress" as judged by a posttest immediately following the phonemic awareness intervention. District X provided the percentage of students in specific grade levels that were considered to be at a suitable level of reading performance. Because this was a binary variable (i.e., either a student was considered to be reading proficiently or they were not), we collapsed the "At Risk" and "Disabled" categories in the meta-analysis into a single category to represent "Insufficient Progress." Across the grade levels in District X's dataset,

---

[1] As mentioned in Ehri et al. (2001), some of the 96 effect sizes came from cases within studies that used the same treatment or control group more than once, thus creating multiple group dependency.

[2] All Iowa state data were publicly available from http://reports.educateiowa.gov/

an average of 29% of students were not reading proficiently, whereas the percentage of participants in the Ehri et al. meta-analysis categorized as exhibiting "Insufficient Progress" was 49%. It seems that there were only slightly fewer students with reading difficulties in District X than among the participants included in the meta-analysis. This may indicate decent alignment between the sampled studies and schools in District X, but caution is needed. As discussed next, the grade levels that were used to calculate these proficiencies were only somewhat aligned.

For the grade-level evidence, only a portion of the grades in the two datasets overlapped. The meta-analysis looked at studies including students in preschool through grade 6, while District X targeted the intervention for grades 3 through 6. The format of the district data separated achievement levels by individual grade level. Thus, we were able to look at mean achievement across the four grade levels by assessing average proficiency. On the other hand, data from the meta-analysis grouped grades 2, 3, 4, 5, and 6 together. The overall effect of the District X intervention for grades 3–6 cannot parcel out the effect, if any, of grade 2 as it is reported in the meta-analysis.

Similarly, the two datasets displayed differences by the socioeconomic status (SES) of the participants. Among the studies in the meta-analysis measuring reading outcomes and reporting SES, only 11 of 40 (28%) had "low" SES samples. Using the available data from District X, one possible proxy for "low" SES would be the percentage of participants receiving free or reduced-price lunch. Those students made up 72% of the participants, so the discrepancy between the meta-analysis and District X information is quite large in this respect. The average SES of study participants in the meta-analysis was considerably higher than the SES of students in District X.

In addition, District X provided several demographic variables (e.g., race, ethnicity). Unfortunately, these were not included in the meta-analysis. As a result, no comparisons on this source of evidence can be made.

Treatments Intervention and treatment characteristics in the meta-analysis had mixed alignment compared to District X. The delivery unit variable refers to whether an intervention was given to individual students, small groups, or whole classes. Given the focus on students with reading disabilities, District X would be implementing its phonemic awareness instruction to small groups of students in a supplemental intervention. However, only 42 of the 90 (47%) effect sizes in the meta-analysis used small-group instruction, indicating weak alignment between District X and the meta-analysis. Another unit variable consideration is the technology usage in the instruction, or whether or not the instruction will be computer-based. District X intended to use non-computer-based instruction. Rather, teachers would deliver all the lessons. Of the 90 reading outcome effects in the meta-analysis which also reported the technology usage, only 8 of those 90 (9%) used computers. This means that most (91%) of the outcomes were from non-computer-based instruction, in strong alignment with District X's plans.

Table 2.2 The CUTOS appraisal tool (sources of evidence and context, judgment, and rationale)

Sources of evidence and context	Judgments	Rationale
	Units	
Reading proficiency	Somewhat agree	District X has slightly higher levels of proficiency than studies in the meta-analysis.
Grade level	Somewhat agree	Meta-analysis does not separate grades 3–6, instead only reports grades 2–6 as a group.
Socioeconomic status	Mostly disagree	District X has almost three times the percentage of students with low SES as samples in meta-analysis.
Student demographics	No information	Meta-analysis does not provide information on school demographics (e.g., race, ethnicity).
	Treatments	
Delivery unit	Mostly disagree	Less than half the studies in the meta-analysis delivered interventions to small groups of students.
Technology usage	Mostly agree	Majority of studies in the meta-analysis use non-computer-based interventions.
Intervention delivery	Mostly disagree	Most studies in meta-analysis do not use trained classroom teachers to deliver intervention.
Length of instruction	Somewhat agree	For the most part, interventions in meta-analysis are no less than 5 hours in length.
	Observations	
Test type	Mostly disagree	Over half of studies in the meta-analysis do not use standardized tests.
Question type	No information	Meta-analysis does not provide information on question type (e.g., multiple choice, free response).
	Settings	
Study year	Mostly disagree	All studies in the meta-analysis were published prior to the year 2000.
School enrollment	No information	Meta-analysis does not provide information on average school enrollment.
School location	No information	Meta-analysis does not provide information on school location (e.g., urban, rural).

A related aspect of intervention delivery concerns whether the typical classroom teachers were responsible for delivering the intervention, or if other individuals (e.g., researchers, paraprofessionals) were actively implementing the intervention. Of the effect sizes in the meta-analysis which used immediate posttests of reading, only 22 of 90 (24%) had classroom teachers provide the phonemic awareness instruction. Because District X would be relying entirely upon trained classroom teachers delivering the intervention, poor alignment with the meta-analysis is present.

The last source of evidence for the treatments section is the length of the intervention, measured in hours. The phonemic awareness instruction in District X was anticipated to vary to some degree, but the expectation was that no less than 5 hours of instruction would be provided to students. This has fairly good alignment with studies in the meta-analysis, of which 80% of effect sizes came from interventions lasting five or more hours.

Observations Two sources of evidence were examined in the observations section: test type and question type. First, test type refers to whether the instrument used to obtain the reading outcome was standardized or created by researchers for a study. Looking specifically at studies in the meta-analysis which involved tests of word reading, 37 of 95 (39%) effect sizes were computed from standardized tests. Given that District X planned to administer only standardized assessments of students' reading development, we again do not see a good match between District X and the meta-analysis. The second observation source of evidence is question type. This variable refers to what sorts of questions (e.g., multiple choice, true/false, free response) were used to assess students' reading abilities. This particular variable was not discussed in the meta-analysis and, thus, alignment—or lack thereof—with District X cannot be inferred.

Settings Three variables were considered for the settings source of evidence: study year, school enrollment, and school location. All reading comprehension effect sizes in the meta-analysis were published prior to the year 2000, meaning that over a decade and a half has passed since the most recent study in the meta-analysis was published. Given the natural gap in time between data collection and publication, it is possible that even more time has elapsed. A stronger alignment between the meta-analysis and District X intervention would require more recent studies (i.e., more recent applications of the phonemic awareness interventions being considered) to be included in the meta-analysis.

The next setting source of evidence was school enrollment. This concerns the average student population of the individual schools in which the instruction is implemented or studied comparatively. Although the meta-analysis provided information on the average sample sizes receiving the interventions, there were no data on intervention and nonintervention school sizes in general. The final characteristic of the setting, and one that was of high importance to District X, was the school location (e.g., urban, rural). Unfortunately, information on this variable was not available from the meta-analysis and, thus, cannot be assessed for alignment with District X.

Considering all sources of evidence from the CUTOS appraisal tool as a whole, there was not particularly good agreement between implementation of the phonemic awareness instruction found in studies included in the meta-analysis and qualities of District X and its planned intervention. In this application of the CUTOS frameworks, the results from the meta-analysis on phonemic awareness instruction revealed the complexities of interpreting the practical implications of the studies. Despite the overall significant effect of the phonemic awareness instruction found in the collection of studies in the meta-analysis, there likely was not enough overlap in unit, treatment, observation, or setting qualities between the meta-analysis and District X. This lack of overlap means that results from the meta-analysis would not necessarily hold for District X.

Discussion

We presented a framework to systematically assess the relevance of empirical evidence for a particular context or application of an intervention. We based this framework on Cronbach's (1982) generalization framework, but we do not use this framework to make statements about the possible application of interventions or programs in other possible circumstances (i.e., to generalize results). Rather, we rely on the CUTOS framework appraisal tool as mechanisms for researchers and decision makers to work together as they systematically assess the level of alignment between existing empirical evidence and the particular context in which the stakeholders are interested.

We acknowledge that making decisions based on empirical evidence is not an easy task. However, we hope this framework and its associated tool facilitate collaborations between researchers and decision makers in addressing problems of practice and agreeing upon a common language for discussing the issues. We also hope this framework will aid researchers and decision makers in discriminating between relevant and irrelevant differences when considering the empirical evidence and the intended application of the intervention. Finally, and most importantly, we hope that this framework and its appraisal tool contribute to making better informed decisions capable of impacting people's lives in a positive manner.

References

Becker, B. J. (1996). The generalizability of empirical research results. In C. P. Benbow & D. Lubinski (Eds.), *Intellectual talent: Psychometric and social issues* (pp. 362–383). Baltimore, MD: Johns Hopkins Press.

Burchett, H., Umoquit, M., & Dobrow, M. (2011). How do we know when research from one setting can be useful in another? A review of external validity, applicability and transferability frameworks. *Journal of Health Services Research and Policy, 16*, 238–244. https://doi.org/10.1258/jhsrp.2011.010124

Campbell, D., & Stanley, J. (1963). *Experimental and quasi-experimental designs for research.* Chicago, IL: Rand-McNally.

Campbell, D. T. (1986). Relabeling internal and external validity for applied social scientists. *New Directions for Program Evaluation, 31*, 67–77. https://doi.org/10.1002/ev.1434

Chandler, J., Churchill, R., Higgins, J. P. T., Lasserson, T., & Tovey, D. (2013). *Methodological Expectations of Cochrane Intervention Reviews (MECIR).* Methodological standards for the conduct of new Cochrane Intervention Reviews.

Cook, T. D. (1991). Meta-analysis: Its potential for causal description and causal explanation within program evaluation. In G. Albrecht, H. U. Otto, S. Karstedt-Henke, & K. Bollert (Eds.), *Social prevention and the social sciences: Theoretical controversies, research problems and evaluation strategies.*

Cook, T. D., & Campbell, D. T. (1979). *Quasi-experimentation: Design and analysis issues for field settings.* Boston, MA: Houghton Mifflin Company.

Cooper, H. M., Hedges, L. V., & Valentine, J. (2009). *The handbook of research synthesis and meta-analysis* (2nd ed.). New York, NY: The Russell Sage Foundation.

Cronbach, L. J. (1982). *Designing evaluations of educational and social programs*. San Francisco, CA: Jossey-Bass.

Des Jarlais, D. C., Lyles, C., Crepaz, N., & the TREND Group. (2004). Improving the reporting quality of nonrandomized evaluations of behavioral and public health interventions: The TREND statement. *American Journal of Public Health, 94*, 361–366. https://doi.org/10.2105/ajph.94.3.361

Ehri, L. C., Nunes, S. R., Willows, D. M., Schuster, B. V., Yaghoub-Zadeh, Z., & Shanahan, T. (2001). Phonemic awareness instruction helps children learn to read: Evidence from the National Reading Panel's meta-analysis. *Reading Research Quarterly, 36*(3), 250–287. https://doi.org/10.1598/RRQ.36.3.2

Ercikan, K., & Roth, W.-M. (2014). Limits of generalizing in education research: Why criteria for research generalization should include population heterogeneity and uses of knowledge claims. *Teachers College Record, 116*, 1–28.

Glass, G. V. (1976). Primary, secondary, and meta-analysis of research. *Educational Researcher, 5*(10), 3–8. https://doi.org/10.3102/0013189X005010003.

GRADE working group. (n.d.). *Organizations that have endorsed or that are using GRADE*. Available from: www.gradeworkinggroup.org

Guyatt, G., Oxman, A. D., Akl, E. A., Kunz, R., Vist, G., Brozek, J., … Schunemann, H. J. (2011). GRADE guidelines: 1. Introduction-GRADE evidence profiles and summary of findings tables. *Journal of Clinical Epidemiology, 64*, 383–394. https://doi.org/10.1016/j.jclinepi.2010.04.026

Higgins, J. P. T., & Green, S. (2011). *Cochrane handbook for systematic reviews of interventions*. Retrieved from www.cochrane-handbook.org

Innvaer, S. S., Vist, G. G., Trommald, M. M., & Oxman, A. A. (2002). Health policy-makers' perceptions of their use of evidence: A systematic review. *Journal of Health Services Research and Policy, 7*, 239–244. https://doi.org/10.1258/135581902320432778

Moher, D., Liberati, A., Tetzlaff, J., Altman, D. G., & the PRISMA Group. (2009). Preferred reporting items for systematic reviews and meta-analysis: The PRISMA statement. *Physical Therapy, 89*, 873–880. https://doi.org/10.1093/ptj/89.9.873

National Institute of Child Health and Human Development (NICHD). (2000). *Report of the National Reading Panel. Teaching children to read: An evidence-based assessment of the scientific research literature on reading and its implications for reading instruction: Reports of the subgroups (NIH Publication No. 00-4754)*. Washington, DC: U.S. Government Printing Office.

Oliver, K., Innvar, S. S., Lorenc, T., Woodman, J., & Thomas, J. (2014). A systematic review of barriers to and facilitators of the use of evidence by policymakers. *BMC Health Services Research, 14*(2), 1–12. https://doi.org/10.1186/1472-6963-14-2

Richardson, W. S., Wilson, M. C., Nishikawa, J., & Hayward, R. S. A. (1995). The well-built clinical question: A key to evidence-based decisions. *ACP Journal Club, 123*, A-12. https://doi.org/10.7326/ACPJC-1005-123-3-A12.

Schulz, K. F., Altman, D. G., Moher, D., & the CONSORT Group. (2010). CONSORT 2010 statement: Updated guidelines for reporting parallel group randomized trials. *Annals of Internal Medicine, 152*, 726–732.

Shadish, W. R., Cook, T. D., & Campbell, D. T. (2002). *Experimental and quasi-experimental design for generalized causal inference*. Boston, MA: Houghton-Mifflin.

Slavin, R. (2008). Perspectives on evidence-based research in education—What works? Issues in synthesizing educational program evaluation. *Educational Researcher, 37*(1), 5–14. https://doi.org/10.3102/0013189x08314117

Stroup, D. F., Berlin, J. A., Morton, S. C., Olkin, I., Williamson, G. D., Rennie, D., … Thacker, S. B. (2000). Meta-analysis of observational studies in epidemiology: A proposal for reporting. *Journal of the American Medical Association, 283*, 2008–2012. https://doi.org/10.1001/jama.283.15.2008

Wang, S., Moss, J. R., & Hiller, J. E. (2005). Applicability and transferability of interventions in evidence-based public health. *Health Promotion International, 12*, 76–83. https://doi.org/10.1186/1472-6963-14-61

Chapter 3
Making Sense of Implementation Theories, Models, and Frameworks

Per Nilsen

Introduction

Implementation science was born out of a desire to address challenges associated with the use of research to achieve more evidence-based practice (EBP) in health care and other areas of professional practice. Early implementation research was empirically driven and did not always pay attention to the theoretical underpinnings of implementation. Eccles, Grimshaw, Walker, Johnston and Pitts (2005, p. 108) remarked that this research seemed like "an expensive version of trial-and-error". A review of guideline implementation strategies by Davies, Walker and Grimshaw (2003) noted that only 10% of the studies identified provided an explicit rationale for their strategies. Mixed results of implementing EBP in various settings were often attributed to a limited theoretical basis (Davies et al., 2003; Eccles et al., 2005; Kitson, Harvey, & McCormack, 1998; Michie et al., 2005; Sales, Smith, Curran, & Kochevar, 2006). Poor theoretical underpinning makes it difficult to understand and explain how and why implementation succeeds or fails, thus restraining opportunities to identify factors that predict the likelihood of implementation success and develop better strategies to achieve more successful implementation.

However, the last decade of implementation science has seen wider recognition of the need to establish the theoretical bases of implementation and strategies to facilitate implementation. There is mounting interest in the use of theories, models and frameworks to gain insights into the mechanisms by which implementation is

P. Nilsen (✉)
Linköping University, Linköping, Sweden
e-mail: per.nilsen@liu.se

© Springer Nature Switzerland AG 2020
B. Albers et al. (eds.), *Implementation Science 3.0*,
https://doi.org/10.1007/978-3-030-03874-8_3

more likely to succeed. Implementation studies now apply theories borrowed from disciplines such as psychology, sociology and organizational theory as well as theories, models and frameworks that have emerged from within implementation science. There are now so many theoretical approaches that some researchers have complained about the difficulties of choosing the most appropriate (Cane, O'Connor, & Michie, 2012; Godin, Bélanger-Gravel, Eccles, & Grimshaw, 2008; ICEBeRG, 2006; Martinez, Lewis, & Weiner, 2014; Mitchell, Fisher, Hastings, Silverman, & Wallen, 2010; Rycroft-Malone & Bucknall, 2010a).

This chapter seeks to further implementation science by providing a narrative review of the theories, models and frameworks applied in this research field. The aim is to describe and analyze how theories, models and frameworks have been applied in implementation science and propose a taxonomy that distinguishes between different approaches to advance clarity and achieve a common terminology. The ambition is to facilitate appropriate selection and application of relevant approaches in implementation studies and foster cross-disciplinary dialogue among implementation researchers. The importance of a clarifying taxonomy has evolved during the many discussions on theoretical approaches used within implementation science that the author has had over the past few years with fellow implementation researchers, as well as reflection on the utility of different approaches in various situations.

Implementation science is defined as the scientific study of methods to promote the systematic uptake of research findings and other EBPs into routine practice to improve the quality and effectiveness of health services and care (Eccles & Mittman, 2006). The terms knowledge translation, knowledge exchange, knowledge transfer, knowledge integration and research utilization are used to describe overlapping and interrelated research on putting various forms of knowledge, including research, to use (Estabrooks, Thompson, Lovely, & Hofmeyer, 2006; Graham et al., 2006; Mitchell et al., 2010; Rabin & Brownson, 2012; Wilson, Brady, & Lesesne, 2011). Implementation is part of a diffusion-dissemination-implementation continuum: diffusion is the passive, untargeted and unplanned spread of new practices; dissemination is the active spread of new practices to the target audience using planned strategies; and implementation is the process of putting to use or integrating new practices within a setting (Greenhalgh, Robert, Bate, Macfarlane, & Kyriakidou, 2005; Rabin & Brownson, 2012).

A narrative review of selective literature was undertaken to identify key theories, models and frameworks used in implementation science. The narrative review approach gathers information about a particular subject from many sources and is considered appropriate for summarizing and synthesizing the literature to draw conclusions about "what we know" about the subject. Narrative reviews yield qualitative results, with strengths in capturing diversities and pluralities of understanding (Cronin, Ryan, & Coughlan, 2008; Jones, 2004). Six textbooks that provide comprehensive overviews of research regarding implementation science and implementation of EBP were consulted: Rycroft-Malone and Bucknall (2010c), Nutley, Walter, and Davies (2007), Greenhalgh et al. (2005), Grol, Wensing and Eccles (2005), Straus, Tetroe and Graham (2009), and Brownson, Colditz, and Proctor (2012). A few papers presenting overviews of theories, models and frameworks used in implementation science were also used: Estabrooks et al. (2006), Sales et al.

(2006), Graham and Tetroe (2007), Mitchell et al. (2010), Flottorp et al. (2013), Meyers, Durlak, and Wandersman (2012), and Tabak, Khoong, Chambers and Brownson (2012). In addition, *Implementation Science* (first published in 2006) was searched using the terms "theory", "model" and "framework" to identify relevant articles. The titles and abstracts of the identified articles were scanned, and those that were relevant to the study aim were read in full.

Overview of Theoretical Approaches

Theories, Models, and Frameworks in the General Literature

Generally, a theory may be defined as a set of analytical principles or statements designed to structure our observation, understanding and explanation of the world (Carpiano, 2006; Frankfort-Nachmias & Nachmias, 1996; Wacker, 1998). Authors usually point to a theory as being made up of definitions of variables, a domain where the theory applies, a set of relationships between the variables and specific predictions (Bunge, 1967; Dubin, 1969; Hunt, 1991; Reynolds, 1971). A "good theory" provides a clear explanation of how and why specific relationships lead to specific events. Theories can be described on an abstraction continuum. High-abstraction-level theories (general or grand theories) have an almost unlimited scope, middle-abstraction-level theories explain limited sets of phenomena and lower-level abstraction theories are empirical generalizations of limited scope and application (Bluedorn & Evered, 1980; Wacker, 1998).

A model typically involves a deliberate simplification of a phenomenon or a specific aspect of a phenomenon. Models need not be completely accurate representations of reality to have value (Cairney, 2012; Carpiano, 2006). Models are closely related to theory, and the difference between a theory and a model is not always clear. Models can be described as theories with a more narrowly defined scope of explanation; a model is descriptive, whereas a theory is explanatory as well as descriptive (Frankfort-Nachmias & Nachmias, 1996).

A framework usually denotes a structure, overview, outline, system or plan consisting of various descriptive categories, e.g., concepts, constructs or variables and the relations between them that are presumed to account for a phenomenon (Sabatier, 1999). Frameworks do not provide explanations; they only describe empirical phenomena by fitting them into a set of categories (Frankfort-Nachmias & Nachmias, 1996).

Theories, Models and Frameworks in Implementation Science

It was possible to identify three overarching aims of the use of theories, models and frameworks in implementation science: (1) describing and/or guiding the process of translating research into practice, (2) understanding and/or explaining what influences implementation outcomes and (3) evaluating implementation. Theoretical approaches which aim at understanding and/or explaining influences on implementation outcomes (i.e., the second aim) can be further broken down into determinant frameworks, classic theories and implementation theories based on descriptions of their origins, how they were developed, what knowledge sources they drew on, stated aims and applications in implementation science. Thus, five categories of theoretical approaches used in implementation science can be delineated (Fig. 3.1, Table 3.1):

- Process models
- Determinant frameworks
- Classic theories
- Implementation theories
- Evaluation frameworks

Although theories, models, and frameworks are distinct concepts, the terms are sometimes used interchangeably in implementation science (Estabrooks et al., 2006; Kitson et al., 2008; Rycroft-Malone & Bucknall, 2010a). A theory in this field usually implies some predictive capacity (e.g., to what extent do health care practitioners' attitudes and beliefs concerning a clinical guideline predict their adherence to this guideline in clinical practice?) and attempts to explain the causal mechanisms of implementation. Models in implementation science are commonly used to describe and/or guide the process of translating research into practice (i.e. "implementation practice") rather than to predict or analyze what factors influence implementation outcomes (i.e., "implementation research"). Frameworks in implementation science often have a descriptive purpose by pointing to factors

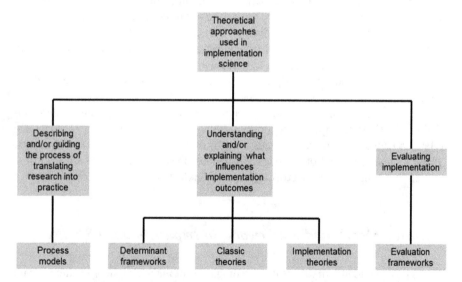

Fig. 3.1 Three aims of the use of theoretical approaches in implementation science and the five categories of theories, models, and frameworks

Table 3.1 Five categories of theories, models, and frameworks used in implementation science

Category	Description	Examples
Process models	Specify steps (stages, phases) in the process of translating research into practice, including the implementation and use of research. The aim of process models is to describe and/or guide the process of translating research into practice. An action model is a type of process model that provides practical guidance in the planning and execution of implementation endeavours and/or implementation strategies to facilitate implementation. Note that the terms "model" and "framework" are both used, but the former appears to be the most common.	Model by Huberman (1994); model by Landry, Amara, and Lamari (2001); model by Davies, Peterson, Helfrich and Cunningham-Sabo (2007); model by Majdzadeh, Sadighi, Nejat, Mahani, and Gholami (2008); the CIHR Model of Knowledge Translation (Canadian Institutes of Health Research, 2014); the K2A Framework; the Stetler Model (Stetler, 2010); the ACE Star Model of Knowledge Transformation (Stevens, 2013); the Knowledge-to-Action Model (Graham et al., 2006); the Iowa Model (Titler et al., 1994, 2001); the Ottawa Model (Logan & Graham, 1998, 2010); model by Grol and Wensing (2004); model by Pronovost, Berenholtz and Needham, (2008); the Quality Implementation Framework (Meyers et al., 2012)
Determinant frameworks	Specify types (also known as classes or domains) of determinants and individual determinants, which act as barriers and enablers (independent variables) that influence implementation outcomes (dependent variables). Some frameworks also specify relationships between some types of determinants. The overarching aim is to understand and/or explain influences on implementation outcomes, e.g., predicting outcomes or interpreting outcomes retrospectively.	PARIHS (Kitson et al., 1998; Rycroft-Malone, 2010), Active Implementation Frameworks (Blasé, Van Dyke, Fixsen, & Bailey, 2012), Understanding User Context Framework, Conceptual Model, framework by Grol et al. (2005), framework by Cochrane et al. (2007), framework by Nutley et al. (2007), Ecological Framework by Durlak and DuPre (2008), CFIR (Damschroder et al., 2009), framework by Gurses et al. (2010), framework by Ferlie and Shortell (2001), Theoretical Domains Framework (Michie, Atkins, & West, 2014)
Classic theories	Theories that originate from fields external to implementation science, e.g., psychology, sociology and organizational theory, which can be applied to provide understanding and/or explanation of aspects of implementation.	Theory of Diffusion (Rogers, 2003), social cognitive theories, theories concerning cognitive processes and decision-making, social networks theories, social capital theories, communities of practice, professional theories, organizational theories

(continued)

Table 3.1 (continued)

Category	Description	Examples
Implementation theories	Theories that have been developed by implementation researchers (from scratch or by adapting existing theories and concepts) to provide understanding and/or explanation of aspects of implementation.	Implementation Climate (Klein & Sorra, 1996), Absorptive Capacity (Zahra & George, 2002), Organizational Readiness (Weiner, 2009), COM-B (Michie, Stralen, & West, 2011), Normalization Process Theory (May & Finch, 2009)
Evaluation frameworks	Specify aspects of implementation that could be evaluated to determine implementation success.	RE-AIM (Glasgow, Vogt, & Boles, 1999), PRECEDE-PROCEED (Green, Kreuter, & Green, 2005), framework by Proctor et al. (2010)

ACE Academic Center for Evidence-Based Practice, *CFIR* Consolidated Framework for Implementation Research, *CIHR* Canadian Institutes of Health Research Knowledge, *COM-B* Capacity-Opportunities-Motivation-Behaviour, *Conceptual Model* Conceptual Model for Considering the Determinants of Diffusion, Dissemination and Implementation of Innovations in Health Service Delivery and Organization (full title), *K2A* Knowledge-to-Action, *PARIHS* Promoting Action on Research Implementation in Health Services, *PRECEDE-PROCEED* Predisposing, Reinforcing and Enabling Constructs in Educational Diagnosis and Evaluation-Policy, Regulatory and Organizational Constructs in Educational and Environmental Development, *RE-AIM* Reach, Effectiveness, Adoption, Implementation, Maintenance

believed or found to influence implementation outcomes (e.g., health care practitioners' adoption of an evidence-based patient intervention). Neither models nor frameworks specify the mechanisms of change; they are typically more like checklists of factors relevant to various aspects of implementation.

Describing and/or Guiding the Process of Translating Research into Practice

Process Models

Process models are used to describe and/or guide the process of translating research into practice. Models by Huberman (1994), Landry et al. (2001), the CIHR (Canadian Institutes of Health Research, 2014), Knowledge Model of Knowledge Translation (Davis et al., 2007; Majdzadeh et al., 2008) and the K2A (Knowledge-to-Action) Framework (Wilson et al., 2011) outline phases or stages of the research-to-practice process, from discovery and production of research-based knowledge to implementation and use of research in various settings.

Early research-to-practice (or Knowledge-to-Action) models tended to depict rational, linear processes in which research was simply transferred from producers to users. However, subsequent models have highlighted the importance of facilitation to support the process and placed more emphasis on the contexts in which research is implemented and used. Thus, the attention has shifted from a focus on production, diffusion and dissemination of research to various implementation aspects (Nutley et al., 2007).

So-called action (or planned action) models are process models that facilitate implementation by offering practical guidance in the planning and execution of implementation endeavours and/or implementation strategies. Action models elucidate important aspects that need to be considered in implementation practice and usually prescribe a number of stages or steps that should be followed in the process of translating research into practice. Action models have been described as active by Graham et al. (2009, p. 185) because they are used "to guide or cause change". It should be noted that the terminology is not fully consistent as some of these models are referred to as frameworks, for instance, the Knowledge-to-Action Framework (Rycroft-Malone & Bucknall, 2010b).

Many of the action models originate from the nursing-led field of research use/ utilization; well-known examples include the Stetler Model (Stetler, 2010), the ACE (Academic Center for Evidence-Based Practice) Star Model of Knowledge Transformation (Stevens, 2013), the Knowledge-to-Action Framework (Graham et al., 2006), the Iowa Model (Titler et al., 1994, 2001) and the Ottawa Model (Logan & Graham, 1998, 2010). There are also numerous examples of similar "how-to-implement" models that have emerged from other fields, including models developed by Grol and Wensing (2004), Pronovost et al. (2008) and the Quality Implementation Framework (Meyers et al., 2012), all of which are intended to provide support for planning and managing implementation endeavours.

The how-to-implement models typically emphasize the importance of careful, deliberate planning, especially in the early stages of implementation endeavours. In many ways, they present an ideal view of implementation practice as a process that proceeds stepwise, in an orderly, linear fashion. Still, authors behind most models emphasize that the actual process is not necessarily sequential. Many of the action models mentioned here have been subjected to testing or evaluation, and some have been widely applied in empirical research, underscoring their usefulness (Field, Booth, Ilott, & Gerrish, 2014; Rycroft-Malone & Bucknall, 2010a).

The process models vary with regard to how they were developed. Models such as the Stetler Model (Stetler, 1994, 2010) and the Iowa Model (Titler et al., 1994, 2001) were based on the originators' own experiences of implementing new practices in various settings (although they were also informed by research and expert opinion). In contrast, models such as the Knowledge-to-Action Framework (Graham et al., 2009) and the Quality Implementation Framework (Meyers et al., 2012) have relied on literature reviews of theories, models, frameworks and individual studies to identify key features of successful implementation endeavours.

Understanding and Explaining What Influences Implementation Outcomes

Determinant Frameworks

Determinant frameworks describe general types (also referred to as classes or domains) of determinants that are hypothesized or have been found to influence implementation outcomes, e.g., health care professionals' behaviour change or adherence to a clinical guideline. Each type of determinant typically comprises a number of individual barriers (hinders, impediments) and/or enablers (facilitators), which are seen as independent variables that have an impact on implementation outcomes, i.e., the dependent variable. Some frameworks also hypothesize relationships between these determinants (e.g., Durlak & Dupre, 2008; Greenhalgh et al., 2005; Gurses et al., 2010), whereas others recognize such relationships without clarifying them (e.g., Cochrane et al., 2007; Damschroder et al., 2009). Information about what influences implementation outcomes is potentially useful for designing and executing implementation strategies that aim to change relevant determinants.

The determinant frameworks do not address how change takes place or any causal mechanisms, underscoring that they should not be considered theories. Many frameworks are multilevel, identifying determinants at different levels, from the individual user or adopter (e.g., health care practitioners) to the organization and beyond. Hence, these integrative frameworks recognize that implementation is a multidimensional phenomenon, with multiple interacting influences.

The determinant frameworks were developed in different ways. Many frameworks (e.g., Cochrane et al., 2007; Durlak & Dupre, 2008; Ferlie & Shortell, 2001; Greenhalgh et al., 2005; Grol et al., 2005; Nutley et al., 2007) were developed by synthesizing results from empirical studies of barriers and enablers for implementation success. Other frameworks have relied on existing determinant frameworks and relevant theories in various disciplines, e.g., the frameworks by Gurses et al. (2010) and CFIR (Consolidated Framework for Implementation Research) (Damschroder et al., 2009).

Several frameworks have drawn extensively on the originator's own experiences of implementing new practices. For instance, the Understanding User Context Framework (Jacobson, Butterill, & Goering, 2003) and Active Implementation Frameworks (Blasé et al., 2012) were both based on a combination of literature reviews and the originators' implementation experiences. Meanwhile, PARIHS (Promoting Action on Research Implementation in Health Services) (Kitson et al., 1998; Rycroft-Malone, 2010) emerged from the observation that successful implementation in health care might be premised on three key determinants (characteristics of the evidence, context and facilitation), a proposition which was then analyzed in four empirical case studies; PARIHS has subsequently undergone substantial research and development work (Rycroft-Malone, 2010) and has been widely applied (Helfrich et al., 2010).

Theoretical Domains Framework represents another approach to developing determinant frameworks. It was constructed on the basis of a synthesis of 128 constructs related to behaviour change found in 33 behaviour change theories, including many social cognitive theories (Cane et al., 2012). The constructs are sorted into 14 theoretical domains (originally 12 domains), e.g., knowledge, skills, intentions, goals, social influences and beliefs about capabilities (Michie et al., 2014). Theoretical Domains Framework does not specify the causal mechanisms found in the original theories, thus sharing many characteristics with determinant frameworks.

The determinant frameworks account for five types of determinants, as shown in Table 3.2 which provides details of eight of the most commonly cited frameworks in implementation science. The frameworks are superficially quite disparate, with a broad range of terms, concepts and constructs as well as different outcomes, yet they are quite similar with regard to the general types of determinants they account for. Hence, implementation researchers agree to a large extent on what the main influences on implementation outcomes are, albeit to a lesser extent on which terms that are best used to describe these determinants.

The frameworks describe "implementation objects" in terms of research, guidelines, interventions, innovations and evidence (i.e., research-based knowledge in a broad sense). Outcomes differ correspondingly, from adherence to guidelines and research use to successful implementation of interventions, innovations, evidence, etc. (i.e., the application of research-based knowledge in practice). The relevance of the end users (e.g., patients, consumers or community populations) of the implemented object (e.g., an EBP) is not explicitly addressed in some frameworks (e.g., Fixsen, Naoom, Blasé, Friedman, & Wallace, 2005; Greenhalgh et al., 2005; Nutley et al., 2007), suggesting that this is an area where further research is needed for better analysis of how various end users may influence implementation effectiveness.

Determinant frameworks imply a systems approach to implementation because they point to multiple levels of influence and acknowledge that there are relationships within and across the levels and different types of determinants. A system can be understood only as an integrated whole because it is composed not only of the sum of its components but also by the relationships among those components (Holmes, Finegood, Riley, & Best, 2012). However, determinants are often assessed individually in implementation studies (e.g., Broyles et al., 2012; Johnson, Jackson, Guillaume, Meier, & Goyder, 2010; Légaré, Ratté, Gravel, & Graham, 2008; Verweij et al., 2012), (implicitly) assuming a linear relationship between the determinants and the outcomes and ignoring that individual barriers and enablers may interact in various ways that can be difficult to predict. For instance, there could be synergistic effects such that two seemingly minor barriers constitute an important obstacle to successful outcomes if they interact. Another issue is whether all relevant barriers and enablers are examined in these studies, which are often based on survey questionnaires, and are thus biased by the researcher's selection of determinants. Surveying the perceived importance of a finite set of predetermined barriers can yield insights into the relative importance of these particular barriers but may overlook factors that independently affect implementation outcomes. Furthermore, there is the issue of whether the barriers and enablers are the actual determinants

Table 3.2 Implementation determinants and outcomes in eight determinant frameworks

	Characteristics of the implementation object	Characteristics of the users/adopters (e.g., health care practitioners)	Characteristics of the end users (e.g., patients)	Characteristics of the context	Characteristics of the strategy or other means of facilitating implementation	Outcomes
PARIHS (Kitson et al., 1998; Rycroft-Malone, 2010)	Characteristics of the evidence	Characteristics of the clinical experience (addressed as an aspect of the evidence element)	Characteristics of the patient experience (addressed as an aspect of evidence element)	Characteristics of the context (comprising culture, leadership and evaluation)	Characteristics of the facilitation, i.e., the process of enabling or making easier the implementation	Successful implementation of research
Conceptual Model (Greenhalgh et al., 2005)	Innovation attributes	Aspects of adopters (e.g., psychological antecedents and nature of the adoption decision) and assimilation by organizations	Not addressed	Features of the inner context (organizational antecedents and organizational readiness for innovation) and outer context (e.g., informal interorganizational networks and political directives)	Influences (e.g., opinion leaders, champions and network structure) lying on a continuum from diffusion to dissemination	Successful diffusion, dissemination and implementation of innovations
Grol et al. (2005)	Features of the innovation	Features of the professionals who should use the innovation	Features of the patients	Features of the social setting (e.g., attitudes of colleagues, culture and leadership) and of the economic, administrative and organizational context	Features of the methods and strategies for dissemination and implementation used	Implementation of new evidence, guidelines and best practices or procedures

	Characteristics of the implementation object	Characteristics of the users/adopters (e.g., health care practitioners)	Characteristics of the end users (e.g., patients)	Characteristics of the context	Characteristics of the strategy or other means of facilitating implementation	Outcomes
Nutley et al. (2007)	Nature of the research to be applied	Personal characteristics of researchers and potential research users and links between research and its users	Not addressed	Context for the use of research	Strategies to improve the use of research	Use of research
Cochrane et al. (2007)	Guidelines and evidence barriers	Cognitive and behavioural barriers, attitudinal and rational-emotional barriers, health care professional and physician barriers	Patient barriers	Support and resource barriers, system and process barriers	Not addressed	Adherence to guidelines or implementation of evidence into clinical practice
Ecological Framework (Durlak & Dupre, 2008)	Characteristics of the innovation	Provider characteristics	Not addressed	Community-level factors (comprising of general organizational features, specific organizational practices and processes and specific staffing considerations)	Features of the prevention support system (comprising of training and technical assistance)	Successful implementation of innovations

(continued)

Table 3.2 (continued)

	Characteristics of the implementation object	Characteristics of the users/adopters (e.g., health care practitioners)	Characteristics of the end users (e.g., patients)	Characteristics of the context	Characteristics of the strategy or other means of facilitating implementation	Outcomes
CFIR (Damschroder et al., 2009)	Intervention characteristics	Characteristics of individuals	Patient needs and resources (addressed as an aspect of the outer setting)	Characteristics of the inner setting (e.g., structural characteristics, networks and communications, culture) and outer setting (e.g., cosmopolitanism, external policies and incentives)	Effectiveness of process by which implementation is accomplished (comprising of planning, engaging, executing, reflection and evaluating)	Successful implementation of interventions
Gurses et al. (2010)	Guideline characteristics	Clinician characteristics	Not addressed	Systems characteristics (e.g., physical environment, organizational characteristics) and implementation characteristics (e.g., tension for change and getting ideas from outside the organization)	Implementation characteristics (e.g., change agents' characteristics, relative strengths of supporters and opponents)	Adherence to guidelines

Conceptual Model Conceptual Model for Considering the Determinants of Diffusion, Dissemination and Implementation of Innovations in Health Service Delivery and Organization (full title, Greenhalgh et al., 2005), *CFIR* Consolidated Framework for Implementation Research, *PARIHS* Promoting Action on Research Implementation in Health Services (i.e., whether they have actually been experienced or encountered) and the extent to which they are perceived to exist (i.e., they are more hypothetical barriers and enablers). The perceived importance of particular factors may not always correspond with the actual importance.

The context is an integral part of all the determinant frameworks. Described as "an important but poorly understood mediator of change and innovation in health care organizations" (Dopson & Fitzgerald, 2005, p. 79), the context lacks a unifying definition in implementation science (and related fields such as organizational behaviour and quality improvement). Still, context is generally understood as the conditions or surroundings in which something exists or occurs, typically referring to an analytical unit that is higher than the phenomena directly under investigation. The role afforded the context varies from studies (e.g., Ashton et al., 2007; Mohr, Lukas, & Meterko, 2008; Scott, Plotnikoff, Karunamuni, Bize, & Rodgers, 2008; Zardo & Collie, 2014) that essentially view the context in terms of a physical "environment or setting in which the proposed change is to be implemented" (Kitson et al., 1998, p. 150) to studies (e.g., Ashton et al., 2007; Gabbay, 2004; Nutley et al., 2007) that assume that the context is something more active and dynamic that greatly affects the implementation process and outcomes. Hence, although implementation science researchers agree that the context is a critically important concept for understanding and explaining implementation, there is a lack of consensus regarding how this concept should be interpreted, in what ways the context is manifested and the means by which contextual influences might be captured in research.

The different types of determinants specified in determinant frameworks can be linked to classic theories. Thus, psychological theories that delineate factors influencing individual behaviour change are relevant for analyzing how user/adopter characteristics affect implementation outcomes, whereas organizational theories concerning organizational climate, culture and leadership are more applicable for addressing the influence of the context on implementation outcomes.

Classic Theories

Implementation researchers also want to apply theories from other fields such as psychology, sociology and organizational theory. These theories have been referred to as classic (or classic change) theories to distinguish them from research-to-practice models (Graham et al., 2009). They might be considered passive in relation to action models because they describe change mechanisms and explain how change occurs without ambitions to actually bring about change.

Psychological behaviour change theories such as the Theory of Reasoned Action (Fishbein & Ajzen, 1975), the Social Cognitive Theory (Bandura, 1977, 1986), the Theory of Interpersonal Behaviour (Triandis, 1979) and the Theory of Planned Behaviour (Ajzen, 2005) have all been widely used in implementation science to study determinants of "clinical behaviour" change (Nilsen, Roback, Broström, & Ellström, 2012). Theories such as the Cognitive Continuum Theory (Hammond, 1981), the Novice-Expert Theory (Benner, 1984), the Cognitive-Experiential

Self-Theory (Epstein, 1994) and habit theories (e.g., Ouellette & Wood, 1998; Verplanken & Aarts, 1999) may also be applicable for analyzing cognitive processes involved in clinical decision-making and implementing EBP, but they are not as extensively used as the behaviour change theories.

Theories regarding the collective (such as health care teams) or other aggregate levels are relevant in implementation science, e.g., theories concerning professions and communities of practice, as well as theories concerning the relationships between individuals, e.g., social networks and social capital (Cunningham et al., 2011; Eccles et al., 2009; Estabrooks et al., 2006; Grol & Wensing, 2004; Mascia & Cicchetti, 2011; Parchman, Scoglio, & Schumm, 2011). However, their use is not as prevalent as the individual-level theories.

There is increasing interest among implementation researchers in using theories concerning the organizational level because the context of implementation is becoming more widely acknowledged as an important influence on implementation outcomes. Theories concerning organizational culture, organizational climate, leadership and organizational learning are relevant for understanding and explaining organizational influences on implementation processes (Chaudoir, Dugan, & Barr, 2013; Durlak & Dupre, 2008; French et al., 2009; Gifford, Davies, Edwards, Griffin, & Lybanon, 2007; Grol & Wensing, 2004; Meijers et al., 2006; Nutley et al., 2007; Parmelli et al., 2011; Wallin, Ewald, Wikblad, Scott-Findlay, & Arnetz, 2006; Wensing, Wollersheim, & Grol, 2006; Yano, 2008). Several organization-level theories might have relevance for implementation science. For instance, Estabrooks et al. (2006) have proposed the use of the Situated Change Theory (Orlikowski, 1996) and the Institutional Theory (DiMaggio & Powell, 1991; Scott, 1995), whereas Plsek and Greenhalgh (2001) have suggested the use of complexity science (Waldrop, 1992) for better understanding of organizations. Meanwhile, Grol et al. (2005) have highlighted the relevance of economic theories and theories of innovative organizations. However, despite increased interest in organizational theories, their actual use in empirical implementation studies thus far is relatively limited.

The Theory of Diffusion, as popularized through Rogers' work on the spread of innovations, has also influenced implementation science. The theory's notion of innovation attributes, i.e., relative advantage, compatibility, complexity, trialability and observability (Rogers, 2003), has been widely applied in implementation science, both in individual studies (e.g., Aubert & Hamel, 2001; Foy et al., 2002; Völlink, Meertens, & Midden, 2002) and in determinant frameworks (e.g., Damschroder et al., 2009; Greenhalgh et al., 2005; Gurses et al., 2010) to assess the extent to which the characteristics of the implementation object (e.g., a clinical guideline) affect implementation outcomes. Furthermore, the Theory of Diffusion highlights the importance of intermediary actors (opinion leaders, change agents and gatekeepers) for successful adoption and implementation (Rogers, 2003), which is reflected in roles described in numerous implementation determinant frameworks (e.g., Blasé et al., 2012; Rycroft-Malone, 2010) and implementation strategy taxonomies (e.g., Grimshaw et al., 2003; Leeman, Baernholdt, & Sandelowski, 2007; Oxman, Thomson, Davis, & Haynes, 1995; Walter, Nutley, & Davies, 2003). The Theory of Diffusion is considered the single most influential theory in the broader field of knowledge utilization of which implementation science is a part (Estabrooks et al., 2008).

Implementation Theories

There are also numerous theories that have been developed or adapted by researchers for potential use in implementation science to achieve enhanced understanding and explanation of certain aspects of implementation. Some of these have been developed by modifying certain features of existing theories or concepts, e.g., concerning organizational climate and culture. Examples include theories such as Implementation Climate (Klein & Sorra, 1996), Absorptive Capacity (Zahra & George, 2002) and Organizational Readiness (Weiner, 2009). The adaptation allows researchers to prioritize aspects considered to be most critical to analyze issues related to the how and why of implementation, thus improving the relevance and appropriateness to the particular circumstances at hand.

COM-B (Capability, Opportunity, Motivation and Behaviour) represents another approach to developing theories that might be applicable in implementation science. This theory began by identifying motivation as a process that energizes and directs behaviour. Capability and opportunity were added as necessary conditions for a volitional behaviour to occur, given sufficient motivation, on the basis of a US consensus meeting of behavioural theorists and a principle of US criminal law (which considers prerequisites for performance of specified volitional behaviours) (Michie et al. 2011). COM-B posits that capability, opportunity and motivation generate behaviour, which in turn influences the three components. Opportunity and capability can influence motivation, while enacting a behaviour can alter capability, motivation and opportunity (Michie et al., 2014).

Another theory used in implementation science, the Normalization Process Theory (May & Finch, 2009), began life as a model, constructed on the basis of empirical studies of the implementation of new technologies (May et al., 2007). The model was subsequently expanded upon and developed into a theory as change mechanisms and interrelations between various constructs were delineated (Finch et al., 2013). The theory identifies four determinants of embedding (i.e., normalizing) complex interventions in practice (coherence or sense-making, cognitive participation or engagement, collective action and reflexive monitoring) and the relationships between these determinants (Murray et al., 2010).

Evaluating Implementation

Evaluation Frameworks

There is a category of frameworks that provide a structure for evaluating implementation endeavours. Two common frameworks that originated in public health are RE-AIM (Reach, Effectiveness, Adoption, Implementation, Maintenance) (Glasgow et al., 1999) and PRECEDE-PROCEED (Predisposing, Reinforcing and Enabling Constructs in Educational Diagnosis and Evaluation-Policy, Regulatory and Organizational Constructs in Educational and Environmental Development) (Green et al., 2005). Both frameworks specify implementation aspects that should be evaluated as part of intervention studies.

Proctor et al. (2010) have developed a framework of implementation outcomes that can be applied to evaluate implementation endeavours. On the basis of a narrative literature review, they propose eight conceptually distinct outcomes for potential evaluation: acceptability, adoption (also referred to as uptake), appropriateness, costs, feasibility, fidelity, penetration (integration of a practice within a specific setting) and sustainability (also referred to as maintenance or institutionalization).

Although evaluation frameworks may be considered in a category of their own, theories, models and frameworks from the other four categories can also be applied for evaluation purposes because they specify concepts and constructs that may be operationalized and measured. For instance, Theoretical Domains Framework (e.g., Fleming, Bradley, Cullinan, & Byrne, 2014; Phillips et al., 2015), Normalization Process Theory (McEvoy et al., 2014) and COM-B (e.g., Connell, McMahon, Redfern, Watkins, & Eng, 2015; Praveen et al., 2014) have all been widely used as evaluation frameworks. Furthermore, many theories, models and frameworks have spawned instruments that serve evaluation purposes, e.g., tools linked to PARIHS (Estabrooks, Squires, Cummings, Birdsell, & Norton, 2009; McCormack, McCarthy, Wright, & Coffey, 2009), CFIR (Damschroder & Lowery, 2013) and Theoretical Domains Framework (Dyson, Lawton, Jackson, & Cheater, 2013). Other examples include the EBP Implementation Scale to measure the extent to which EBP is implemented (Melnyk, Fineout-Overholt, & Mays, 2008) and the BARRIERS Scale to identify barriers to research use (Kajermo et al., 2010), as well as instruments to operationalize theories such as Implementation Climate (Jacobs, Weiner, & Bunger, 2014) and Organizational Readiness (Gagnon et al., 2011).

Discussion

Implementation science has progressed towards increased use of theoretical approaches to address various implementation challenges. While this chapter is not intended as a complete catalogue of all individual approaches available in implementation science, it is obvious that the menu of potentially useable theories, models and frameworks is extensive. Researchers in the field have pragmatically looked into other fields and disciplines to find relevant approaches, thus emphasizing the interdisciplinary and multiprofessional nature of the field.

This chapter proposes a taxonomy of five categories of theories, models and frameworks used in implementation science. These categories are not always recognized as separate types of approaches in the literature. For instance, systematic reviews and overviews by Graham and Tetroe (2007), Mitchell et al. (2010), Flottorp et al. (2013), Meyers et al. (2012) and Tabak et al. (2012) have not distinguished between process models, determinant frameworks or classic theories because they all deal with factors believed or found to have an impact on implementation processes and outcomes. However, what matters most is not how an individual approach is labelled; it is important to recognize that these theories, models and frameworks differ in terms of their assumptions, aims and other characteristics, which have implications for their use.

There is considerable overlap between some of the categories. Thus, determinant frameworks, classic theories and implementation theories can also help to guide implementation practice (i.e., functioning as action models), because they identify potential barriers and enablers that might be important to address when undertaking an implementation endeavour. They can also be used for evaluation because they describe aspects that might be important to evaluate. A framework such as the Active Implementation Frameworks (Holmes et al., 2012) appears to have a dual aim of providing hands-on support to implement something and identifying determinants of this implementation that should be analyzed. Somewhat similarly, PARIHS (Kitson et al., 1998) can be used by "anyone either attempting to get evidence into practice, or anyone who is researching or trying to better understand implementation processes and influences" (Rycroft-Malone, 2010, p. 120), suggesting that it has ambitions that go beyond its primary function as a determinant framework.

Despite the overlap between different theories, models and frameworks used in implementation science, knowledge about the three overarching aims and five categories of theoretical approaches is important to identify and select relevant approaches in various situations. Most determinant frameworks provide limited "how-to" support for carrying out implementation endeavours since the determinants may be too generic to provide sufficient detail for guiding users through an implementation process. While the relevance of addressing barriers and enablers to translating research into practice is mentioned in many process models, these models do not identify or systematically structure specific determinants associated with implementation success. Another key difference is that process models recognize a temporal sequence of implementation endeavours, whereas determinant frameworks do not explicitly take a process perspective of implementation since the determinants typically relate to implementation as a whole.

Theories applied in implementation science can be characterized as middle level. Higher-level theories can be built from theories at lower abstraction levels, so-called theory ladder climbing (Osigweh Yg, 1989). May (2013) has discussed how a "general theory of implementation" might be constructed by linking the four constructs of Normalization Process Theory with constructs from relevant sociology and psychology theories to provide a more comprehensive explanation of the constituents of implementation processes. Still, it seems unlikely that there will ever be a grand implementation theory since implementation is too multifaceted and complex a phenomenon to allow for universal explanations. There has been debate in the policy implementation research field for many years whether researchers should strive to produce a theory applicable to public policy as a whole (Sabatier, 1999). However, policy implementation researchers have increasingly argued that it would be a futile undertaking because "the world is too complex and there are too many causes of outcomes to allow for parsimonious explanation" (Cairney, 2012, p. 31). Determinant frameworks in implementation science clearly suggest that many different theories are relevant for understanding and explaining the many influences on implementation.

The use of a single theory that focuses only on a particular aspect of implementation will not tell the whole story. Choosing one approach often means placing weight on some aspects (e.g., certain causal factors) at the expense of others, thus offering only partial understanding. Combining the merits of multiple theoretical approaches may offer more complete understanding and explanation, yet such combinations may mask contrasting assumptions regarding key issues. For instance, are people driven primarily by their individual beliefs and motivation, or does a pervasive organizational culture impose norms and values that regulate how people behave and make individual characteristics relatively unimportant? Is a particular behaviour primarily influenced by reflective thought processes, or is it an automatically enacted habit? Furthermore, different approaches may require different methods based on different epistemological and ontological assumptions.

There is a current wave of optimism in implementation science that using theoretical approaches will contribute to reducing the research-practice gap (Blasé et al., 2012; Cane et al., 2012; Martinez et al., 2014; Michie, Abraham, et al., 2011; Sales et al., 2006). Although the use of theories, models and frameworks has many advocates in implementation science, there have also been critics (Bhattacharyya, Reeves, Garfinkel, & Zwarenstein, 2006; Oxman, Fretheim, & Flottorp, 2005) who have argued that theory is not necessarily better than common sense for guiding implementation. Common sense has been defined as a group's shared tacit knowledge concerning a phenomenon (Fletcher, 1984). One could argue that common sense about how or why something works (or does not) also constitutes a theory, albeit an informal and non-codified one. In either case, empirical research is needed to study how and the extent to which the use of implementation theories, models and frameworks contributes to more effective implementation and under what contextual conditions or circumstances they apply (and do not apply). It is also important to explore how the current theoretical approaches can be further developed to better address implementation challenges. Hence, both inductive construction of theory and deductive application of theory are needed.

While the use of theory does not necessarily yield more effective implementation than using common sense, there are certain advantages to applying formal theory over common sense (i.e., informal theory). Theories are explicit and open to question and examination; common sense usually consists of implicit assumptions, beliefs and ways of thinking and is therefore more difficult to challenge. If deductions from a theory are incorrect, the theory can be adapted, extended or abandoned. Theories are more consistent with existing facts than common sense, which typically means that a hypothesis based on an established theory is a more educated guess than one based on common sense. Furthermore, theories give individual facts a meaningful context and contribute towards building an integrated body of knowledge, whereas common sense is more likely to produce isolated facts (Cacioppo, 2004; Fletcher, 1984). On the other hand, theory may serve as blinders, as suggested by Kuhn (1970) and Greenwald, Pratkanis, Leippe, and Baumgardner (1986), causing us to ignore problems that do not fit into existing theories, models and frameworks or hindering us from seeing known problems in new ways. Theorizing about implementation should therefore not be an abstract academic exercise unconnected with the real world of implementation practice. In the words of Immanuel Kant, "Experience without theory is blind, but theory without experience is mere intellectual play".

Acknowledgments I am grateful to Bianca Albers, Susanne Bernhardsson, Dean L. Fixsen, Karen Grimmer, Ursula Reichenpfader and Kerstin Roback for constructive comments on drafts of this chapter. Also, thanks are due to Margit Neher, Justin Presseau and Jeanette Wassar Kirk for their input.

References

Ajzen, I. (2005). *Attitudes, personality and behavior*. Maidenhead, England: Open University Press.

Ashton, C. M., Khan, M. M., Johnson, M. L., Walder, A., Stanberry, E., Beyth, R. J., … Wray, N. P. (2007). A quasi-experimental test of an intervention to increase the use of thiazide-based treatment regimens for people with hypertension. *Implementation Science, 2*(1). https://doi.org/10.1186/1748-5908-2-5

Aubert, B. A., & Hamel, G. (2001). Adoption of smart cards in the medical sector: The Canadian experience. *Social Science & Medicine, 53*(7), 879–894. https://doi.org/10.1016/s0277-9536(00)00388-9

Bandura, A. (1977). Self-efficacy: Toward a unifying theory of behavioral change. *Psychological Review, 84*(2), 191–215. https://doi.org/10.1037//0033-295x.84.2.191

Bandura, A. (1986). *Social foundations of thought and action a social cognitive theory*. Upper Saddle River, NJ: Prentice Hall.

Benner, P. E. (1984). *From novice to expert: Excellence and power in clinical nursing practice*. Menlo Park, CA: Addison-Wesley.

Bhattacharyya, O., Reeves, S., Garfinkel, S., & Zwarenstein, M. (2006). Designing theoretically-informed implementation interventions: Fine in theory, but evidence of effectiveness in practice is needed. *Implementation Science, 1*(1). https://doi.org/10.1186/1748-5908-1-5

Blasé, K. A., Van Dyke, M., Fixsen, D. L., & Bailey, F. W. (2012). Implementation science: Key concepts, themes and evidence for practitioners in educational psychology. In B. Kelly & D. F. Perkins (Eds.), *Handbook of implementation science for psychology in education* (pp. 13–34). Cambridge, UK: Cambridge University Press.

Bluedorn, A. C., & Evered, R. D. (1980). Middle range theory and the strategies of theory construction. In C. C. Pinder & L. F. Moore (Eds.), *Middle range theory and the study of organizations* (pp. 19–32). Boston, MA: Martinus Nijhoff.

Brownson, R. C., Colditz, G. A., & Proctor, E. K. (2012). *Dissemination and implementation research in health: Translating science to practice.* Oxford, UK: Oxford University Press.

Broyles, L., Rodriguez, K. L., Kraemer, K. L., Sevick, M., Price, P. A., & Gordon, A. J. (2012). A qualitative study of anticipated barriers and facilitators to the implementation of nurse-delivered alcohol screening, brief intervention, and referral to treatment for hospitalized patients in a Veterans Affairs medical center. *Addiction Science & Clinical Practice, 7*(1), 7. https://doi.org/10.1186/1940-0640-7-7

Bunge, M. (1967). *Scientific research 1 (The search for system).* Berlin, Germany: Springer.

Cacioppo, J. T. (2004). Common sense, intuition, and theory in personality and social psychology. *Personality and Social Psychology Review, 8*(2), 114–122. https://doi.org/10.1207/s15327957pspr0802_4

Cairney, P. (2012). *Understanding public policy: Theories and issues.* Houndmills, Basingstoke, Hampshire, England: Palgrave Macmillan.

Canadian Institutes of Health Research (CIHR). About knowledge translation. [http://www.cihr-irsc.gc.ca/e/29418.html]. Accessed 18 Dec 2014.

Cane, J., O'Connor, D., & Michie, S. (2012). Validation of the theoretical domains framework for use in behaviour change and implementation research. *Implementation Science, 7*(1). https://doi.org/10.1186/1748-5908-7-37

Carpiano, R. M. (2006). A guide and glossary on postpositivist theory building for population health. *Journal of Epidemiology & Community Health, 60*(7), 564–570. https://doi.org/10.1136/jech.2004.031534

Chaudoir, S. R., Dugan, A. G., & Barr, C. H. (2013). Measuring factors affecting implementation of health innovations: A systematic review of structural, organizational, provider, patient, and innovation level measures. *Implementation Science, 8*(1). https://doi.org/10.1186/1748-5908-8-22

Cochrane, L. J., Olson, C. A., Murray, S., Dupuis, M., Tooman, T., & Hayes, S. (2007). Gaps between knowing and doing: Understanding and assessing the barriers to optimal health care. *Journal of Continuing Education in the Health Professions, 27*(2), 94–102. https://doi.org/10.1002/chp.106

Connell, L. A., McMahon, N. E., Redfern, J., Watkins, C. L., & Eng, J. J. (2015). Development of a behaviour change intervention to increase upper limb exercise in stroke rehabilitation. *Implementation Science, 10*(1). https://doi.org/10.1186/s13012-015-0223-3

Cronin, P., Ryan, F., & Coughlan, M. (2008). Undertaking a literature review: A step-by-step approach. *British Journal of Nursing, 17*(1), 38–43. https://doi.org/10.12968/bjon.2008.17.1.28059

Cunningham, F. C., Ranmuthugala, G., Plumb, J., Georgiou, A., Westbrook, J. I., & Braithwaite, J. (2011). Health professional networks as a vector for improving healthcare quality and safety: A systematic review. *BMJ Quality & Safety, 21*(3), 239–249. https://doi.org/10.1136/bmjqs-2011-000187

Damschroder, L. J., Aron, D. C., Keith, R. E., Kirsh, S. R., Alexander, J. A., & Lowery, J. C. (2009). Fostering implementation of health services research findings into practice: A consolidated framework for advancing implementation science. *Implementation Science, 4*(1). https://doi.org/10.1186/1748-5908-4-50

Damschroder, L. J., & Lowery, J. C. (2013). Evaluation of a large-scale weight management program using the consolidated framework for implementation research (CFIR). *Implementation Science, 8*(1). https://doi.org/10.1186/1748-5908-8-51

Davies, P., Walker, A., & Grimshaw, J. (2003). Theories of behavior change in studies of guideline implementation. *Proceedings of the British Psychological Society, 11*, 120.

Davis, S. M., Peterson, J. C., Helfrich, C. D., & Cunningham-Sabo, L. (2007). Introduction and conceptual model for utilization of prevention research. *American Journal of Preventive Medicine, 33*(1). https://doi.org/10.1016/j.amepre.2007.04.004

DiMaggio, P. J., & Powell, W. W. (1991). *The new institutionalism and organizational analysis.* Chicago, IL: University of Chicago Press.

Dopson, S., & Fitzgerald, L. (2005). The active role of context. In S. Dopson & L. Fitzgerald (Eds.), *Knowledge to action? Evidence-based health care in context* (pp. 79–103). New York, NY: Oxford University Press.

Dubin, R. (1969). *Theory building.* New York, NY: Free Press.

Durlak, J. A., & Dupre, E. P. (2008). Implementation matters: A review of research on the influence of implementation on program outcomes and the factors affecting implementation. *American Journal of Community Psychology, 41*(3–4), 327–350. https://doi.org/10.1007/s10464-008-9165-0

Dyson, J., Lawton, R., Jackson, C., & Cheater, F. (2013). Development of a theory-based instrument to identify barriers and levers to best hand hygiene practice among healthcare practitioners. *Implementation Science, 8*(1). https://doi.org/10.1186/1748-5908-8-111

Eccles, M. P., Grimshaw, J., Walker, A., Johnston, M., & Pitts, N. (2005). Changing the behavior of healthcare professionals: The use of theory in promoting the uptake of research findings. *Journal of Clinical Epidemiology, 58*(2), 107–112. https://doi.org/10.1016/j.jclinepi.2004.09.002

Eccles, M. P., Hrisos, S., Francis, J. J., Steen, N., Bosch, M., & Johnston, M. (2009). Can the collective intentions of individual professionals within healthcare teams predict the team's performance: Developing methods and theory. *Implementation Science, 4*(1). https://doi.org/10.1186/1748-5908-4-24

Eccles, M. P., & Mittman, B. S. (2006). Welcome to implementation science. *Implementation Science, 1*(1). https://doi.org/10.1186/1748-5908-1-1

Epstein, S. (1994). Integration of the cognitive and the psychodynamic unconscious. *American Psychologist, 49*(8), 709–724. https://doi.org/10.1037//0003-066x.49.8.709

Estabrooks, C. A., Derksen, L., Winther, C., Lavis, J. N., Scott, S. D., Wallin, L., & Profetto-McGrath, J. (2008). The intellectual structure and substance of the knowledge utilization field: A longitudinal author co-citation analysis, 1945 to 2004. *Implementation Science, 3*(1). https://doi.org/10.1186/1748-5908-3-49

Estabrooks, C. A., Squires, J. E., Cummings, G. G., Birdsell, J. M., & Norton, P. G. (2009). Development and assessment of the Alberta context tool. *BMC Health Services Research BMC Health Serv Res, 9*(1). https://doi.org/10.1186/1472-6963-9-234

Estabrooks, C. A., Thompson, D. S., Lovely, J. J., & Hofmeyer, A. (2006). A guide to knowledge translation theory. *Journal of Continuing Education in the Health Professions, 26*(1), 25–36. https://doi.org/10.1002/chp.48

Ferlie, E. B., & Shortell, S. M. (2001). Improving the quality of health care in the United Kingdom and the United States: A framework for change. *The Milbank Quarterly, 79*(2), 281–315. https://doi.org/10.1111/1468-0009.00206

Field, B., Booth, A., Ilott, I., & Gerrish, K. (2014). Using the knowledge to action framework in practice: A citation analysis and systematic review. *Implementation Science, 9*(1). https://doi.org/10.1186/s13012-014-0172-2

Finch, T. L., Rapley, T., Girling, M., Mair, F. S., Murray, E., Treweek, S., … May, C. R. (2013). Improving the normalization of complex interventions: Measure development based on normalization process theory (NoMAD): Study protocol. *Implementation Science, 8*(1). https://doi.org/10.1186/1748-5908-8-43

Fishbein, M., & Ajzen, I. (1975). *Belief, attitude, intention, and behaviour.* New York, NY: John Wiley.

Fixsen, D. L., Naoom, S. F., Blasé, K. A., Friedman, R. M., & Wallace, F. (2005). *Implementation research: A synthesis of the literature.* Tampa, FL: National Implementation Research Network.

Fleming, A., Bradley, C., Cullinan, S., & Byrne, S. (2014). Antibiotic prescribing in long-term care facilities: A qualitative, multidisciplinary investigation. *BMJ Open, 4*(11). https://doi.org/10.1136/bmjopen-2014-006442

Fletcher, G. J. (1984). Psychology and common sense. *American Psychologist, 39*(3), 203–213. https://doi.org/10.1037//0003-066x.39.3.203

Flottorp, S. A., Oxman, A. D., Krause, J., Musila, N. R., Wensing, M., Godycki-Cwirko, M., ... Eccles, M. P. (2013). A checklist for identifying determinants of practice: A systematic review and synthesis of frameworks and taxonomies of factors that prevent or enable improvements in healthcare professional practice. *Implementation Science, 8*(1). https://doi.org/10.1186/1748-5908-8-35

Foy, R., Maclennan, G., Grimshaw, J., Penney, G., Campbell, M., & Grol, R. (2002). Attributes of clinical recommendations that influence change in practice following audit and feedback. *Journal of Clinical Epidemiology, 55*(7), 717–722. https://doi.org/10.1016/s0895-4356(02)00403-1

Frankfort-Nachmias, C., & Nachmias, D. (1996). *Research methods in the social sciences* (p. 1996). London, England: Arnold.

French, B., Thomas, L. H., Baker, P., Burton, C. R., Pennington, L., & Roddam, H. (2009). What can management theories offer evidence-based practice? A comparative analysis of measurement tools for organisational context. *Implementation Science, 4*(1). https://doi.org/10.1186/1748-5908-4-28

Gabbay, J. (2004). Evidence based guidelines or collectively constructed "mindlines?" Ethnographic study of knowledge management in primary care. *BMJ, 329*(7473), 1013. https://doi.org/10.1136/bmj.329.7473.1013

Gagnon, M., Labarthe, J., Légaré, F., Ouimet, M., Estabrooks, C. A., Roch, G., ... Grimshaw, J. (2011). Measuring organizational readiness for knowledge translation in chronic care. *Implementation Science, 6*(1). https://doi.org/10.1186/1748-5908-6-72

Gifford, W., Davies, B., Edwards, N., Griffin, P., & Lybanon, V. (2007). Managerial leadership for nurses' use of research evidence: An integrative review of the literature. *Worldviews on Evidence-Based Nursing, 4*(3), 126–145. https://doi.org/10.1111/j.1741-6787.2007.00095.x

Glasgow, R. E., Vogt, T. M., & Boles, S. M. (1999). Evaluating the public health impact of health promotion interventions: The RE-AIM framework. *American Journal of Public Health, 89*(9), 1322–1327. https://doi.org/10.2105/ajph.89.9.1322

Godin, G., Bélanger-Gravel, A., Eccles, M., & Grimshaw, J. (2008). Healthcare professionals' intentions and behaviours: A systematic review of studies based on social cognitive theories. *Implementation Science, 3*(1). https://doi.org/10.1186/1748-5908-3-36

Graham, I. D., Logan, J., Harrison, M. B., Straus, S. E., Tetroe, J., Caswell, W., & Robinson, N. (2006). Lost in knowledge translation: Time for a map? *Journal of Continuing Education in the Health Professions, 26*(1), 13–24. https://doi.org/10.1002/chp.47

Graham, I. D., & Tetroe, J. (2007). Some theoretical underpinnings of knowledge translation. *Academic Emergency Medicine, 14*(11), 936–941. https://doi.org/10.1197/j.aem.2007.07.004

Graham, I. D., Tetroe, J., & KT Theories Group. (2009). Planned action theories. In S. E. Straus, J. Tetroe, & I. D. Graham (Eds.), *Knowledge translation in health care: Moving from evidence to practice* (pp. 185–195). Chichester, UK: Wiley-Blackwell/BMJ.

Green, L. W., Kreuter, M. W., & Green, L. W. (2005). *Health program planning: An educational and ecological approach*. New York, NY: McGraw-Hill.

Greenhalgh, T., Robert, G., Bate, P., Macfarlane, F., & Kyriakidou, O. (2005). *Diffusion of innovations in service organisations: A systematic literature review*. Malden, MA: Blackwell.

Greenwald, A. G., Pratkanis, A. R., Leippe, M. R., & Baumgardner, M. H. (1986). Under what conditions does theory obstruct research progress? *Psychological Review, 93*(2), 216–229. https://doi.org/10.1037//0033-295x.93.2.216

Grimshaw, J., McAuley, L. M., Bero, L. A., Grilli, R., Oxman, A. D., Ramsay, C., ... Zwarenstein, M. (2003). Systematic reviews of effectiveness of quality improvement strategies and programmes. *Quality and Safety in Health Care, 12*(4), 298–303. https://doi.org/10.1136/qhc.12.4.298

Grol, R., & Wensing, M. (2004). What drives change? Barriers to and incentives for achieving evidence-based practice. *Medical Journal of Australia, 180*, S57–S60.

Grol, R., Wensing, M., & Eccles, M. (2005). *Improving patient care: The implementation of change in clinical practice*. Edinburgh, Scotland: Elsevier Butterworth Heinemann.

Gurses, A. P., Marsteller, J. A., Ozok, A. A., Xiao, Y., Owens, S., & Pronovost, P. J. (2010). Using an interdisciplinary approach to identify factors that affect clinicians' compliance with evidence-based guidelines. *Critical Care Medicine, 38*(8 Suppl), S282–S291. https://doi.org/10.1097/ccm.0b013e3181e69e02

Hammond, K. R. (1981). *Principles of organization in intuitive and analytical cognition.* Ft. Belvoir, VA: Defense Technical Information Center.

Helfrich, C. D., Damschroder, L. J., Hagedorn, H. J., Daggett, G. S., Sahay, A., Ritchie, M., … Stetler, C. B. (2010). A critical synthesis of literature on the promoting action on research implementation in health services (PARIHS) framework. *Implementation Science, 5*(1). https://doi.org/10.1186/1748-5908-5-82

Holmes, B. J., Finegood, D. T., Riley, B. L., & Best, A. (2012). Systems thinking in dissemination and implementation research. In R. C. Brownson, G. A. Colditz, & E. K. Proctor (Eds.), *Dissemination and implementation research in health* (pp. 192–212). Oxford, UK: Oxford University Press.

Huberman, M. (1994). Research utilization: The state of the art. *Knowledge and Policy, 7*(4), 13–33. https://doi.org/10.1007/bf02696290

Hunt, S. D. (1991). *Modern marketing theory: Critical issues in the philosophy of marketing science.* Cincinnati, OH: South-Western Publishing.

ICEBeRG. (2006). Designing theoretically-informed implementation interventions. *Implementation Science, 1*(1). https://doi.org/10.1186/1748-5908-1-4

Jacobs, S. R., Weiner, B. J., & Bunger, A. C. (2014). Context matters: Measuring implementation climate among individuals and groups. *Implementation Science, 9*(1). https://doi.org/10.1186/1748-5908-9-46

Jacobson, N., Butterill, D., & Goering, P. (2003). Development of a framework for knowledge translation: Understanding user context. *Journal of Health Services Research & Policy, 8*(2), 94–99. https://doi.org/10.1258/135581903321466067

Johnson, M., Jackson, R., Guillaume, L., Meier, P., & Goyder, E. (2010). Barriers and facilitators to implementing screening and brief intervention for alcohol misuse: A systematic review of qualitative evidence. *Journal of Public Health, 33*(3), 412–421. https://doi.org/10.1093/pubmed/fdq095

Jones, K. (2004). Mission drift in qualitative research, or moving toward a systematic review of qualitative studies, moving back to a more systematic narrative review. *The Qualitative Report, 9,* 95–112.

Kajermo, K. N., Boström, A., Thompson, D. S., Hutchinson, A. M., Estabrooks, C. A., & Wallin, L. (2010). The BARRIERS scale – The barriers to research utilization scale: A systematic review. *Implementation Science, 5*(1). https://doi.org/10.1186/1748-5908-5-32

Kitson, A. L., Harvey, G., & McCormack, B. (1998). Enabling the implementation of evidence based practice: A conceptual framework. *Quality and Safety in Health Care, 7*(3), 149–158. https://doi.org/10.1136/qshc.7.3.149

Kitson, A. L., Rycroft-Malone, J., Harvey, G., McCormack, B., Seers, K., & Titchen, A. (2008). Evaluating the successful implementation of evidence into practice using the PARiHS framework: Theoretical and practical challenges. *Implementation Science, 3*(1). https://doi.org/10.1186/1748-5908-3-1

Klein, K. J., & Sorra, J. S. (1996). The challenge of innovation implementation. *Academy of Management Review, 21*(4), 1055–1080. https://doi.org/10.5465/amr.1996.9704071863

Kuhn, T. S. (1970). *The structure of scientific revolutions.* Chicago, IL: University of Chicago Press.

Landry, R., Amara, N., & Lamari, M. (2001). Climbing the ladder of research utilization: Evidence from social science research. *Science Communication, 22*(4), 396–422. https://doi.org/10.1177/1075547001022004003

Leeman, J., Baernholdt, M., & Sandelowski, M. (2007). Developing a theory-based taxonomy of methods for implementing change in practice. *Journal of Advanced Nursing, 58*(2), 191–200. https://doi.org/10.1111/j.1365-2648.2006.04207.x

Légaré, F., Ratté, S., Gravel, K., & Graham, I. D. (2008). Barriers and facilitators to implementing shared decision-making in clinical practice: Update of a systematic review of health professionals' perceptions. *Patient Education and Counseling, 73*(3), 526–535. https://doi.org/10.1016/j.pec.2008.07.018

Logan, J., & Graham, I. (2010). The Ottawa Model of research use. In J. Rycroft-Malone & T. Bucknall (Eds.), *Models and frameworks for implementing evidence-based practice: Linking evidence to action* (pp. 83–108). Chichester, West Sussex, England: Wiley-Blackwell.

Logan, J., & Graham, I. D. (1998). Toward a comprehensive interdisciplinary model of health care research use. *Science Communication, 20*(2), 227–246. https://doi.org/10.1177/1075547098020002004

Majdzadeh, R., Sadighi, J., Nejat, S., Mahani, A. S., & Gholami, J. (2008). Knowledge translation for research utilization: Design of a knowledge translation model at Tehran University of Medical Sciences. *Journal of Continuing Education in the Health Professions, 28*(4), 270–277. https://doi.org/10.1002/chp.193

Martinez, R. G., Lewis, C. C., & Weiner, B. J. (2014). Instrumentation issues in implementation science. *Implementation Science, 9*(1). https://doi.org/10.1186/s13012-014-0118-8

Mascia, D., & Cicchetti, A. (2011). Physician social capital and the reported adoption of evidence-based medicine: Exploring the role of structural holes. *Social Science & Medicine, 72*(5), 798–805. https://doi.org/10.1016/j.socscimed.2010.12.011

May, C. (2013). Towards a general theory of implementation. *Implementation Science, 8*(1). https://doi.org/10.1186/1748-5908-8-18

May, C., & Finch, T. (2009). Implementing, embedding, and integrating practices: An outline of normalization process theory. *Sociology, 43*(3), 535–554. https://doi.org/10.1177/0038038509103208

May, C., Finch, T., Mair, F., Ballini, L., Dowrick, C., Eccles, M., ... Heaven, B. (2007). Understanding the implementation of complex interventions in health care: The normalization process model. *BMC Health Services Research, 7*, 148. https://doi.org/10.1186/1472-6963-7-148

McCormack, B., McCarthy, G., Wright, J., & Coffey, A. (2009). Development and testing of the context assessment index (CAI). *Worldviews on Evidence-Based Nursing, 6*(1), 27–35. https://doi.org/10.1111/j.1741-6787.2008.00130.x

McEvoy, R., Ballini, L., Maltoni, S., O'Donnell, C. A., Mair, F. S., & Macfarlane, A. (2014). A qualitative systematic review of studies using the normalization process theory to research implementation processes. *Implementation Science, 9*(1). https://doi.org/10.1186/1748-5908-9-2

Meijers, J. M., Janssen, M. A., Cummings, G. G., Wallin, L., Estabrooks, C. A., & Halfens, R. Y. (2006). Assessing the relationships between contextual factors and research utilization in nursing: Systematic literature review. *Journal of Advanced Nursing, 55*(5), 622–635. https://doi.org/10.1111/j.1365-2648.2006.03954.x

Melnyk, B. M., Fineout-Overholt, E., & Mays, M. Z. (2008). The evidence-based practice beliefs and implementation scales: Psychometric properties of two new instruments. *Worldviews on Evidence-Based Nursing, 5*(4), 208–216. https://doi.org/10.1111/j.1741-6787.2008.00126.x

Meyers, D. C., Durlak, J. A., & Wandersman, A. (2012). The quality implementation framework: A synthesis of critical steps in the implementation process. *American Journal of Community Psychology, 50*(3–4), 462–480. https://doi.org/10.1007/s10464-012-9522-x

Michie, S., Abraham, C., Eccles, M. P., Francis, J. J., Hardeman, W., & Johnston, M. (2011). Strengthening evaluation and implementation by specifying components of behaviour change interventions: A study protocol. *Implementation Science, 6*(1). https://doi.org/10.1186/1748-5908-6-10

Michie, S., Atkins, L., & West, R. (2014). *The behaviour change wheel: A guide to designing interventions*. Manchester, UK: Silverback.

Michie, S., Johnston, M., Abraham, C., Lawton, R., Parker, D., & Walker, A. (2005). Making psychological theory useful for implementing evidence based practice: A consensus approach. *Quality and Safety in Health Care, 14*(1), 26–33. https://doi.org/10.1136/qshc.2004.011155

Michie, S., Stralen, M. M., & West, R. (2011). The behaviour change wheel: A new method for characterising and designing behaviour change interventions. *Implementation Science, 6*(1). https://doi.org/10.1186/1748-5908-6-42

Mitchell, S. A., Fisher, C. A., Hastings, C. E., Silverman, L. B., & Wallen, G. R. (2010). A thematic analysis of theoretical models for translational science in nursing: Mapping the field. *Nursing Outlook, 58*(6), 287–300. https://doi.org/10.1016/j.outlook.2010.07.001

Mohr, D. C., Lukas, C. V., & Meterko, M. (2008). Predicting healthcare employees' participation in an office redesign program: Attitudes, norms and behavioral control. *Implementation Science, 3*(1). https://doi.org/10.1186/1748-5908-3-47

Murray, E., Treweek, S., Pope, C., Macfarlane, A., Ballini, L., Dowrick, C., … May, C. (2010). Normalisation process theory: A framework for developing, evaluating and implementing complex interventions. *BMC Medicine, 8*(1). https://doi.org/10.1186/1741-7015-8-63

Nilsen, P., Roback, K., Broström, A., & Ellström, P. (2012). Creatures of habit: Accounting for the role of habit in implementation research on clinical behaviour change. *Implementation Science, 7*(1). https://doi.org/10.1186/1748-5908-7-53

Nutley, S. M., Walter, I., & Davies, H. T. (2007). *Using evidence: How research can inform public services*. Bristol, UK: Policy Press.

Orlikowski, W. J. (1996). Improvising organizational transformation over time: A situated change perspective. *Information Systems Research, 7*(1), 63–92. https://doi.org/10.1287/isre.7.1.63

Osigweh Yg, C. A. B. (1989). Concept fallibility in organizational science. *Academy of Management Review, 14*(4), 579–594. https://doi.org/10.5465/amr.1989.4308390

Ouellette, J. A., & Wood, W. (1998). Habit and intention in everyday life: The multiple processes by which past behavior predicts future behavior. *Psychological Bulletin, 124*(1), 54–74. https://doi.org/10.1037//0033-2909.124.1.54

Oxman, A. D., Fretheim, A., & Flottorp, S. (2005). The OFF theory of research utilization. *Journal of Clinical Epidemiology, 58*(2), 113–116. https://doi.org/10.1016/j.jclinepi.2004.10.002

Oxman, A. D., Thomson, M. A., Davis, D. A., & Haynes, R. B. (1995). No magic bullets: A systematic review of 102 trials of interventions to improve professional practice. *CMAJ, 153*, 1423–1431.

Parchman, M. L., Scoglio, C. M., & Schumm, P. (2011). Understanding the implementation of evidence-based care: A structural network approach. *Implementation Science, 6*(1). https://doi.org/10.1186/1748-5908-6-14

Parmelli, E., Flodgren, G., Beyer, F., Baillie, N., Schaafsma, M. E., & Eccles, M. P. (2011). The effectiveness of strategies to change organisational culture to improve healthcare performance: A systematic review. *Implementation Science, 6*(1). https://doi.org/10.1186/1748-5908-6-33

Phillips, C. J., Marshall, A. P., Chaves, N. J., Lin, I. B., Loy, C. T., Rees, G., … Michie, S. (2015). Experiences of using theoretical domains framework across diverse clinical environments: A qualitative study. *Journal of Multidisciplinary Healthcare, 8*, 139–146. https://doi.org/10.2147/JMDH.S78458

Plsek, P. E., & Greenhalgh, T. (2001). Complexity science: The challenge of complexity in health care. *BMJ, 323*(7313), 625–628. https://doi.org/10.1136/bmj.323.7313.625

Praveen, D., Patel, A., Raghu, A., Clifford, G. D., Maulik, P. K., Abdul, A. M., … Peiris, D. (2014). SMARTHealth India: Development and field evaluation of a mobile clinical decision support system for cardiovascular diseases in rural India. *JMIR mHealth and uHealth, 2*(4). https://doi.org/10.2196/mhealth.3568

Proctor, E., Silmere, H., Raghavan, R., Hovmand, P., Aarons, G., Bunger, A., … Hensley, M. (2010). Outcomes for implementation research: Conceptual distinctions, measurement challenges, and research agenda. *Administration and Policy in Mental Health and Mental Health Services Research, 38*(2), 65–76. https://doi.org/10.1007/s10488-010-0319-7

Pronovost, P. J., Berenholtz, S. M., & Needham, D. M. (2008). Translating evidence into practice: A model for large scale knowledge translation. *BMJ, 337*. https://doi.org/10.1136/bmj.a1714

Rabin, B. A., & Brownson, R. C. (2012). Developing the terminology for dissemination and imple-mentation research. In R. C. Brownson, G. A. Colditz, & E. K. Proctor (Eds.), *Dissemination and implementation research in health* (pp. 23–51). New York, NY: Oxford University Press.

Reynolds, P. D. (1971). *A primer in theory construction*. Indianapolis, IN: Bobbs-Merrill.

Rogers, E. M. (2003). *Diffusion of innovations* (5th ed.). New York, NY: Free Press.

Rycroft-Malone, J. (2010). Promoting action on research implementation in health services (PARIHS). In J. Rycroft-Malone & T. Bucknall (Eds.), *Models and frameworks for imple-menting evidence-based practice: Linking evidence to action* (pp. 10–136). Chichester, West Sussex, England: Wiley-Blackwell.

Rycroft-Malone, J., & Bucknall, T. (2010a). Theory, frameworks, and models: Laying down the groundwork. In J. Rycroft-Malone & T. Bucknall (Eds.), *Models and frameworks for imple-menting evidence-based practice: Linking evidence to action* (pp. 23–50). Chichester, West Sussex, England: Wiley-Blackwell.

Rycroft-Malone, J., & Bucknall, T. (2010b). Analysis and synthesis of models and frameworks. In J. Rycroft-Malone & T. Bucknall (Eds.), *Models and frameworks for implementing evidence-based practice: Linking evidence to action* (pp. 223–245). Chichester, West Sussex, England: Wiley-Blackwell.

Rycroft-Malone, J., & Bucknall, T. (2010c). *Models and frameworks for implementing evidence-based practice: Linking evidence to action*. Chichester, West Sussex, England: Wiley-Blackwell.

Sabatier, P. A. (1999). *Theories of the policy process*. Boulder, CO: Westview Press.

Sales, A., Smith, J., Curran, G., & Kochevar, L. (2006). Models, strategies, and tools: Theory in implementing evidence-based findings into health care practice. *Journal of General Internal Medicine, 21*(S2). https://doi.org/10.1007/s11606-006-0274-x

Scott, S. D., Plotnikoff, R. C., Karunamuni, N., Bize, R., & Rodgers, W. (2008). Factors influenc-ing the adoption of an innovation: An examination of the uptake of the Canadian Heart Health Kit (HHK). *Implementation Science, 3*(1). https://doi.org/10.1186/1748-5908-3-41

Scott, W. R. (1995). *Institutions and organizations*. Thousand Oaks, CA: Sage.

Stetler, C. B. (1994). Refinement of the Stetler/Marram model for application of research findings to practice. *Nursing Outlook, 42*(1), 15–25. https://doi.org/10.1016/0029-6554(94)90067-1

Stetler, C. B. (2010). Stetler model. In J. Rycroft-Malone & T. Bucknall (Eds.), *Models and frame-works for implementing evidence-based practice: Linking evidence to action* (pp. 51–82). Chichester, West Sussex, England: Wiley-Blackwell.

Stevens, K. R. (2013). The impact of evidence-based practice in nursing and the next big ideas. *The Online Journal of Issues in Nursing, 18*(2), 4.

Straus, S. E., Tetroe, J., & Graham, I. D. (2009). *Knowledge translation in health care: Moving from evidence to practice*. Chichester, UK: Wiley-Blackwell/BMJ.

Tabak, R. G., Khoong, E. C., Chambers, D. A., & Brownson, R. C. (2012). Bridging research and practice: Models for dissemination and implementation research. *American Journal of Preventive Medicine, 43*, 337–350.

Titler, M. G., Kleiber, C., Steelman, V., Goode, C., Rakel, B., Barry-Walker, J., … Buckwalter, K. (1994). Infusing research into practice to promote quality care. *Nursing Research, 43*(5). https://doi.org/10.1097/00006199-199409000-00009

Titler, M. G., Kleiber, C., Steelman, V. J., Rakel, B. A., Budreau, G., Everett, L. Q., … Goode, C. J. (2001). The Iowa Model of evidence-based practice to promote quality care. *Critical Care Nursing Clinics of North America, 13*, 497–509.

Triandis, H. C. (1979). Values, attitudes, and interpersonal behaviour. In M. M. Page, & H. E. Howe (Eds.), (1980). *Nebraska Symposium on Motivation, 1979: Beliefs, attitudes and values* (pp. 195–259). Lincoln, NE: University of Nebraska Press.

Verplanken, B., & Aarts, H. (1999). Habit, attitude, and planned behaviour: Is habit an empty construct or an interesting case of goal-directed automaticity? *European Review of Social Psychology, 10*(1), 101–134. https://doi.org/10.1080/14792779943000035

Verweij, L. M., Proper, K. I., Leffelaar, E. R., Weel, A. N., Nauta, A. P., Hulshof, C. T., & Mechelen, W. V. (2012). Barriers and facilitators to implementation of an occupational health guideline aimed at preventing weight gain among employees in the Netherlands. *Journal of Occupational and Environmental Medicine, 54*(8), 954–960. https://doi.org/10.1097/jom.0b013e3182511c9f

Völlink, T., Meertens, R., & Midden, C. J. (2002). Innovating 'diffusion of innovation' theory: Innovation characteristics and the intention of utility companies to adopt energy conservation interventions. *Journal of Environmental Psychology, 22*(4), 333–344. https://doi.org/10.1006/jevp.2001.0237

Wacker, J. (1998). A definition of theory: Research guidelines for different theory-building research methods in operations management. *Journal of Operations Management, 16*(4), 361–385. https://doi.org/10.1016/s0272-6963(98)00019-9

Waldrop, M. M. (1992). *Complexity: The emerging science at the edge of order and chaos.* New York, NY: Simon & Schuster.

Wallin, L., Ewald, U., Wikblad, K., Scott-Findlay, S., & Arnetz, B. B. (2006). Understanding work contextual factors: A short-cut to evidence-based practice? *Worldviews on Evidence-Based Nursing, 3*(4), 153–164. https://doi.org/10.1111/j.1741-6787.2006.00067.x

Walter, I., Nutley, S. M., Davies, H, T, O. (2003). Developing a taxonomy of interventions used to increase the impact of research. St. Andrews: University of St Andrews. Discussion Paper 3, Research Unit for Research Utilisation, University of St. Andrews.

Weiner, B. J. (2009). A theory of organizational readiness for change. *Implementation Science, 4*(1). https://doi.org/10.1186/1748-5908-4-67

Wensing, M., Wollersheim, H., & Grol, R. (2006). Organizational interventions to implement improvements in patient care: A structured review of reviews. *Implementation Science, 1*(1). https://doi.org/10.1186/1748-5908-1-2

Wilson, K. M., Brady, T. J., Lesesne, C., & on behalf of the NCCDPHP Work Group on Translation. (2011). An organizing framework for translation in public health: The knowledge to action framework. *Preventing Chronic Disease, 8*, A46.

Yano, E. M. (2008). The role of organizational research in implementing evidence-based practice: QUERI series. *Implementation Science, 3*(1). https://doi.org/10.1186/1748-5908-3-29

Zahra, S. A., & George, G. (2002). Absorptive capacity: A review, reconceptualization, and extension. *Academy of Management Review, 27*(2), 185–203. https://doi.org/10.5465/amr.2002.6587995

Zardo, P., & Collie, A. (2014). Predicting research use in a public health policy environment: Results of a logistic regression analysis. *Implementation Science, 9*(1). https://doi.org/10.1186/s13012-014-0142-8

Chapter 4
Factors Associated with Effective Implementation: Research and Practical Implications

Melanie Barwick, Raluca Dubrowski, and Laura Damschroder

Introduction

Implementation of evidence into practice is a complex endeavor, and new evidence, resources, and tools have emerged steadily over the last decade. Those working in service provision are in great need of knowledge and resources to support the work they are increasingly compelled to take on by policy makers, payers, and care recipients (e.g., in Canada, Ontario's Comprehensive Mental Health and Addictions Strategy, Excellent Care for All Act, Government of Ontario, 2011; in the United States, Achieving the Promise: Transforming Mental Health Care in America, 2003; in the United Kingdom, Improving Access to Psychological Therapies, 2007; in Australia, Better Outcomes in Mental Health Care scheme, 2001). Researchers of implementation science are working from many angles to develop theory, models, and frameworks (see reviews by Moulin, Sabater-Hernández, Fernandez-Llimos & Benrimoj, 2015; Nilsen, 2015; Tabak, Khoong, Chambers, & Brownson, 2012); to identify processes and strategies that can guide and support the work (Meyers, Durlak & Wandersman, 2012); to identify key constructs that can inform successful and sustainable evidence-based implementation (Damschroder et al., 2009); and to map psychometrically sound and practical measures to these constructs for use by researchers and practitioners alike (Lewis et al., 2015).

In all of these areas of development, there is tremendous value in considering the utility of theories and conceptual frameworks to inform research and practice (Davidoff, Dixon-Woods, Leviton & Michie, 2015). Research demonstrates that the use of theories and frameworks in dissemination and implementation research

M. Barwick (✉) · R. Dubrowski
Hospital for Sick Children, Toronto, ON, Canada
e-mail: melanie.barwick@sickkids.ca

L. Damschroder
Ann Arbor VA Center for Clinical Management Research, Washington, DC, USA

© Springer Nature Switzerland AG 2020
B. Albers et al. (eds.), *Implementation Science 3.0*,
https://doi.org/10.1007/978-3-030-03874-8_4

can enhance the interpretability of study findings and ensure that effective implementation constructs, strategies, and processes are considered in implementation
work (Mitchell, Fisher, Hastings, Silverman, & Wallen, 2010; Sales, Smith, Curran,
& Kochevar, 2006; Van Achterberg, Schoonhoven, & Grol, 2008). To this end, this
chapter pertains to the Consolidated Framework for Implementation Research
(Damschroder et al., 2009) and reviews research highlighting the factors associated
with implementation success based on findings from studies across a diverse array
of settings and interventions. These include a weight management program in a
large integrated US healthcare system; an e-health application in Norway; and a
Canadian study of a maternal and child health intervention undertaken in Mali and
Ethiopia. Our goal is to review how these studies identify contextual factors that
are associated with effective implementation and, thus, help to differentiate
between high and low implementers as well as to highlight factors that can be
manipulated throughout the implementation process to improve success. Through
a review of these studies, we document how use of this framework propels our
understanding of successful implementation in a way that informs both research
and practice.

Organization of the Chapter

This chapter extends on *Concepts, Theories and Frameworks* (Nilsen, 2020, this
volume) by advancing our knowledge about contextual factors influencing the
implementation process and drilling down to explore those that are implicated in
successful implementation, providing greater specificity for the implementation and
making the endeavor that much more concrete. This chapter also helps to set the
stage for the chapter on *Advancing Implementation Science Measurement* (Lewis &
Dorsey, 2020, this volume). We first provide a brief introduction on types of implementation frameworks and classify the framework that will be highlighted in this
chapter, the Consolidated Framework for Implementation Research (CFIR;
Damschroder et al., 2009). We then move to discuss methodological considerations
related to the value of qualitative content analysis that is guided by a framework like
the CFIR, identify empirical studies that have used the CFIR, and show how the
knowledge base can be systematically built upon by use of a common framework
across diverse settings. Finally, we discuss methodological, conceptual, and practical implications of this comparative analysis.

Written with both the researcher and practitioner in mind, we provide an overview of the key elements of effective implementation, what we have learned from
research in different sectors, and where future research in this line of investigation
needs to go. For the practitioner, the utility of this emerging evidence is discussed to
provide support for how implementation of evidence in real-world practice settings
might be structured and improved upon.

Theory in Implementation Science and Practice

To realize intended health outcomes, interventions found to be both effective and cost-effective must then be implemented and adopted as part of clinical or public health practice. However, few studies or systematic reviews of effective interventions exist to guide practitioners and policy makers with the "how" of implementing evidence-based treatments or programs in usual care settings, whether they be in health, behavioral health, education, or other social or human services. Most studies are focused on establishing internal validity (i.e., ensuring that the intervention being evaluated is indeed the cause of observed outcomes) in highly controlled randomized clinical trials (RCTs). By design, the complexity of context, so critical to effective implementation, is minimized to the extent possible in these RCT studies, and this truncates their usefulness for real-world implementation.

More recently, new hybrid designs for implementation science (e.g., Curran, Bauer, Mittman, Pyne & Stetler, 2012) have been proposed that seek to incorporate this complexity with the aim of establishing external validity and generating knowledge about how to scale up, disseminate, and implement interventions that worked in a controlled clinical trial. These designs blend design components of clinical effectiveness and implementation research to focus on understanding not just what works but *how*, *where*, and *why* (Bauer, Damschroder, Hagedorn, Smith & Kilbourne, 2015).

In addition to advancements in research designs, consistent use of theory can be efficient, even essential, to creating new knowledge (Foy et al., 2011). However, achieving this envisioned efficiency is challenging given the multitude of theoretical frameworks (Tabak et al., 2012), constructs (Chaudoir, Dugan & Barr, 2013; Damschroder et al., 2009), and measures (Lewis et al., 2015). Implementation researchers are faced with a "Tower of Babel" (McKibbon et al., 2010; Shojania et al., 2009), a disorganized and inconsistently applied array of terms and definitions that are used to explicate, report, and assess models used in research studies. This chaos has contributed to a lack of clarity between researchers that undermines the development of psychometrically sound and feasible quantitative measures and approaches and creates a formidable barrier to advancing implementation science (Martinez, Lewis & Weiner, 2014).

An approach that could counter this situation would be to systematically base investigation on a common framework of consistently described and labeled constructs (or factors, with the two terms being used interchangeably here) implicated in implementation. Doing so would provide a shared understanding from which theories, constructs, and measures can be developed, adapted, applied, and described. This approach would benefit the field by identifying constructs that are associated with implementation success and thereby enabling identified constructs to be mapped to measures and/or to be prospectively considered in the implementation planning process; both advances would promote synthesis of knowledge across diverse studies and settings. This chapter illustrates such an approach by using the CFIR as an organizing conceptual framework.

The Consolidated Framework for Implementation Research (CFIR)

Among the types of theories common to implementation science – process models, determinant frameworks, classic theories, implementation theories, and evaluation frameworks – it is the determinant theories that lend themselves to the aim of establishing external validity (Nilsen, 2015). The purpose of these frameworks is to identify factors and explain the nature of their influence on implementation outcomes, ideally, as predictors of outcomes or to help interpret outcomes retrospectively. As a *determinant* type framework, CFIR (Damschroder et al., 2009) specifies and defines domains and individual factors within those domains that may act as barriers or enablers (independent variables) that influence implementation outcomes (dependent variables).

CFIR is a meta-theoretical framework that provides a repository of standardized implementation-related constructs that can be applied across the spectrum of implementation research. CFIR comprises 39 constructs organized across 5 major domains (outer setting, inner setting, intervention characteristics, process, and characteristics of the individuals involved), all of which interact to influence implementation and implementation effectiveness. CFIR provides a common language by which determinants of implementation can be articulated, as well as a comprehensive, standardized list of constructs to serve as a guide for researchers as they identify variables that are most salient to implementation of a particular innovation. CFIR can be used to develop data collection approaches (e.g., interview guide, codebook) and as a guide for analyzing, interpreting, and/or reporting implementation-related findings. CFIR can be applied at any phase of implementation (i.e., pre-, during, or post-implementation), and its constructs can be used as building blocks for developing testable hypothetical models that focus on specific constructs and their interrelationships. At the macro level, the CFIR provides a standardized structure for building on findings across studies.

A review by Kirk et al. (2016) explored the breadth of CFIR use, its application, and contribution to implementation research. Among 429 unique articles, 26 met inclusion criteria and demonstrated a great breadth of application over a wide variety of study objectives, settings, and units of analysis. Very few of these studies noted a justification for the use of CFIR constructs, and the majority of studies used the CFIR to guide data analysis only. Fewer still sought to specifically evaluate the CFIR, demonstrating a need for more studies to assess and further develop CFIR's ability to explain what and how factors influence implementation success and to determine which factors are more important than others.

Method

Using the CFIR to Distinguish Between High and Low Implementers

As noted in the introduction, a great advantage in using a determinant framework such as CFIR across different studies is that it allows for a common conceptualization, analysis, and interpretation of the variables of interest – that is, contextual factors – and for elucidating how they contribute to implementation success. This common conceptual thread facilitates meaningful comparisons across interventions and settings and, ultimately, the accumulation of a robust body of knowledge about the interaction between interventions and contexts and what makes the difference between high and low implementers (i.e., above average versus below average process and outcomes, with study-specific examples of operationalization of high/low implementers being described below). Applying CFIR to this end, to identify contextual factors that distinguish between different degrees of implementation success, goes beyond using the framework merely as a conceptual guide to inform data collection and interpretation. Using a systematic, well-defined analytic approach, described in detail by Damschroder and Lowery (2013), yields rich findings about contextual factors influencing implementation effectiveness that can be combined with findings from across diverse studies. To illustrate application of the CFIR, in the following sections, we review this analytic approach using three published studies that all used the CFIR consistently, following methods recommended by the original authors.

Brief Description of the Studies

The three studies selected here for review offer examples of implementing different evidence-based interventions in diverse settings. They all have in common the use of CFIR as a guiding conceptual framework, as well as similar methods for data analyses, as documented by Damschroder and Lowery (2013). The original study by Damschroder and Lowery (2013) discussed the implementation of MOVE!, a weight management program disseminated nationally to the Veteran Affairs medical centers in the United States. Barwick, Barac, and Zlotkin (2015) evaluated the implementation of exclusive breastfeeding (EBF), a public health intervention for improving maternal and child health, in two low-income countries, Ethiopia and Mali (Barwick et al., 2015). Varsi, Ekstedt, Gammon, and Ruland (2015) examined the implementation of an e-health intervention, Internet-based patient-provider communication (IPPC), in five hospitals in Norway (Varsi et al., 2015). Table 4.1 summarizes study characteristics as well as how CFIR domains and implementation

Table 4.1 Study characteristics and operationalization of the CFIR

	Damschroder and Lowery (2013)	Barwick et al. (2015)	Varsi et al. (2015)
Study design	Mixed methods	Mixed methods	Qualitative methods
Data collection techniques	Phone semi-structured interviews (24 transcripts)	In-person semi-structured interviews and focus groups (32 transcripts)	In-person semi-structured interviews (17 transcripts)
Duration of interviews and focus groups	60 minutes	90 to 120 minutes	10 to 75 minutes
Setting	Health; high income (USA)	Global health; low income (Ethiopia, Mali)	e-Health; high income (Norway)
Intervention	MOVE! (weight management)	Exclusive breastfeeding (EBF)	Internet-based patient-provider communication (IPPC)
Inner setting	5 Veteran Affairs medical centers delivering the MOVE!	2 international NGOs delivering a package of interventions to increase maternal, newborn, and child health	5 units treating patients with cancer or diagnoses within internal medicine
Outer setting	The Veterans Heath Administration and veterans who were offered the program	The villages where the interventions were implemented	The patients who were offered IPPC
Characteristics of the individuals involved	Regional and local facility MOVE! coordinators ($n = 24$)	(a) NGO staff, government staff, and community health workers delivering the intervention ($n = 67$) (b) Mothers who received the intervention ($n = 53$)	The nurses, physicians, and the nutritionist who operated the IPPC service ($n = 17$)
Characteristics of the intervention recipients[a]		Mothers who received the EBF intervention in selected villages in Mali and Ethiopia	
Process	The process of implementing MOVE!	The process of implementing the EBF intervention	The process through which IPPC was implemented
Implementation success	Operationalized as the proportion of candidate Veterans participating in the programs as well as program components actually implemented	Operationalized as changes in EBF rates from pre- to post-implementation of the EBF program	Operationalized as the proportion of available patients who were offered information about IPPC

Note. [a]This is a 6th domain added to the CFIR by Barwick et al. (2015)

outcomes were operationalized in each study. From this snapshot it is apparent that the three studies differ in many respects that highlight the universal, versatile use of the framework to examine implementation context and how it relates to implementation success across a variety of settings and interventions.

Data Collection Procedures

The three studies followed a similar data collection procedure, using a comprehensive, semi-structured interview guide (see published Additional File 1 and Appendix A Table 1 for the complete interview guides used in the Damschroder and Lowery (2013) and Barwick et al. (2015) studies, respectively). Each guide was developed based on the CFIR and included questions that mapped onto CFIR domains and constructs. Among these studies, only two evaluated all CFIR constructs (Barwick et al., 2015; Varsi et al., 2015), whereas Damschroder and Lowery (2013) did not include the *characteristics of the individuals* domain because it was not relevant to the study research questions. Each CFIR construct was addressed through one or multiple questions. For instance, in the Barwick study, based on Damschroder and Lowery's study (2013), information about complexity was elicited through the following questions: "On a scale from 0 to 10, with 0 being very easy and 10 nearly impossible, how difficult has it been to implement the EBF intervention in your region? a. Why? b. What barriers are you experiencing in implementing EBF? c. What factors support the implementation of EBF?"

In addition, the Barwick et al. (2015) study included questions exploring a sixth domain, *characteristics of intervention recipients*, or in this case, mothers who received EBF instruction. This was done to accommodate the unique multi-level nature of the context within which the intervention was implemented; essentially, implementation interventions were targeted to NGO staff and community health workers who themselves intervened with mothers, who in turn carried out the exclusive breastfeeding with their babies. As such, the intervention recipients played a central role in the design and delivery of the EBF intervention. Based on a review of past behavior change research in low- and middle-income countries, four constructs were included under this domain: maternal education and literacy; family composition (e.g., number of children, co-habitation with mother-in-law); religious and cultural beliefs; and socioeconomic status (e.g., Prost et al., 2013). In all three studies, interviews and focus group discussions were digitally recorded and transcribed verbatim, with the exception of one interview in the Varsi et al. (2015) study where the respondent did not allow the use of a voice recorder and the interviewer took detailed notes during the interview instead.

Analytic Approach

In all three studies, data were analyzed using a deductive content analysis approach guided by consensual qualitative research methods. *Content analysis* refers to a set of systematic, rule-guided techniques used to analyze the informational content of textual data (Forman & Damschroder, 2008; Mayring, 2000). There is no one single way of doing qualitative content analysis, and authors disagree with respect to the precise definition and what the analysis actually entails, namely, the extent to which it includes quantitative techniques such as counting words or categories to identify patterns in the data. Despite these differences, there is general agreement that qualitative content analysis (a) examines data coming from open-ended questions; (b) focuses on the informational content of the data from an atheoretical angle, which makes it a generic type of analysis; and (c) has the goal of understanding a phenomenon in detail and depth, as opposed to using statistical inferences to generalize from a sample to the population, which is characteristic of quantitative analyses (Forman & Damschroder, 2008).

Second, *deductive* refers to the fact that data are categorized or coded based on a priori or predetermined categories. In other words, this is a top-down analytic approach because data are coded against pre-set categories rather than emerging from the actual data set, and the authors can decide what these categories are even before they collect data based on a review of the literature or existing theories and frameworks. In this case, these a priori categories are the CFIR constructs.

Third, being guided by *consensual qualitative methods* means that (a) data are collected through open-ended questions; (b) multiple judges are used at all stages of data analysis to incorporate multiple perspectives; (c) consensual validation is achieved through deliberation and consensus; and d) a qualitative expert who is largely external to the study reviews the process to ensure rigor and to maximize validity of the findings (Damschroder & Lowery, 2013).

Having defined the main terms, we review the steps involved in this analytic approach. This is intended to be a high-level summary, as it is beyond the scope of this chapter to delve into qualitative methods. Readers who are unfamiliar with qualitative research will need to consult additional sources (e.g., Coffey & Atkinson, 1996; Miles & Huberman, 1994).

Step 1: Data coding and memo writing Coding refers to indexing or organizing qualitative data according to certain categories (i.e., codes) in order to facilitate the identification of meaningful patterns or concepts that answer the research questions guiding the study. But where do codes come from? Given that this is a deductive type of analysis, as mentioned above, codes are established a priori and represent CFIR constructs. Thus, this step starts by developing a codebook where the codes are derived from the CFIR constructs of interest. For instance, Damschroder and Lowery (2013) assessed 31 CFIR constructs under 4 domains, Barwick et al. (2015) assessed 42 constructs (including all original CFIR constructs plus constructs related to characteristics of intervention recipients) under 6 domains, and Varsi et al. (2015) examined 39 constructs falling under 5 domains. It is important to note that although this is primarily a deductive type of analysis, researchers are advised to remain open to new concepts emerging from the data which have the potential to refine or add to the existing CFIR constructs. For instance, in one of the studies (Barwick et al., 2015), while coding for the CFIR construct *planning*, it became apparent that *planning for sustainability* was a salient aspect of planning and was proposed by the authors as a distinct CFIR factor and a sub-construct of *planning*. As noted above, in contrast to this inductive addition of the *planning for sustainability* construct to the CFIR, other constructs, such as *family composition; socioeconomic status; religious, traditional beliefs and practices*; and *maternal education* – all under a 6th domain, *characteristics of intervention recipients* – were derived following a literature review and then applied deductively in the qualitative analysis.

Qualitative codebooks typically organize codes in a hierarchical structure with parent or superordinate codes (i.e., CFIR domains) and child or subordinate codes (i.e., CFIR constructs and sub-constructs) and include detailed definitions and examples in order to ensure consistent interpretation of the codes. Guidance for coding each construct is available online at www.cfirguide.org. In all three studies, coding was done by pairs of coders – part of the consensual approach to analysis mentioned above – who coded transcripts independently using a qualitative analysis software, e.g., NVivo (QSR International, Australia), met and compared coding, discussed discrepancies, and reached consensus regarding final codes.

The coded data form the basis for the next level of analysis – writing memos. Memos are summary statements organized by CFIR construct and illustrated with supporting quotes, typically developed for each case (with a case referring to each of the units of analysis being compared). Specifically, a case is a health facility in the Damschroder and Lowery (2013) study, an NGO/country in the Barwick et al. (2015) study, and a medical unit in the Varsi et al. (2015) study, for a total of five, two, and five cases, respectively. A memo template and memo examples are available online at http://www.cfirguide.org/qual.html.

Step 2: Rating the CFIR constructs After case memos are finalized, team members independently assign a rating to all CFIR constructs within each case. Table 4.2 lists the criteria used to guide assignments of the ratings. The ratings reflect the valence (positive or negative influence) and the magnitude or strength of each construct within each case relative to implementation success. Briefly, each construct is rated with a score of −2 to +2, with a negative valence indicating a negative influence on implementation and a positive valence indicating a facilitative influence. Different degrees of the strength of the influence are reflected in a score of 0, 1, or 2. Constructs rated as 0 either had a neutral influence on implementation or a blend of positive and negative influences.

Similar to coding and memo writing, ratings are assigned following a consensual approach. For instance, in the Barwick et al. (2015) study, the research team included four members, and consensus was defined as perfect agreement among three or four raters. For both cases, about 70% of the ratings were identical for at least three of

Table 4.2 Criteria used to rate the CFIR constructs

Rating	Criteria
−2	The construct is a negative influence in the organization, an impeding influence in work processes, and/or an impeding influence in implementation efforts. The majority of interviewees (at least two) describe explicit examples of how the key or all aspects (or the absence) of a construct manifests itself in a negative way.
−1	The construct is a negative influence in the organization, an impeding influence in work processes, and/or an impeding influence in implementation efforts. Interviewees make general statements about the construct manifesting in a negative way but without concrete examples: (a) the construct is mentioned only in passing or at a high level without examples or evidence of actual, concrete descriptions of how that construct manifests; (b) there is a mixed effect of different aspects of the construct but with a general overall negative effect; (c) there is sufficient information to make an indirect inference about the generally negative influence; and/or (d) judged as weakly negative by the absence of the construct.
0	A construct has neutral influence if (a) it appears to have neutral effect (purely descriptive) or is only mentioned generically without valence; (b) there is no evidence of positive or negative influence; (c) credible or reliable interviewees contradict each other; (d) there are positive and negative influences at different levels in the organization that balance each other out; and/or (e) different aspects of the construct have positive influence, while others have negative influence, and overall, the effect is neutral.
+1	The construct is a positive influence in the organization, a facilitating influence in work processes, and/or a facilitating influence in implementation efforts. Interviewees make general statements about the construct manifesting in a positive way but without concrete examples: (a) the construct is mentioned only in passing or at a high level without examples or evidence of actual, concrete descriptions of how that construct manifests; (b) there is a mixed effect of different aspects of the construct but with a general overall positive effect; and/or (c) there is sufficient information to make an indirect inference about the generally positive influence.
+2	The construct is a positive influence in the organization, a facilitating influence in work processes, and/or a facilitating influence in implementation efforts. The majority of interviewees (at least two) describe explicit examples of how the key or all aspects of a construct manifests itself in a positive way.
Missing	Interviewee(s) were not asked about the presence or influence of the construct; or if asked about a construct, their responses did not correspond to the intended construct and were instead coded to another construct. Interviewee(s) lack of knowledge about a construct does not necessarily indicate missing data and may instead indicate the absence of the construct.

Taken from Damschroder and Lowery (2013)

the four raters. When there was no consensus among the four raters, that is, fewer than three of the raters assigned the same rating, two of the raters reviewed the memos, resolved discrepancies, and assigned a final rating. Table 4.3 presents an excerpt from a memo developed in the Barwick et al. (2015) study for the *patient needs and resources* construct, which received a +2 rating for the case in Ethiopia.

Step 3: Interpretation of ratings Once a rating is assigned for each CFIR construct and for each of the cases, the final step entails comparing and contrasting these ratings. This is facilitated by creating a matrix that lists the ratings for each

Table 4.3 Extract from a memo for the patient needs and resources construct from the Barwick et al. (2015) study

Summary statement	Prior to implementation, the NGO staff conducted a situational analysis and identified the areas with high food insecurity in Ethiopia where they planned to implement the EBF intervention. In these areas, they found very low rates of breastfeeding, high rates of malnutrition in children under the age of 2, and very high rates of maternal malnourishment and anemia and thus designed the intervention and the delivery strategy to target populations with low socioeconomic status and pregnant and lactating females in each of the households. In addition to identifying the target population, in order to inform the implementation approach, the NGO looked at cultural practices regarding feeding habits, traditional and religious beliefs, gender issues, and major decision-makers at the level of village and household.
Supporting quotes	"So we are not talking about working at the margins. We are not trying to increase EBF rates from the 85% to the 95%. We are looking at ...EBF rates below 50%, so you've got a huge cohort of people who are in that area, who are ...able to make those kinds of changes."
	"We have taken a lot of time to think of how to approach nutrition and breast feeding programming, and being sensitive to the fact that if you [are] asking women to breast feed who are starving, who really don't have enough to eat. What does that look like, and how do you talk to families about that?"
	"This area is a highly populated area, the terrain is not good for cultivation, crop productivity is very low, land is degraded, and these are the major issues -especially the land they have, they cannot support themselves and their families from the land they have...the average land holding is below half a hectare."
	"And also men are always given priority. Men, the husband should get the lion's share of the meat, they have to eat first, after they eat meat first, and then boys, then girls, then mothers, last."

Note. Patient needs and resources refers to the extent to which patient needs, as well as barriers and facilitators to meet those needs, are accurately known and prioritized by the organization

CFIR construct for each of the cases of interest (see Table 4.4 for a table excerpt from Damschroder and Lowery (2013) study). The purpose of this exercise is to identify patterns in the data, specifically CFIR constructs distinguishing high from low implementers. In other words, once implementers are categorized as high or low effectiveness, it is possible to identify the CFIR constructs that are more frequently endorsed by participants as having a positive influence in the organization and a facilitating influence in work processes and implementation efforts.

Implementation effectiveness or success can be operationalized in different ways. For instance, Damschroder and Lowery (2013) operationalized success based on the number of Veterans participating in the MOVE! intervention, as well as the number of program components actually being implemented. Similarly, in the Varsi et al. (2015) study, implementation effectiveness was operationalized as the proportion of available patients who were offered information about the IPPC intervention. And, finally, Barwick et al. (2015) measured implementation success as changes in EBF rates from the beginning to the end of the implementation (i.e., the percentage of infants aged 0–5 months who were exclusively breastfed). Based on these operational definitions of implementation effectiveness, in two of the three studies, the

Table 4.4 Ratings assigned to CFIR constructs by case

Construct[a]	Low implementation facilities		Transition facility	High implementation facilities		
Tension for change	0	0	+2	+1	+1	b
Compatibility	−2	+1	0	+1	+2	
Relative priority	−1	−2	−2	+1	+2	b
Organizational incentives and rewards	0	−1	0	0	+1	
Goals and feedback	−2	−1	+1	+1	+2	b
Learning climate	Missing	−1	Missing	+1	+2	b

Note. Excerpt from Table 3, Damschroder and Lowery (2013) study, reproduced with journal permission

[a]All constructs listed are part of the inner setting domain

[b]Constructs listed strongly distinguish between low and high implementation effectiveness

authors could clearly categorize their cases as high and low implementers: two high and two low implementers in the Damschroder and Lowery (2013) study and four high and one low implementer in the Varsi et al. (2015) study. For these two studies, CFIR constructs were characterized as (a) having insufficient information to discern a pattern, labeled as "missing"; (b) not distinguishing between low and high implementers; (c) weakly distinguishing between implementers; and (d) strongly distinguishing between implementers.

However, in the Barwick et al. (2015) study, the two cases could not be meaningfully categorized as high and low implementers based on the changes in the EBF rates from the beginning to the end of the implementation. For one of the cases, Mali, EBF rates were very low at baseline (27%) and increased significantly post-implementation (66%). For the second case, Ethiopia, EBF rates were moderate at baseline (69%), and they were maintained and increased slightly post-implementation (75%). Thus, the implementation task with respect to EBF was different for the two cases, rendering a categorization into high and low implementers as artificial. In this study, given that both implementing entities were effective in their implementation, CFIR constructs were used to identify the contextual factors that were most common across the two cases which both had relatively high implementation effectiveness.

Table 4.5 summarizes the CFIR constructs distinguishing between high and low implementers in two of the three studies selected for review where this distinction was possible (Damschroder & Lowery, 2013; Varsi et al., 2015) and the CFIR constructs associated with success in the Barwick et al. (2015) study where both implementing entities were effective. Overall, this summary table exemplifies the value of using a common framework and a consistent analytic approach across studies – it allows systematic knowledge building because the same language, encapsulated by constructs, is used across the studies even though they evaluated a diverse array of interventions across diverse settings. For instance, this summary highlights three constructs associated with implementation effectiveness in all three studies: *relative*

Table 4.5 Qualitative associations between CFIR constructs and implementation success

CFIR domains and constructs	Damschroder and Lowery (2013)	Varsi et al. (2015)	Barwick et al. (2015)
	Constructs distinguishing between high and low implementers		*Constructs associated with implementation success*
1. Intervention characteristics			
Relative advantage[a]	Yes	Yes	Yes
Trialability		Yes	
Adaptability			Yes
Complexity			Yes
2. Outer setting			
Patient needs and resources[a]	Yes	Yes	Yes
Cosmopolitanism			Yes
External policies and incentives	Yes		Yes
3. Inner setting			
Structural characteristics		Yes	
Networks and communications	Yes		
Culture		Yes	
Implementation climate			
Tension for change[a]	Yes	Yes	Yes
Compatibility		Yes	
Relative priority	Yes	Yes	
Goals and feedback	Yes		
Learning climate	Yes		
Readiness for implementation			
Leadership engagement	Yes		
Available resources	Yes	Yes	
Access to information and knowledge			Yes
4. Characteristics of individuals			
Knowledge and beliefs about the intervention		Yes	Yes
5. Process			
Planning	Yes	Yes	
Planning for sustainability[b]			Yes
Formally appointed internal implementation leaders		Yes	
Champions			Yes
Reflecting and evaluating	Yes		
6. Characteristics of intervention recipients[b]			
Family composition			Yes
Spiritual, religious, traditional beliefs and practices			Yes
Key constructs in each study (n)	12	12	13

[a]Measured only in the Barwick et al. (2015) study
[b]Constructs strongly associated with implementation effectiveness in all three studies reviewed

advantage (i.e., stakeholders' perception of the advantage of implementing the intervention versus an alternative solution; part of the *intervention characteristics* domain); *patient needs and resources* (i.e., the extent to which patient needs and barriers and facilitators to meet those needs are accurately known and prioritized by the organization; part of *outer setting* domain); and *tension for change* (i.e., the degree to which stakeholders perceive the current situation as intolerable or needing change; part of *inner setting* domain). Other constructs may be key depending on type of intervention and setting. For instance, *relative priority* and *available resources* distinguish between high and low implementers in two of the three studies conducted in high-income countries, in health settings (Damschroder & Lowery, 2013; Varsi et al., 2015).

Discussion

This chapter highlights the advantage of using conceptual frameworks to inform research and practice as demonstrated in a qualitative comparative analysis across three studies that utilized the CFIR in a similarly analytical way. Although the sample of studies in this analysis is small, we were able to identify factors that appear to be associated with implementation success across a diverse array of settings and interventions, including weight management in a large integrated US healthcare system, an e-health application in Norway, and a Canadian study of a maternal and child health intervention undertaken in Mali and Ethiopia. This synthesis contributes to our understanding of the circumstances under which some constructs may play a significant role in influencing implementation and clinical outcomes, over time and with the addition of more studies, could be used by implementers for predictive and planning purposes.

Which CFIR Factors Are Strongly Associated with Implementation Success?

Our comparative analysis identified three factors that were strongly related to implementation success across three different studies: *relative advantage, tension for change*, and *patient needs and resources*. These three constructs appear to have mattered most for implementation effectiveness in the three studies, transcending the very real differences between studies related to intervention type and setting. Practically, these constructs had greater weight in our analysis and indicate that they should be taken seriously when planning, delivering strategies for implementation, and evaluating. CFIR is not prescriptive about how to achieve implementation objectives. Rather, it provides a list of factors that that may be important and should be measured. For more guidance on strategies, the reader will benefit from reading the compilation of implementation strategies generated by Powell and colleagues as part of the Expert Recommendations for Implementing Change (ERIC) study (Boyd, Powell, Endicott & Lewis, 2018; Leeman, Birken, Powell, Rohweder & Shea, 2017; Powell et al., 2015).

Similar to other studies (e.g., Greenhalgh, Robert, Macfarlane, Bate & Kyriakidou, 2004), *relative advantage* appears to be a sine qua non condition for successful adoption and implementation (Gustafson et al., 2003). This means that if users perceive a clear, unambiguous advantage in the effectiveness or efficiency of the intervention, our study finds that it is more likely that the implementation will be successful. Benefits of the intervention must be clearly observable to stakeholders, and thus, efforts to demonstrate benefits of the intervention will help implementation (Denis, Hebert, Langley, Lozeau, & Trottier, 2002; Greenhalgh et al., 2004; Grol, Bosch, Hulscher, Eccles, Wensing, 2007). Strategically, planning for implementation would benefit from paying attention to *relative advantage* early on, during the intervention selection process, possibly by working through implementation process tools like the Hexagon tool (Kiser, Blasé & Fixsen, 2013) or the Checklist for Assessing Readiness for Implementation (CARI; Barwick, Unpublished).

In addition, successful implementers displayed high levels of *tension for change*. As such, staff in these implementing organizations have to really "feel the need to change" (Heath & Heath, 2010) and generate sustainable motivation for this effort. Whether or not stakeholders who are involved in local implementation actually feel a tension for change has been shown to be an important antecedent for successful implementation (e.g., Lukas et al., 2007). Practically, this means that, if, for instance, *tension for change* does not exist before implementing a new intervention, strategies should be designed to build that tension to help heighten receptivity for the intervention among key stakeholders. To this end, effective communication (captured by the CFIR construct, *networks and communications*) can foster tension for change by building dissatisfaction with status quo as well as announcing a change, cultivating commitment, and reducing resistance (Greenhalgh et al., 2004). Similarly, when stakeholders have firsthand experience with the problem, implementation is especially more likely to be successful (Gustafson et al., 2003). Strategically, creating a strong perception of *tension for change* within an organization can be greatly facilitated by leadership. Leadership support in terms of commitment and active interest can lead to a stronger implementation climate that, in turn, can positively influence implementation effectiveness.

Patient needs and resources, knowing and prioritizing patient needs, as well as barriers and facilitators to meet those needs, was strongly associated with successful implementation across the three studies reviewed. In other types of settings, such as educational settings, one might consider the needs of students. For instance, our own research has shown that teachers are more likely to implement an intervention if it maps onto the needs of a preponderance of students in the classroom, rather than for a select few (Barwick, Barac, Akrong, Johnson & Chaban, 2014). This finding is pertinent in a service culture that increasingly stresses the importance of consumer engagement (see, e.g., Clancy, 2011). Along the same line, consumer-centered organizations are more likely to implement change effectively in healthcare (Shortell et al., 2004). This means that, strategically, implementers might consider early on the key elements of consumer-centered care that delineate the extent to which consumers are at the center of organizational processes and decisions, such as those articulated by the Practical, Robust Implementation and Sustainability Model (PRISM) in healthcare: patient choices are provided, patient barriers are addressed, transition between program elements is seamless, complexity and costs are minimized, and patients have high satisfaction with service and degree of access and receive feedback (Feldstein & Glasgow, 2008).

Other CFIR Factors Distinguishing Between High and Low Implementers

In addition to the three CFIR factors that characterized successful implementation in all three studies reviewed (*relative advantage, tension for change* and *patient needs and resources*), in two of the studies (Damschroder & Lowery, 2013; Varsi et al., 2015) – both conducted in high-income settings – CFIR-based coding identified three other factors that strongly distinguished between high and low implementers: *relative priority, available resources*, and *planning*. Two of these factors (*relative priority; available resources*) are associated with the internal working of the organizations suggesting that the *inner setting* is highly salient for preparing the stage for successful implementation and central to success in the practice change endeavor.

In contrast to *relative advantage*, which is an intervention characteristic, *relative priority* relates to the inner setting and reflects the stakeholders' perception of the importance of the implementation within the organization. If employees perceive that implementation of a certain intervention is a key organizational priority, then implementation climate is likely to be strong (Klein, Conn & Sorra, 2001) and employees will perceive the intervention as important rather than a distraction from their "real work." Past research has shown that the higher the relative priority of implementing an intervention, the more effective the implementation is likely to be (Klein et al., 2001; Helfrich, Weiner, McKinney & Minasian, 2007). Importantly, the ability of an organization to fully implement an intervention may be a function of how many other initiatives or changes have been rolled out in the recent past which may lead to being overwhelmed with yet another initiative (Greenhalgh et al., 2004; Gustafson et al., 2003) and a low priority being assigned. This is an important consideration for funders and governments who may not have sufficient appreciation for the complexities and real-world timelines of implementation initiatives stemming from policy and who often push out interventions without sufficient regard for both individual and organizational absorptive capacity to take on the additional work (Barwick et al., 2019).

Available resources (the level of resources dedicated for implementation and ongoing operations including money, training, education, physical space, and time, and planning) appeared as critical to successful implementation. The key role played by these factors may stem from the fact that they contribute to the readiness and preparedness of an organization for implementation.

Strategically, the *relative priority* of implementing an intended intervention, the *planning* and *available resources* dedicated to implementation should be considered early on in the implementation process and require consideration of the *inner* and *outer settings* in which the intervention is to be adopted. We again highlight the role of leaders and middle managers in considering these key constructs from the implementation onset through networking and communication and negotiating for resources.

Methodological Recommendations and Future Research

The present exercise illustrates the value of using a common conceptual framework and analytic method across studies. Methodological consistency ensures study rigor and comparability; monitoring, testing, and validation of context-specific additions or revisions to the CFIR; as well as systematically documenting conceptual overlaps, coding difficulties, and definitional ambiguities. Researchers interested in using CFIR to guide implementation and evaluate outcomes are encouraged to use the full CFIR coding methodology, as described here and in the CFIR Guide (http://cfirguide.org/index.html).

With respect to CFIR additions, as noted in the Method section, in the Barwick et al. (2015) study, the authors added a 6th domain related to the recipients of the program because past research in low- and middle-income countries emphasized the importance of considering these characteristics as part of the implementation (Prost et al., 2013). Essentially, this addition does not propose a construct that is not conceptually covered by the CFIR but rather magnifies or expands on the *patient needs and resources* construct, which appeared as critical to implementation success in two of the three studies reviewed. Moreover, this is in line with the observation by Varsi et al. (2015) that CFIR is an institution-centric framework with patients being placed under the outer setting, which was interpreted by the authors to suggest that the patients play a "peripheral role in the implementation process." The authors argued that this was in contrast with the increasing emergence of patient-centric models of care and the salience of the healthcare providers, represented in two of the five CFIR domains (*inner setting, characteristic of individuals*).

Importantly, this point of discussion does not highlight a framework limitation but identifies the role and value of using the same framework to guide various research studies across different contexts. CFIR was not intended to be a static, once-and-for-all answer to all implementation questions but rather a tool – a "pragmatic structure for identifying potential influences on implementation and organizing findings across studies" (Damschroder et al., 2009). As the authors noted in the original article outlining the CFIR (Damschroder et al., 2009), the utility and validity of the framework needs to ultimately be judged through systematic research, answering questions such as "Does the CFIR promote comparison of results across contexts and studies over time? Does the CFIR stimulate new theoretical developments?" These points are all relevant for the continued evolution of CFIR in future research and evaluation efforts to systematically examine the rich, dynamic role played by contextual factors in implementation and ultimately contributing to providing more specificity to the types of implementation activities needed to foster implementation success.

References

Barwick, M. (Unpublished). Checklist for assessing readiness for implementation. Retrieved 4 July 2016 from http://melaniebarwick.com/implementation.php

Barwick, M., Barac, R., Akrong, L. M., Johnson, S., & Chaban, P. (2014). Bringing evidence to the classroom: Exploring educator notions of evidence and preferences for practice change. *International Education Research, 2*(4), 1–15. https://doi.org/10.12735/ier.v2i4p01

Barwick M, Kimber M, Akrong L, Johnson S, Cunningham CE, Bennett K, Ashbourne G, Godden T. (2019). Advancing Implementation Frameworks with a Mixed Methods Multi-Case Study in Child Behavioral Health. Translational Behavioral Medicine, ibz005, https://doi.org/10.1093/tbm/ibz005

Barwick, M., Barac, R., & Zlotkin, S. (2015). Evaluation of effective implementation of exclusive breastfeeding in Ethiopia and Mali using the Consolidated Framework for Implementation Research. Canada: Hospital for Sick Children. http://melaniebarwick.com/wp-content/uploads/dlm_uploads/2019/02/EBF-Research-Report-FINAL-July-29-2015.pdf.

Bauer, M. S., Damschroder, L., Hagedorn, H., Smith, J., & Kilbourne, A. M. (2015). An introduction to implementation science for the non-specialist. *BMC Psychology, 3*(1), 1.

Boyd, M. R., Powell, B. J., Endicott, D., & Lewis, C. C. (2018). A method for tracking implementation strategies: An exemplar implementing measurement-based care in community behavioral health clinics. *Behaviour Therapy, 49*(4), 525–537.

Chaudoir, S. R., Dugan, A. G., & Barr, C. H. (2013). Measuring factors affecting implementation of health innovations: A systematic review of structural, organizational, provider, patient, and innovation level measures. *Implementation Science, 8*(1), 22.

Clancy, C. M. (2011). Patient engagement in health care. *Health Services Research, 46*(2), 389–393. https://doi.org/10.1111/j.1475-6773.2011.01254.x

Coffey, A., & Atkinson, P. (1996). *Making sense of qualitative data, complementary research strategies*. London, Thousand Oaks, CA and New Delhi: Sage Publications.

Curran, G. M., Bauer, M., Mittman, B., Pyne, J. M., & Stetler, C. (2012). Effectiveness-implementation hybrid designs: Combining elements of clinical effectiveness and implementation research to enhance public health impact. *Medical Care, 50*(3), 217–226. https://doi.org/10.1097/MLR.0b013e3182408812

Damschroder, J. L., & Lowery, J. C. (2013). Evaluation of a large-scale weight management program using the Consolidated Framework for Implementation Research (CFIR). *Implementation Science, 8*, 51.

Damschroder, L., Aron, D., Keith, R., Kirsh, S., Alexander, J., & Lowery, J. (2009). Fostering implementation of health services research findings into practice: A consolidated framework for advancing implementation science. *Implementation Science, 4*(1), 50.

Davidoff, F., Dixon-Woods, M., Leviton, L., & Michie, S. (2015). Demystifying theory and its use in improvement. *BMJ Quality & Safety, 24*, 228–238.

Denis, J.-L., Hébert, Y., Langley, A., Lozeau, D., & Trottier, L.-H. (2002). Explaining diffusion patterns for complex health care innovations. *Health Care Management Review, 27*, 60–73.

Department of Health United Kingdom. (2007). *Improving access to psychological therapies*. Retrieved from http://iapt.nhs.uk/silo/files/specification-for-the-commissionerled-pathfinder-programme.pdf

Feldstein, A. C., & Glasgow, R. E. (2008). A practical, robust implementation and sustainability model (PRISM) for integrating research findings into practice. *The Joint Commission Journal on Quality and Patient Safety, 34*(4), 228–243.

Forman, J., & Damschroder, L. J. (2008). Qualitative content analysis. In L. Jacoby & L. A. Siminoff (Eds.), *Empirical methods for bioethics: A primer* (pp. 39–62). Oxford, UK: Elsevier.

Foy, R., Ovretveit, J., Shekelle, P. G., Pronovost, P. J., Taylor, S. L., Dy, S., … Wachter, R. M. (2011). The role of theory in research to develop and evaluate the implementation of patient safety practices. *Quality & Safety in Health Care, 20*(5), 453–459. https://doi.org/10.1136/bmjqs.2010.047993. Epub 2011 Feb 11.

Government of Australia. (2001). *Australian General Practice Network. National primary care initiative. Better outcomes in mental health care initiative.* Retrieved from http://www.health.gov.au/internet/main/publishing.nsf/Content/mental-boimhc

Government of Ontario. (2011). *Open minds, healthy minds: Ontario's comprehensive mental health and addictions strategy.* Retrieved from http://www.health.gov.on.ca/en/common/ministry/publications/reports/mental_health2011/mentalhealth_rep2011.pdf

Greenhalgh, T., Robert, G., Macfarlane, F., Bate, P., & Kyriakidou, O. (2004). Diffusion of innovations in service organizations: Systematic review and recommendations. *Milbank Quarterly, 82*, 581–629. https://doi.org/10.1111/j.0887-378X.2004.00325.x

Grol, R. P., Bosch, M. C., Hulscher, M. E., Eccles, M. P., & Wensing, M. (2007). Planning and studying improvement in patient care: The use of theoretical perspectives. *The Milbank Quarterly, 85*, 93–138.

Gustafson, D. H., Sainfort, F., Eichler, M., Adams, L., Bisognano, M., & Steudel, H. (2003). Developing and testing a model to predict outcomes of organizational change. *Health Services Research, 38*, 751–776. https://doi.org/10.1111/1475-6773.00143

Heath, C., & Heath, D. (2010). *Switch: How to change things when change is hard.* New York, NY: Broadway Books.

Helfrich, C. D., Weiner, B. J., McKinney, M. M., & Minasian, L. (2007). Determinants of implementation effectiveness: Adapting a framework for complex innovations. *Medical Care Research and Review, 64*(3), 279–303.

Kirk, M. A., Kelley, C., Yankey, N., Birken, S. A., Abadie, B., & Damschroder, L. (2016). A systematic review of the use of the consolidated framework for implementation research. *Implementation Science, 11*, 72. https://doi.org/10.1186/s13012-016-0437-z

Kiser, L., Blasé, K., & Fixsen, D. (2013). The hexagon tool: Exploring context. Chapel Hill, NC: The National Implementation Research Network. Retrieved 4 July 2016 from http://implementation.fpg.unc.edu/sites/implementation.fpg.unc.edu/files/resources/NIRN-Education-TheHexagonTool.pdf

Klein, K. J., Conn, A. B., & Sorra, J. S. (2001). Implementing computerized technology: An organizational analysis. *The Journal of Applied Psychology, 86*, 811–824.

Leeman, J., Birken, S. A., Powell, B. J., Rohweder, C., & Shea, C. M. (2017). Beyond "implementation strategies": Classifying the full range of strategies used in implementation science and practice. *Implementation Science, 12*(1), 125. https://doi.org/10.1186/s13012-017-0657-x

Lewis, C., & Dorsey, C. (2020). Advancing implementation science measurement. In R. Mildon, B. Albers, & A. Shlonsky (Eds.), *The Science of Implementation* (pp.). Cham: Springer.

Lewis, C. C., Stanick, C. F., Martinez, R. G., Weiner, B. J., Kim, M., Barwick, M., & Comtois, K. A. (2015). The Society for Implementation Research Collaboration instrument review project: A methodology to promote rigorous evaluation. *Implementation Science, 10*, 2. https://doi.org/10.1186/s13012-014-0193-x

Lukas, C. V., Holmes, S. K., Cohen, A. B., Restuccia, J., Cramer, I. E., Shwartz, M., & Charns, M. P. (2007). Transformational change in health care systems: An organizational model. *Health Care Management Review, 32*, 309–320.

Martinez, R., Lewis, C., & Weiner, B. (2014). Instrumentation issues in implementation science. *Implementation Science, 9*(1), 118.

Mayring, P. (2000). Qualitative content analysis. Forum: *Qualitative Social Research*, 1.

McKibbon, K. A., Lokker, C., Wilczynski, N. L., Ciliska, D., Dobbins, M., Davis, D. A., ... Straus, S. E. (2010). A cross-sectional study of the number and frequency of terms used to refer to knowledge translation in a body of health literature in 2006: A Tower of Babel? *Implementation Science, 5*, 16. https://doi.org/10.1186/1748-5908-5-16

Meyers, D. C., Durlak, J. A., & Wandersman, A. (2012). The quality implementation framework: A synthesis of critical steps in the implementation process. *American Journal of Community Psychology, 50*(3–4), 462–480. https://doi.org/10.1007/s10464-012-9522-x

Miles, M. B., & Huberman, A. M. (1994). *Qualitative data analysis* (2nd ed.). Thousand Oaks, CA: Sage Publications.

Mitchell, S. A., Fisher, C. A., Hastings, C. E., Silverman, L. B., & Wallen, G. R. (2010). A thematic analysis of theoretical models for translational science in nursing: Mapping the field. *Nursing Outlook, 58*(6), 287–300.

Moulin, J., Sabater-Hernandez, D., Fernandez-Llimos, F., & Benrimoj, S. (2015). A systematic review of implementation frameworks of innovations in healthcare and resulting generic implementation framework. *Health Research Policy and Systems, 13*(16). https://doi.org/10.1186/s12961-015-0005-z

New Freedom Commission on Mental Health. (2003). *Achieving the promise: Transforming mental health in America – Final report.* Retrieved from http://govinfo.library.unt.edu/mental-healthcommission/reports/FinalReport/downloads/FinalReport.pdf

Nilsen, P. (2015). Making sense of implementation theories, models and frameworks. *Implementation Science, 10*, 53.

Nilsen, P. (2020). Making sense of implementation theories, models, and frameworks. In R. Mildon, B. Albers, & A. Shlonsky (Eds.), *The Science of Implementation* (pp.). Cham: Springer.

Powell, B. J., Waltz, T. J., Chinman, M. J., Damschroder, L. J., Smith, J. L., Matthieu, M. M., ... Kirchner, J. E. (2015). A refined compilation of implementation strategies: Results from the Expert Recommendations for Implementing Change (ERIC) project. *Implementation Science, 10*, 21. https://doi.org/10.1186/s13012-015-0209-1

Prost, A., Colbourn, T., Seward, N., Azad, K., Coomarasamy, A., Copas, A., ... Costello, A. (2013). Women's groups practising participatory learning and action to improve maternal and newborn health in low-resource settings: A systematic review and meta-analysis. *Lancet, 381*, 1736–1746.

Sales, A., Smith, J., Curran, G., & Kochevar, L. (2006). Models, strategies, and tools. Theory in implementing evidence-based findings into health care practice. *Journal of General Internal Medicine, 21*(Suppl 2), S43–S49.

Shojania, K. G., Jennings, A., Mayhew, A., Ramsay, C. R., Eccles, M. P., & Grimshaw, J. (2009). The effects of on-screen, point of care computer reminders on processes and outcomes of care. *Cochrane Database Systematic Reviews*, (3), CD001096.

Shortell, S. M., Marsteller, J. A., Lin, M., Pearson, M. L., Wu, S. Y., Mendel, P., ... Rosen, M. (2004). The role of perceived team effectiveness in improving chronic illness care. *Medical Care, 42*(11), 1040–1048.

Tabak, R. G., Khoong, E. C., Chambers, D. A., & Brownson, R. C. (2012). Bridging research and practice: Models for dissemination and implementation research. *American Journal of Preventive Medicine, 43*(3), 337–350.

Van Achterberg, T., Schoonhoven, L., & Grol, R. (2008). Nursing implementation science: How evidence based nursing requires evidence based implementation. *Journal of Nursing Scholarship, 40*(4), 302–310.

Varsi, C., Ekstedt, M., Gammon, D., & Ruland, C. M. (2015). Using the consolidated framework for implementation research to identify barriers and facilitators for the implementation of an internet-based patient-provider communication service in five settings: A qualitative study. *Journal of Medical Internet Research, 17*(11), e262.

Chapter 5
Organizational Readiness for Change: What We Know, What We Think We Know, and What We Need to Know

Bryan J. Weiner, Alecia S. Clary, Stacey L. Klaman, Kea Turner, and Amir Alishahi-Tabriz

Organizational readiness for change is considered a critical precursor to successful implementation. Indeed, some claim that half of all implementation failures occur because organizational leaders do not sufficiently prepare organizational members for change (Kotter, 1996). Although management consultants have written for decades about organizational readiness and how to create it, social scientists have only recently focused attention on the importance of organizational readiness in supporting the adoption and implementation of innovation and evidence-based practices in health and human service settings. Eight years ago, a review was published of how organizational readiness for change had been defined and measured in health services research and other fields (Weiner, Amick, & Lee, 2008). Since then, social scientists have written a great deal about, developed measures of, and studied the antecedents and consequences of organizational readiness. However, this work spans many disciplinary fields, focuses on different types of change, and appears in specialized journals. Further advances in theory, research, and practice would profit from an updated review of this growing, but scattered, body of work.

This chapter takes stock of what we know, what we think we know, and what we need to know about what organizational readiness is, why it matters, and how you create it. Those new to the field of implementation science will find this chapter a useful entry point into the scientific discussion about organizational readiness.

B. J. Weiner (✉)
Departments of Global Health and Health Services, University of Washington, Seattle, WA, USA
e-mail: bjweiner@uw.edu

A. S. Clary · K. Turner · A. Alishahi-Tabriz
Department of Health Policy and Management, University of North Carolina at Chapel Hill, Chapel Hill, NC, USA

S. L. Klaman
Department of Maternal and Child Health, University of North Carolina at Chapel Hill, Chapel Hill, NC, USA

© Springer Nature Switzerland AG 2020
B. Albers et al. (eds.), *Implementation Science 3.0*,
https://doi.org/10.1007/978-3-030-03874-8_5

Those already engaged in the scientific discussion might find thought-provoking the chapter's critical reflections on the current state of the field and recommendations for future directions in research and practice.

What Is Organizational Readiness for Change?

An earlier review of the literature noted several conceptual ambiguities in the meaning of organizational readiness for change (Weiner et al., 2008). Is organizational readiness a psychological construct referring to organizational members' attitudes, beliefs, and intentions, or it is a structural construct referring to organizational capabilities and resources? Is readiness an individual-level phenomenon, a collective phenomenon, or both? Is readiness relevant only prior to change initiation or is it relevant throughout the change process?

Like many social science constructs, readiness is a concept borrowed from everyday language. Before examining how social scientists have defined readiness, it is useful to ask what readiness means in everyday discourse. This is especially worthwhile since many social scientists writing about readiness do not define the concept but rather draw upon—and ask their readers to draw upon—common sense meanings of the term (Weiner et al., 2008).

What do we mean when we ask: Are they ready to go to the party? Are these children ready to learn to read? Are employees ready for the big news about the management shake-up? In all of these cases, we are asking how prepared they are to do something or how prepared they are for something to happen. Sometimes we use the term "ready" to indicate that some group is poised to, or about to, do something (e.g., "They are ready to quit."). This use also implies preparedness. Even the statement, "Dinner is ready," indicates that the meal is prepared for eating. There are, of course, many different ways in which someone or some group can be prepared. There is certainly a behavioral component (e.g., are you prepared to execute a course of action?), but there is also a psychological component (e.g., are you mentally or emotionally prepared to initiate action or respond to an event?). When we ask if a basketball team is ready for the big game or if a military unit is ready for battle, we are inquiring not only into the team's preparedness behaviorally but also psychologically (e.g., are they "psyched up"?). In sum, the concept of readiness in everyday discourse connotes a *state* of *preparedness* for *future* action, either proactive or responsive. This future orientation is important. It does not make sense in ordinary discourse to ask if some group is ready to do something when they have already done it or are currently doing it. When we inquire during or after some action whether a group *was* ready, we are asking about how prepared they were *before* they acted or responded to an event.

With this common sense meaning in mind, one can examine how social scientists have defined readiness and whether more recent conceptual work has resolved any of the aforementioned ambiguities in the meaning of readiness. Although social scientists are not obliged to adopt or adhere to common sense meanings when they develop scientific constructs, common sense meanings can serve as a useful touchstone for gauging whether something important has been lost or preserved when social scientists assign formal definitions to concepts borrowed from everyday discourse.

A quick perusal of the various definitions of organizational readiness for change that have been offered over the years (see Table 5.1) reveals a growing consensus that readiness is a psychological construct rather than a structural one. Many recent definitions of readiness draw upon the psychologically based definition of the construct offered more than 20 years ago by Armenakis, Harris, and Mossholder (1993). Holt, Helfrich, Hall, and Weiner (2010) and Scaccia and colleagues (2015) differ in that they view readiness as a construct that has both psychological and structural dimensions. Despite consensus on the psychological nature of the construct, disagreement persists concerning the psychological content of the construct. For example, although definitions generally include a cognitive component, the specific beliefs and ideas that comprise this cognitive component vary. Efficacy, or the belief in one's individual or collective capabilities, is a common cognitive component. Principal support, or the belief that the organization will provide tangible support for change in the form of resources and information, is not. Some see valence, or the belief that the change is valued, as an aspect of readiness (Armenakis & Bedeian, 1999; Holt, Armenakis, Harris, & Feild, 2006), whereas others see it as a determinant (Weiner, 2009).

Disagreement also exists about whether or not readiness includes an intention component. An intention is a determination to act in a certain way, something one plans to do or achieve, a psychological leaning toward some specific action. Some definitions explicitly include intention as a component of readiness (Armenakis et al., 1993; Bouckenooghe, 2010), while others implicitly include it through motivational components like change commitment (Weiner, 2009). In contrast, Rafferty, Jimmieson, and Armenakis (2013) argue that it is not appropriate to include intentions as a component of readiness. As they see it, readiness is an evaluative summary judgment that precedes and influences intention, much like attitudes determine behavioral intentions in the Theory of Planned Behavior (Ajzen, 1991).

Lack of agreement about the content domain of readiness has frustrated efforts to distinguish readiness from related constructs like acceptance of change, openness to change, commitment to change, coping with change, cynicism about change, and resistance to change. Bouckenooghe (2010) and Choi et al. (2011) have observed that these constructs not only overlap in their psychological content (e.g., ideas, beliefs, and intentions) but also share similar antecedent conditions (e.g., leadership, trust, and communication). Part of the problem is that social scientists have treated readiness as an attitude and tried to situate it within a broader class of change attitudes or change reactions. This conceptual move does not seem helpful for two reasons. First, social scientists do not agree on what constitutes an attitude. Citing competing definitions, some see attitudes as including an intentional component (Bouckenooghe, 2010), whereas others do not (Rafferty et al., 2013). Second, using common sense meanings as a touchstone, something is lost or distorted in regarding readiness as an attitude. When I inquire about a group's readiness for change, I am not inquiring about their attitude toward change. I am not asking how they evaluate

Table 5.1 Definitions and facets of organizational readiness for change

Authors	Definition	Components	Level
Armenakis et al. (1993), and Armenakis and Bedeian (1999)	An individual's beliefs, attitudes, and intentions regarding the extent to which changes are needed and the organization's capacity to successfully undertake those changes	Discrepancy Efficacy Appropriateness Principal support Personal valence	Individual
Eby et al. (2000)	An individual's perception of a specific facet of his or her work environment—the extent to which the organization is perceived to be ready to take on large-scale change (p. 422)	Not specified	Individual
Jones et al. (2005)	Extent to which employees hold positive views about the need for organizational change (i.e., change acceptance), as well as the extent to which employees believe that such changes are likely to have positive implications for themselves and the wider organization (p. 362)	Openness to change Looking forward to change Personal valence	
Holt et al. (2007)	A comprehensive attitude that is influenced by the content process, context, and individuals involved and collectively reflects the extent to which an individual or collection of individuals is cognitively and emotionally inclined to accept, embrace, or adopt a particular change (p. 326)	Appropriateness Management support Change efficacy Personal valence	Individual
Weiner et al. (2008), and Weiner (2009)	Extent to which organizational members are psychologically and behaviorally prepared to implement change	Change commitment Change efficacy	Organization
Kwahk and Lee (2008)	Extent to which organizational members hold positive views about the need for organizational change, as well as their belief that changes are likely to have positive implications for them and the organization	Not specified	Individual

(continued)

Table 5.1 (continued)

Authors	Definition	Components	Level
Bouckenooghe (2010)	An attitude toward change, that is, a tridimensional state composed of cognitive, affective, and intentional/behavioral reactions toward episodic or continuous change (p. 518)	Feelings toward change Opinions about advantages, disadvantages, and necessity of change Knowledge required to handle change Actions already taken or will be taken in the future for or against change	Individual
Holt et al. (2010)	Readiness for change is comprised of both psychological and structural factors, reflecting the extent to which the organization and its members are inclined to accept, embrace, and adopt a particular plan to purposefully alter the status quo (p. S51).	Individual psychological factors (e.g., appropriateness, principal support, change efficacy, valence) Organizational psychological factors (e.g., collective commitment, collective efficacy) Individual structural factors (e.g., knowledge and skills) Organizational structural factors (e.g., discrepancy, support climate, facilitation strategies)	Individual organization
Rafferty et al. (2013)	An individual's beliefs, attitudes, and intentions regarding the extent to which changes are needed and the organization's capacity to successfully undertake those changes (p. 111)	Cognitive (need for change, efficacy, personal valence) Emotional responses to specific change event	Individual group organization
Stevens (2013)	A positive and proactive response to change over time as a function of contextualized affective and cognitive reactions (p. 346)	Not specified	
Scaccia et al. (2015)	Readiness refers to the extent to which an organization is both willing and able to implement a particular innovation	Motivation General capacity Innovation-specific capacity	Organization

or judge the change (i.e., how they think and feel about it) but rather how prepared they are to act or respond to support change implementation. Likewise, lumping readiness with related constructs obscures their distinctive meanings. In everyday discourse, the statements, we are open to change, we accept change, and we are committed to change, are not semantically interchangeable with the statement, we are ready for change. One interesting possibility is that these related constructs share similar antecedent conditions because they represent different states or levels along a continuum ranging from resistance, reluctance, openness, acceptance, willingness, and readiness. This continuum varies from negative to positive responses, with the bias toward action increasing toward each pole. More theorizing is needed to clarify the conceptual content of, and relations among, these constructs.

Three recent developments in how readiness has been conceptualized merit attention. First, social scientists have begun including an affective component in definitions of readiness (Bouckenooghe, 2010; Holt et al., 2006; Rafferty et al., 2013). Affect simply means the experience of feelings or emotions. Authors have noted that organizational change can generate a wide range of emotions such as hope, fear, excitement, anger, happiness, sorrow, delight, and disgust. These emotions, they argue, are important aspects of readiness that can profoundly shape the extent to which organizational members accept, embrace, and engage in the change effort. Moreover, Rafferty et al. (2013) contend that affective components of readiness are not only conceptually and empirically distinguishable from cognitive components but could also have differential effects on organization members' change-related behaviors. In everyday discourse, we often inquire or make statements about our own or other people's emotional readiness to engage in some action or respond to some event. This is one aspect, and often an important one, of being prepared. Thus, the inclusion of an affective component in scientific constructions of readiness is consistent with common sense meanings of the term. Further investigation is needed as to which emotions are integral to readiness, how affective and cognitive components of readiness interact to constitute readiness, and how affective components of readiness influence change-related behavior and outcomes.

Second, social scientists increasingly regard readiness as a multilevel phenomenon relevant at the individual, group, and organizational level of analysis. Although most scientists focus on a single level of analysis, many recognize that readiness can be conceptualized, measured, studied, and influenced at more than one level (Holt et al., 2010; Rafferty et al., 2013; Vakola, 2013; Weiner, 2009). Opinion differs as to whether readiness means the same thing at multiple levels. Rafferty et al. (2013) argue that that the definition and components of readiness do not differ across levels; they regard readiness as a "shared team property" at the group or organizational level, and as such, readiness can be measured at the group or organizational level by aggregating individuals' readiness perceptions if statistical tests indicate sufficient inter-rater reliability and agreement. By contrast, Vakola (2013) contends that readiness has different meanings at different levels. At the organizational level, readiness refers to the organization's capability of implementing change. At the group level, readiness refers to a group's capacity and decision to support change. At the individual level, readiness refers to individual's perceptions of change. By implication, measures of readiness would differ at each level. Also unsettled is whether the relationships between readiness and other variables differ at multiple levels. Rafferty et al. (2013) have developed a multilevel framework that depicts similar, although not identical, antecedents and consequences of readiness at individual, workgroup, and organizational levels. This is an important conceptual advance, although more work is needed to refine the framework into a theory that specifies the independent effects of readiness at each level and the cross-level effects of readiness at multiple levels.

Finally, some social scientists advocate conceptualizing readiness as an ongoing process rather a state (Stevens, 2013). This perspective is girded by three insights. First, readiness is not a steady state: it can increase or decrease over time as a function of changing circumstances (Scaccia et al., 2015). Second, readiness itself can be regarded as a flow of activity situated in time rather than as a discrete event (e.g., readying or preparing). Third, readiness is a relevant construct not only prior to change initiation but also throughout the change process (Scaccia et al., 2015). In adopting a process-based perspective on readiness, it is important to remember that when assessing readiness in research or practice, time is "bracketed" and readiness is treated as a state exhibiting various levels. Thus, readiness can be construed as either a process or state depending one's purposes. Moreover, it is important not to lose sight of the common sense meaning of readiness as a *state* of *preparedness* for *future* action. While we can inquire about or assess readiness at multiple points in the process of change, when we do so, we are inquiring about or assessing readiness for the next stage in the change process (e.g., ready *for*, ready *to*). Unlike change acceptance, change commitment, or other change attitudes or change reactions, readiness inherently invokes the future; in everyday discourse, readiness is considered a precursor to action or response.

How Do We Assess Organizational Readiness for Change?

The earlier review of the literature noted that many publicly available measures of organizational readiness for change exhibited limited reliability and validity (Weiner et al., 2008). A more recently published review of measures to assess organizational readiness for knowledge translation reported similar findings (Gagnon et al., 2014). However, both reviews simply reported whether or not psychometric information was available for the measure. Moreover, both reviews examined only the source article in which the measure first appeared. The discussion that follows moves beyond the checklist approach to psychometric assessment by rating the level of evidence or psychometric quality of readiness measures. In addition, its moves beyond the source article by including all subsequent articles that used the measure in whole or in part. It also includes many measures not previously identified, including those developed as recently as 2016.

Method Several published reviews were used to identify measures of organizational readiness for change (Chaudoir, Dugan, & Barr, 2013; Chor, Wisdom, Olin, Hoagwood, & Horwitz, 2015; Gagnon et al., 2014; Weiner et al., 2008). These reviews varied in the bibliographic databases, search strings, and inclusion and exclusion criteria that they employed; as a result, the search began with 27 measures of organizational readiness that have been used in health care, business, education, child welfare, substance use, criminal justice, and other settings. Measures that assessed related constructs, such as change commitment (Herscovitch & Meyer, 2002) or team climate (Anderson & West, 1998), were excluded. The bibliographic database Scopus was then used to conduct a forward citation search to identify articles that cited the source article for the readiness measure. Two authors independently reviewed the titles and abstracts of retrieved articles using pre-determined screening criteria. To be included for further review, articles had to be published in English in a peer-reviewed journal, report original empirical research, and use quantitative or mixed research methods. Book chapters, conference proceedings, commentaries, editorials, systematic reviews, study protocols, and articles using only qualitative methods were excluded. When disagreements occurred, the lead author examined the full text of the article and made the final decision. Two authors independently reviewed the full text of articles passing the title and abstract screening criteria to determine whether the readiness measure was used in its original form, adapted, or not used. Measures were considered used in original form when the whole measure or any of its scales were used without adaptation. Measures were considered adapted if they differed from the original form in the number of items, scales, or response options. Adapted measures were treated as new measures of readiness and subjected to the same forward citation search. Articles where original or adapted measures were used to assess constructs other than readiness (e.g., organizational needs) were retained if they provided psychometric information about the measure. When disagreements occurred, the lead author reviewed the full text of the article and made the final decision. Additional readiness measures discovered through full-text review were subjected to citation search, screening, and review using the abovementioned procedures.

Two authors independently abstracted for each measure the number of times the measure had been used in published research, the number of scales and items comprising the measure, the types of settings in which measure has been used, the level of measurement of readiness, the type of implementation outcomes assessed (if any), and the level of measurement of implementation outcomes (if assessed). Table 5.2 describes how the abstracted information was coded. When disagreements occurred, the lead author reviewed the full text of the article and made the final decision.

In addition, two authors independently evaluated the psychometric properties of measures using evidence-based assessment (EBA) criteria developed by Hunsley and Mash and adapted by Lewis and colleagues (Lewis, Fischer, et al., 2015; Lewis, Stanick, et al., 2015; Lewis, Weiner, Stanick, & Fischer, 2015) (see Table 5.3). For measures used multiple times, the EBA ratings assigned for each use of the measure

Table 5.2 Descriptive coding form

Measure name	Name of measure used by authors
Originating authors	Citation of article where measure first appeared
Number of uses	Number of published articles, including originating article, using the measure (articles using one or more subscales included)
Number of scales	Number of scales (or subscales) in the measure
Setting type	Organizational setting in which readiness was assessed: H = Heath care B = Business E = Education CW = Child welfare SU = Substance use treatment MH = Mental health CJ = Criminal justice O = Other (e.g., unspecified or mixed settings)
Level of readiness assessment	The level at which the construct was measured: I = Individual level of analysis O = Organizational level of analysis B = Individual and organizational level of analysis
Implementation outcomes assessed	The stage in the organizational change process to which the construct applies: ADO = Adoption (e.g., reported use of or offering of service) IMP = Implementation (e.g., extent of implementation or frequency of use) ATT = Change-related attitudes (e.g., change commitment) OTH = Other outcomes (e.g., turnover, job satisfaction) NONE = No outcomes
Level of outcomes assessment	The level at which outcomes were measured: I = Individual level of analysis O = Organizational level of analysis B = Individual and organizational level of analysis NA = Not applicable (no outcome assessed)

Note: Setting type refers to the organizational setting in which the sample of respondents work, not the evidence-based practice or treatment. For example, a study examining the adoption of mental health treatment in schools is coded "E" for education

(i.e., for each article) were averaged for each psychometric property and rounded up ($\geq$.50) or down ($\leq$.49) to the nearest whole number. For multi-scale measures, reliability is rated using the "worst counts" method (Lewis, Stanick, et al., 2015), meaning the measure received an overall rating equal to the rating for the scale with the lowest reliability.

A total of 2639 articles were retrieved from forward citation searches for the 27 readiness measures identified in previous reviews and additional measures discovered through full-text review. Of these, 597 were excluded based on article type (e.g., book chapters, editorials, commentaries, and conference proceedings), and 766 were excluded based on research type (e.g., systematic reviews, study protocols, qualitative methods only). Of the remaining 1276 articles, 181 could not be obtained in electronic or print format, and 948 cited the source article of a measure

Table 5.3 Evidence-based assessment criteria guidelines

	Reliability information
NA	Not applicable: Consistency measures not applicable (e.g., single items)
0	None: α values not yet tested or not reported
1	Minimal/emerging: α values of <.60
2	Adequate: α values of .60–.69
3	Good: α values of .70–.79
4	Excellent: α values of $\geq$ .80

	Structural validity
0	None: No exploratory or confirmatory analysis has yet been performed, nor have any item response theory tests of dimensionality have been conducted. OR, percent variance explained is not reported
1	Minimal/emerging: The sample consisted of less than five times the number of items, AND an exploratory factor analysis explained less than 25% of the variance
2	Adequate: The sample consisted of five times the number of items but is less than 100 in total, AND an exploratory factor analysis explained less than 50% of the variance, OR a confirmatory factor analysis revealed an RMSEA or SRMR of .08 to .05 or CFI or GFI = .90 to .95
3	Good: The sample consisted of five times the number of items and is greater than or equal to 100 in total, OR the sample consisted of five to seven times the number of items but is less than 100 in total, AND in either case, an exploratory factor analysis explained less than 50% of the variance, OR a confirmatory factor analysis revealed an RMSEA or SRMR of .05 to .03 OR CFI or GFI = .95 to .97
4	Excellent: The sample consisted of seven times the number of items and is greater than 100 in total, AND an exploratory factor analysis explained greater than 50% of the variance, OR a confirmatory factor analysis revealed an RMSEA or SRMR of < .03 or a GFI or CFI of > .97

	Known-groups validity information
0	None: Known-groups validity failed to be detected in evaluation or known-groups validity not yet tested (NY)
1	Minimal: Statistically significant difference between groups detected, but no hypothesis tested
2	Adequate: Two or more statistically significant difference between groups detected, but no hypotheses tested
3	Good: Statistically significant difference between groups detected AND hypothesis tested
4	Excellent: Two or more statistically significant differences between groups detected AND hypotheses tested

	Predictive validity information
0	None: Predictive validity failed to be detected in evaluation, or predictive validity for adoption or implementation outcomes not yet tested (NY)
1	Minimal/emerging: Evidence of small correlation (range, 0.1–0.29) between instrument and scores on another test (measuring a distinct construct of interest or outcome) administered at some point in the future
2	Adequate: Evidence of medium correlation (range, 0.3–0.49) between instrument and scores on another instrument (measuring a distinct construct of interest or outcome) administered at some point in the future

(continued)

Table 5.3 (continued)

	Reliability information
3	Good: Evidence of strong correlation (range, 0.5–1.00) between instrument and scores on another instrument (measuring a distinct construct of interest or outcome) administered at some point in the future
4	Excellent: Evidence of medium strong correlation (0.3 or higher) between instrument and scores on at least two other instruments (measuring a distinct construct of interest or outcome) administered at some point in the future

but did not actually use the measure. Of the 181 articles that could not be obtained in print or electronic form, only 25 mentioned readiness or its synonyms in the title or abstract; of these 25, 7 were published in journals in health, mental health, or substance use. The remaining 107 articles represented additional uses of one of the 27 original measures or one of the 49 additional measures identified through full-text review. In sum, the search found 183 uses of 76 readiness measures (76 source articles plus 107 additional uses). Although most (84%) of the 183 articles in which a readiness measure was used focused on high-income countries (e.g., the United States, Canada, Australia, and the United Kingdom), some (11%) focused on upper middle-income countries (e.g., China, Malaysia, Turkey, and South Africa), and a few (2%) focused on lower middle-income countries (e.g., Pakistan and Syria). Six articles (3%) focused on multiple countries.

Description Table 5.4 summarizes the characteristics of the 76 readiness measures identified in the review. Most strikingly, 72% of readiness measures were used once by the authors who developed them and never used again. Sixteen measures (21%) have been used between two and five times, either wholly or partly. Only five measures (7%) have been used six times or more. The Texas Christian University Organizational Readiness for Change (TCU-ORC) measure developed by Lehman, Greener, and Simpson (2002) holds the record for number of uses (63 times) of the whole measure or some of its scales. The Individual Readiness for Organizational Change (IROC) (Holt, Armenakis, Feild, & Harris, 2007), the Organizational Readiness to Change Assessment (ORCA) (Helfrich, Li, Sharp, & Sales, 2009), and the National Criminal Justice Treatment Practices (NCJTP) Training and Resources scales (Friedmann, Taxman, & Henderson, 2007) have been used wholly or partly 11, 8, and 6 times, respectively. Older measures were more likely to be used more than once, but not much more likely. Thirty percent of those developed before 2011 have been used more than once, compared to 17% of those developed after 2011.

Readiness measures varied widely in number of scales and number of items. Seven measures (9%) had no scales, only individual items. Thirty-two measures (42%) had one scale, 19 measures (26%) had two to five scales, and 18 measures (22%) had six or more scales. The Functional Organizational Readiness for Change Evaluation (FORCE) (Devereaux et al., 2006) topped out with 22 scales, followed by the ORCA (Helfrich et al., 2009) with 19 scales and the TCU-ORC (Lehman et al., 2002) with 18 scales. Eight measures (11%) had 1–5 items,

Table 5.4 Description of organizational readiness for change measures

	Number	Frequency (%)
Number of uses		
1	55	72
2–5	16	21
6 or more	5	7
Number of scales		
1	32	42
2–5	20	26
6 or more	17	22
Number of items		
1–5	8	11
6–10	21	28
11 or more	43	57
Setting types		
Heath care	22	29
Business	31	41
Education	4	5
Child welfare	3	4
Substance use treatment	4	5
Mental health	0	0
Criminal justice	3	4
Multiple	4	5
Other (e.g., unspecified or mixed settings)	5	7
Level of readiness assessment		
Individual	34	45
Organizational	37	49
Both	5	7
Implementation outcomes assessed		
Adoption	8	11
Implementation	6	8
Change-related attitudes	6	8
Other outcomes	15	20
Multiple outcomes	6	8
No outcomes	35	46
Level of outcome assessment		
Individual	17	22
Organizational	22	29
Both	2	3

21 measures (28%) had 6–10 items, and 43 measures (57%) had 11 or more items. The TCU-ORC (Lehman et al., 2002) had the most items (118). The ORCA (Helfrich et al., 2009) ranked third with 77 items. While it is not surprising that measures with more scales tended to have more items, it is surprising that two of the most frequently used measures are long. However, many authors using these measures did not use all of the scales but rather only some of them.

Most measures have been used to assess readiness in business settings (41%) or health-care settings (29%). A fourth (25%) of measures have been used to assess readiness in a variety of other not-for-profit settings, including education, child welfare, substance use treatment, and criminal justice settings. These figures are somewhat understated since four measures (5%) have been used in multiple settings, including those listed above. For example, the TCU-ORC (Lehman et al., 2002) has been used to assess readiness in health-care settings (3 times), educational settings (once), child welfare settings (twice), substance use treatment settings (39 times), mental health settings (9 times), and criminal justice settings (7 times). In some instances, the TCU-ORC was used to assess readiness in multiple settings in the same study.

Although readiness is increasingly regarded as a multilevel phenomenon, most measures have been used to assess readiness at only one level of analysis. Forty-five percent have been used at the individual level. Slightly less than half of the measures (49%) have been used at the organizational level. Only five measures (7%) have been used at both the individual and organizational levels, although not always in the same study. For example, the TCU-ORC (Lehman et al., 2002) has been used 21 times at the individual level, 24 times at the organizational level, and 9 times at both levels.

Readiness is considered a critical precursor to successful organizational change; yet often readiness assessment has been a goal in and of itself. Nearly half of the measures identified in this review (46%) have been used to predict no outcome; rather they have been used to describe the readiness of organizations, explore group differences in readiness, or examine the conditions that promote readiness. Whether readiness predicts adoption or implementation is a question of great interest. Yet only eight measures (11%) have been used to predict adoption, and six measures (9%) have been used to predict implementation. These figures are somewhat understated since six measures (8%) that have been used to study multiple outcomes have also been used to predict adoption, implementation, or both. Examples include the TCU-ORC (Lehman et al., 2002) and the IROC (Holt et al., 2007). The predictive validity of readiness measures with regard to adoption and implementation is examined below. Six measures (8%) have been used to study change-related attitudes, such as adoption intentions or change commitment, while another 15 measures (20%) have been used to predict other outcomes, such as job satisfaction, employee turnover, or perceived impact.

Psychometric Properties Eighteen measures (24%) reported no information about scale reliability or reported reliabilities for subscales but not the full scale used (see Table 5.5). Four measures (5%) included one or more one-item scales for which inter-item consistency could not be calculated. Fourteen measures (18%) included one or more scales with "minimal" or "adequate" reliability, meaning an alpha coefficient less than .70. The TCU-ORC (Lehman et al., 2002), for example, includes one scale with an average rating of "minimal" reliability based on 20 reported alpha coefficients (autonomy) and eight scales with an "adequate" rating based on 18–23 reported alpha coefficients (staffing, training, computer access, e-communication, growth, efficacy, adaptability, and change). The ORCA (Helfrich et al., 2009) and the IROC (Holt et al., 2007) also have at least one scale with "adequate" reliability based on multiple reported alphas. Forty-one measures (54%) exhibited "good" or "excellent" ratings for reliability.

Table 5.5 Evidence-based assessment of psychometric properties of readiness measures

	Number	Frequency (%)
Reliability		
NA	4	5
None (or not yet tested)	18	24
Minimal	5	7
Adequate	8	11
Good	18	24
Excellent	23	30
Structural validity		
None (or not yet tested)	37	49
Minimal	10	13
Adequate	1	1
Good	11	14
Excellent	17	22
Known-groups validity		
None (or not yet tested)	54	71
Minimal	8	11
Adequate	8	11
Good	4	5
Excellent	2	3
Predictive validity		
None (or not yet tested)	60	79
Minimal	3	4
Adequate	5	7
Good	1	1
Excellent	7	9

Structural validity information has not been reported for nearly half of the readiness measures identified in this review (49%). The lack of such information for multi-scale measures of readiness is particularly worrisome, as it suggests that authors constructed these scales without checking whether they are empirically distinct from related concepts. Also troubling, authors calculated inter-item consistency for scales without first checking their unidimensionality. Ten measures (13%), including the TCU-ORC (Lehman et al., 2002) and the ORCA (Helfrich et al., 2009), exhibited "minimal" structural validity: they employed principal components analysis or exploratory factor analysis with five or fewer observations per variable. One measure (1%) exhibited "adequate" structural validity, 11 measures (14%) exhibited "good" structural validity, and 17 measures (22%) exhibited "excellent" structural validity.

Known-groups validity information has not been reported for 51 measures (67%). Known-group differences were tested but not detected for additional three measures (4%). Fifteen measures (20%) have been used to compare levels of readiness among different types of organizations (e.g., correctional facilities versus treatment facilities). Measures have also been used to compare levels of readiness among individuals holding different organizational or professional roles (e.g., staff versus administrators), having different demographic characteristics (e.g., women versus men), or participating in different intervention conditions (e.g., social network versus knowledge-building interventions). In most cases, no specific hypothesis was offered, making the test of group differences exploratory. Only four measures (5%) tested a hypothesized difference between known groups (Bouckenooghe, Devos, & Van Den Broeck, 2009; Holt et al., 2007; Sen, Sinha, & Ramamurthy, 2006; Taxman, Henderson, Young, & Farrell, 2014). Although not often tested, significant differences in readiness perceptions have been reported between administrative staff and clinical staff (Bohman et al., 2008; Devereaux et al., 2006; Helfrich et al., 2009; Lehman et al., 2002) and between managers and employees (Bouckenooghe et al., 2009). These findings should discourage the practice of relying on single respondents—often administrative staff or managers—to describe the readiness of organizations, especially when perceptual measures of readiness are employed. Indeed, caution is warranted in interpreting predictive validity when a single respondent supplies information not only readiness but also about adoption, implementation, or other outcomes.

Predictive validity information for adoption or implementation outcomes has not been reported for 55 measures and has not been demonstrated for 5 additional measures (79%). Three measures (4%) exhibited "minimal" predictive validity for these outcomes, five measures (7%) exhibited adequate predictive validity, and one measure (1%) exhibited "good" predictive validity. Seven measures (9%) exhibited "excellent" predictive validity; however, caution is warranted in interpreting this finding. Measures that have been used repeatedly or have multiple scales have greater chances of achieving an "excellent" rating, meaning two or more medium strong correlations or associations between the measure, or the scales that comprise it, and adoption or implementation outcomes. However as discussed below, the evidence for predictive validity of adoption and implementation outcomes for the most frequently used, multi-scale measures is limited, mixed, and confusing.

The 2008 literature review concluded that most publicly available measures of organizational readiness exhibited limited evidence of reliability and validity (Weiner et al., 2008). Unfortunately, time has not altered this conclusion. Of the seven measures identified in the earlier review as having undergone a systematic development and testing process, only one seems promising for those seeking to assess organizational readiness in health and human service settings. The IROC (Holt et al., 2007) has "excellent" structural validity, "excellent" known-groups validity, and an "adequate" rating for only one of the four scales comprising the measure (the other three scales exhibited "good" or "excellent" reliability). By comparison, the TCU-ORC (Lehman et al., 2002), despite frequent use, continues to have "minimal" structural validity, "minimal" known-groups validity, and "minimal" or "adequate" reliability ($\alpha < .70$) for 9 of the 18 scales. The TCU-ORC (Lehman et al., 2002) exhibits some predictive validity with regard to adoption and implementation; however, as discussed below, no discernible pattern of significant associations can be observed across multiple studies.

The current review identified four additional measures that have promising psychometric properties and therefore merit consideration. The Organizational Readiness for Implementing Change, or ORIC (Shea, Jacobs, Esserman, Bruce, & Weiner, 2014), has "excellent" structural validity, "good" known-groups validity, and "excellent" reliability. The Perceived Organizational Readiness for Change, or PORC (Cinite, Duxbury, & Higgins, 2009), has "excellent" structural validity and "good" reliability; it has not been tested for known-groups validity. The Organizational Change Recipients' Beliefs Scale or OCRBS (Armenakis, Bernerth, Pitts, & Walker, 2007) has "excellent" structural validity, "minimal" known-groups validity, and "good" reliability. Finally, the Organizational Change Questionnaire-Process, Context, and Readiness, or OCQ-PCR, (Bouckenooghe et al., 2009) has "excellent" structural validity, "good" known-groups validity, and "adequate" reliability for one of the three readiness scales (the other two had "excellent" reliability). All four of these promising measures have yet to be tested for predictive validity, particularly for adoption and implementation outcomes.

What Conditions Promote Organizational Readiness for Change?

What do we know about the conditions that promote organizational readiness for change? As Rafferty et al. (2013) observe, we know far less than we think we know because (a) relatively few studies have examined the antecedents of readiness and (b) those that have done so have defined and measured readiness in different, inconsistent, ways. Given the state of measurement in the field, additional caution is warranted in interpreting research findings. With these caveats in mind, it is possible to review what we know, or think we know, using a framework by Holt et al. (2006). They propose that readiness is influenced by the content (i.e., what is being changed), the process (i.e., how the change is being implemented), the context (i.e., circumstances under which the change is occurring), and the individuals (i.e., characteristics of those being asked to change).

Of these four categories of influencers, we know the least about how the content of change affects readiness. It is reasonable to expect that change attributes such as relative advantage, compatibility, complexity, trialability, observability, cost, and risk would positively or negatively influence readiness. While these change attributes are known to affect change attitudes (Rafferty et al., 2013), their effect on readiness has not been studied. What has been shown is that the radical or incremental nature of the change moderates the effect of the context of change. Rafferty and Simons (2006) observed, for example, that for corporate transformation changes, trust in leadership was significantly, positively associated with readiness; for corporate fine-tuning changes, it was not. Change attributes might also explain the effects of some aspects of the context of change. Vakola (2014), for example, found that the perceived impact of change fully mediated the effect of trust in leadership on readiness.

One reason why we know so little about the influence of the content of change on readiness is that readiness is often conceived and measured in terms of beliefs about or perceptions of the change (Armenakis et al., 2007; Brink et al., 1995; Holt et al., 2007; Kurnia, Choudrie, Mahbubur, & Alzougool, 2015; Lai & Ong, 2010). This way of thinking about readiness is inconsistent with the meaning of readiness in everyday discourse. When we ask a group of employees if they are ready to change, we are not asking if they believe the change is appropriate, better than current practice, or likely to produce good outcomes. We are asking how prepared they are to change or for change. These beliefs might well influence their readiness, but they do not directly indicate their readiness. We will learn much more about the influence of the content of change when we cease conflating the construct of readiness with its potential determinants, including perceived change attributes.

In terms of the context of change, research shows that trust in leadership (Bouckenooghe et al., 2009; Kondakçi, Zayim, & Çalişkan, 2013; Zayim & Kondakci, 2015), trust in peers (Eby, Adams, Russell, & Gaby, 2000; Kondakçi et al., 2013; Lai, Kan, & Ulhas, 2013; Zayim & Kondakci, 2015), social relationships in the workplace (Kondakçi et al., 2013; Madsen, Miller, & John, 2005; Shah & Shah, 2010), participatory management (Lai et al., 2013), organizational culture and climate (Becan, Knight, & Flynn, 2012; Bouckenooghe et al., 2009; Claiborne, Auerbach, Lawrence, & Schudrich, 2013; Haffar, Al-Karaghouli, & Ghoneim, 2013, 2014; Jones, Jimmieson, & Griffiths, 2005; Shah & Shah, 2010), perceived organizational support (Ming-Chu & Meng-Hsiu, 2015; Rafferty & Simons, 2006), and flexible organizational policies and procedures (Rafferty & Simons, 2006) are significantly, positively associated with readiness. Although some findings are not consistently observed across studies (cf. Eby et al., 2000), generally speaking, a supportive organizational context enhances readiness. This statement needs to be qualified in two ways. First, readiness is often conceptually and operationally defined in terms of the contextual factors that influence or determine it (Bohman et al., 2008; Helfrich et al., 2009; Lehman et al., 2002; Molla & Licker, 2005; Snyder-Halpern, 2002; Tan, Tyler, & Manica, 2007). In fact, some readiness measures, such as the TCU-ORC (Lehman et al., 2002), include organizational climate scales and have been used to assess organizational functioning, which raises some construct validity concerns. Second, the broad contextual features mentioned above describe general states of affairs that are likely to have distal, indirect, or even weak effects on readiness compared to more situationally specific factors like the timing or content of change. Rafferty and Simons (2006) observed, for example, that perceived organizational support was positively, significantly associated with readiness for corporate transformation changes, but not with readiness for corporate fine-tuning changes. The content of the change might matter as much as, or even more than, the context of the change.

Armenakis et al. (1993) argued long ago that the process of change strongly influences readiness. Evidence suggests that high-quality, timely, and accurate communication about the change is significantly, positively associated with readiness (Caldwell, Roby-Williams, Rush, & Ricke-Kiely, 2009; Claiborne et al., 2013; Holt et al., 2007). Whether change communication has direct or indirect effects on readiness is unclear. In one study, at least, the effect of the change communication was fully mediated by the perceived impact of change (Vakola, 2014). Employee involvement in the change process and employee perceptions of management's involvement in, support of, and ability to lead the change are also significantly, positively associated with readiness (Bouckenooghe et al., 2009; Holt et al., 2007; Trzcinski & Sobeck, 2012). Some caution is warranted in interpreting these findings since change processes and change contexts are likely to be confounded. A few studies have tried to disentangle their effects. For example, Rafferty and Simons (2006) found that participation in change was not significantly associated with readiness for corporate transformation changes once trust in peers and trust in leaders were taken into account. Similarly, Caldwell et al. (2009) found that transformational leadership—a contextual factor—was no longer significantly, positively associated with readiness once procedural justice (operationally defined in terms of change communication) was taken into account. We need to know more about how change process and change context interact. It could be the case, for example, that transformational leaders generate readiness by communicating more effectively about the change or inviting employee participation in the change effort (Caldwell et al., 2009).

Finally, we know quite a bit about how the characteristics of individuals influence readiness. Individual characteristics significantly, positively associated with readiness include organizational commitment (Hameed, Roques, & Arain, 2013; Kwahk & Lee, 2008; Madsen et al., 2005; Nordin, 2012), change efficacy (Caldwell et al., 2009; Kwahk & Lee, 2008; Lai & Ong, 2010; Rafferty & Simons, 2006; Vakola, 2014), psychological ownership (Armenakis et al., 2007), job satisfaction (Kondakçi et al., 2013; Vakola, 2014), and personality traits like locus of control (Holt et al., 2007). Again, the characteristics of individuals, the content of change, and the context of change can interact in complex ways. Nordin (2012), for example, found that organizational commitment moderated the effect of transformational leadership on readiness. Similarly, Vakola (2014) observed that the perceived impact of change fully mediated the effect of job satisfaction on readiness for change. Definitional differences also make it difficult to interpret these findings. Some see change-related self-efficacy as an integral aspect of readiness (Armenakis et al., 2007; Holt et al., 2007; Shea et al., 2014), whereas others see it as an antecedent condition (Rafferty & Simons, 2006). Lastly, some have argued (Rafferty et al., 2013), and one study shows (Eby et al., 2000), that organizational readiness is influenced less by characteristics of individuals than by the context and process of change.

Does Organizational Readiness for Change Matter?

Given the limited number of studies that have examined the effects of readiness on adoption and implementation, the differences in the ways that readiness has been measured across studies, and the paucity of psychometric information for most readiness measures, the best answer to the question of whether organizational readiness for change matters is a heavily qualified yes. Whether readiness is a critical *precursor* to successful organizational change cannot be answered because no study has prospectively assessed readiness and its consequences. Instead, studies have examined the association of readiness with innovations or evidence-based practices that have already been adopted or implemented. This is a significant shortcoming that needs to be addressed.

In business settings, several studies show that organizational readiness is positively associated with the adoption or implementation of e-commerce technologies by small- to medium-size firms in China, Saudi Arabia, Iran, Malaysia, South Africa, and Australia (Al-Somali, Gholami, & Clegg, 2015; Ghobakhloo, Hong, & Standing, 2014; Hung, Chang, Lin, & Hsiao, 2014; Kurnia et al., 2015; Molla & Licker, 2005; Ram, Corkindale, & Wu, 2013; Tan et al., 2007). In all of these studies, a single respondent, usually the owner or manager, described the readiness of the organization. As noted earlier, administrators tend to report higher levels of readiness than employees or clinical staff do; hence, some caution is warranted in interpreting these study results. Moreover, not all studies report positive results. In a study of family-run small- to medium-size business in the United Kingdom, for example, organizational readiness was not associated with e-commerce technologies (Wang & Ahmed, 2009). Other studies of the effects of readiness on e-commerce adoption and implementation also report null results (Molla, Peszynski, & Pittayachawan, 2010; Yan Xin, Ramayah, Soto-Acosta, Popa, & Ai Ping, 2014).

In health, human service, and criminal justice settings, organizational readiness is significantly, positively associated with adoption or implementation of evidence-based treatments in some studies (Chang et al., 2013; Henderson, Young, Farrell, & Taxman, 2009; Henderson et al., 2007; Herbeck, Hser, & Teruya, 2008; Jippes et al., 2015; Noe, Kaufman, Kaufmann, Brooks, & Shore, 2014; Oser, Tindall, & Leukefeld, 2007; Young, Farrell, Henderson, & Taxman, 2009) but not in others (Guerrero, He, Kim, & Aarons, 2014; Guerrero & Kim, 2013; McCrae, Scannapieco, Leake, Potter, & Menefee, 2014; Smith & Manfredo, 2011; Taxman, Cropsey, Melnick, & Perdoni, 2008). It is difficult to make sense of these mixed results given differences across studies in measures, settings, and innovations or evidence-based practices. Yet, mixed results have also been reported within the same study. For example, using the ORCA (Helfrich et al., 2009), Noe et al. (2014) found that leaders' practices were positively associated with greater implementation of services for American Indians and Alaska Natives in the Veterans Health Administration. However, leadership, performance measures, opinion leaders, and Veteran Integrated Service Network (VISN) support were not.

Unfortunately, the picture is not much clearer in studies using the same measure in the same or similar settings. For example, the availability of funding for new programs—one of the NCJTP scales adapted from the TCU-ORC (Lehman et al., 2002)—was positively associated with the provision of intensive substance use treatment services and the adoption of HIV testing in correctional facilities (Oser et al., 2007; Young et al., 2009). Yet, funding availability was not significantly associated with the adoption of HIV testing in community substance use treatment programs (Oser et al., 2007), nor was it significantly associated with the availability and capacity of substance use treatment programs in correctional facilities (Taxman & Kitsantas, 2009) or the provision of detoxification services and medication-based treatments in correctional institutions (Oser, Knudsen, Staton-Tindall, Taxman, & Leukefeld, 2009). Moreover, funding availability was negatively associated with the use of evidence-based substance use treatment practices in community and institutional settings for juvenile offenders (Henderson et al., 2007). A mixed pattern of results similarly occurs for the availability of staff training and development programs, another NCJTP scale derived from the TCU-ORC (Henderson, Taxman, & Young, 2008; Henderson et al., 2007; Herbeck et al., 2008; Oser et al., 2007).

The TCU-ORC (Lehman et al., 2002) has been the most frequently used measure for assessing the effect of organizational readiness on adoption and implementation. Only two studies have used all 18 scales to examine implementation-related outcomes. Lundgren et al. (2012) found that 16 of the 18 scales were not significantly associated with staff ratings of barriers to implementing evidence-based practices in substance use treatment settings. The two that were significantly, positively associated with staff ratings of implementation barriers were stress and program needs. In another study, Lundgren et al. (2013) found that 1 of the 18 ORC scales was significantly associated with evidence-based practice modification during implementation. Specifically, staff who reported having a higher level of influence in their organization reported a significantly higher level of modifications to the specified evidence-based practice in the implementation process. Becan et al. (2012) found that all four staff attributes (growth, efficacy, adaptability, and influence) were significantly, positively associated with innovation adoption in substance use treatment settings. Others, though, have found mixed results for various ORC scales. Simpson et al. (2007), for example, found that mission and openness to change were significantly, positively associated with trial use of an innovation following a workshop; however, cohesiveness, autonomy, stress, and communication were not significantly associated with trial use. Likewise, Baer et al. (2009) found that agencies where staff perceived more autonomy and staff efficacy retained less motivational interviewing (MI) spirit and improved less and retained less reflection skill following a training workshop; by comparison, agencies where staff perceived greater openness to organizational change achieved or sustained higher levels on these two implementation fidelity measures.

Four studies have used the TCU-ORC super-scales (organizational climate, motivation for change, staff attributes, and resource adequacy) and found null or mixed results. Beidas et al. (2012) found that none of the super-scales was significantly associated with changes in therapists' adherence, skills, or knowledge of cognitive behavioral therapy (CBT) following a training workshop and consultation. In a related study, Beidas et al. (2014) observed that one of the four super-scales (organizational climate) was significantly, positively associated with therapists adherence to CBT but none of the super-scales is significantly associated with penetration of CBT among youth with anxiety served by the therapists. In two other studies, only one of the four super-scales—organizational climate in one study, motivation for change in the other—was significantly, positively associated with either adoption or implementation of an innovation or evidence-based practice (Guerrero & Kim, 2013; Henggeler et al., 2008). In sum, organizational readiness, whether measured by the TCU-ORC or other instruments, does seem to matter, at least to some extent, when it comes to predicting adoption or implementation; but the evidence supporting this conclusion is limited, mixed, and confusing.

Where Do We Go from Here?

Given what we know, or think we know, about organizational readiness for change, should we try to increase organizational readiness in health and human service settings so that we see greater adoption and higher-quality implementation of innovations and evidence-based practices? If so, how? Intuitively, it seems that we should do whatever we can to prepare clinical and nonclinical staff for organizational change before we initiate it. Yet, given the current state of theory, measurement, and research, we should proceed with caution in our efforts to do so. As a field, we hold different and, to some extent, inconsistent ideas of what it means to be ready; we have few reliable, valid, and practical tools for measuring readiness; we have limited knowledge of the conditions that promote readiness; and we have limited evidence that readiness matters. At this point, most authors would conclude that we need more research in order to guide practice; yet, it seems unreasonable to expect practitioners to wait for evidence to materialize.

Although no one has developed and tested an intervention for increasing organizational readiness, we have some clues about which strategies might work. To increase organizational members' psychological preparedness for change, change agents could employ communications strategies that highlight the need for change and underscore the urgency of change. These strategies prime organizational members for some kind of change, but not for any specific, proposed change. For that, change agents need to persuade organizational members that the proposed change is not only better than the current practice but also likely to produce benefits that matter to them. The more organizational members value the proposed change, the more psychologically prepared they will be to implement it. For organizational members to feel behaviorally prepared for change, they must have the necessary knowledge, skills, and resources and the confidence that they can deploy them effectively. Change agents could take a variety of actions to communicate or ensure that these elements are in place. Finally, change agents can increase organizational members' readiness to embark on a journey that can be a disruptive, difficult, and risky by creating a supportive context characterized by psychological safety.

Before we develop, test, or recommend strategies for increasing organizational readiness, we need more robust, conclusive evidence that readiness matters. Generating such evidence requires assessing organizational readiness *prospectively* using a reliable, valid, and preferably brief measure in order to minimize response burden on busy clinicians. Assessing the impact of organizational readiness (as opposed to individual readiness) also requires a large sample of organizations poised to implement the same or similar innovation or evidence-based practice over roughly the same period of time; moreover, for prospective measurement to occur, these organizations must be willing to initiate implementation shortly after readiness assessment. This is a tall order, but federal governments and philanthropic foundations sometimes fund large-scale demonstration programs that meet these criteria. With more robust, conclusive evidence in hand that readiness matters, scientists can attend to strengthening our understanding of the conditions that promote readiness, with an eye toward developing and testing strategies to increase it.

While we wait for such evidence to accumulate, practitioners could use existing measures to guide implementation efforts. Two relatively new measures illustrate different approaches for doing so. Based on a review of the literature, Scaccia and Wandersman proposed a practical implementation science heuristic, abbreviated as $R = MC^2$, that distills readiness into three main components: (a) motivation to implement an innovation, (b) general capacities of an organization, and (c) innovation-specific capacities needed for a particular innovation (Scaccia et al., 2015). They subsequently developed an organizational readiness tool comprised of 82 items that assesses 16 subcomponents of motivation (e.g., relative advantage), general capacity (e.g., leadership), and innovation-specific capacity (e.g., program champion). While the psychometric properties of this tool have not yet been fully established, the developers report good scale and subscale reliabilities (> .70) and known-groups validity (personal communication). Importantly, they report that, despite the tool's length, the health-care organizations and community coalitions that have used the tool find its comprehensive view of readiness useful for identifying specific areas in which actions could be taken to increase readiness for implementation. In contrast to this "maximalist" approach to readiness assessment, Shea and Weiner have developed a measure, the ORIC, that takes a "minimalist" approach (Shea et al., 2014). As noted earlier, the ORIC is comprised of ten items that assess two dimensions of readiness: change commitment and change efficacy. In addition to being theory-based, the ORIC has "good" to "excellent" reliability, structural validity, and known-groups validity. The ORIC's brevity makes it attractive for practitioners interested in assessing readiness prior to implementation; however, the ORIC is less actionable than the $R = MC^2$ tool in that it does not provide detailed diagnostic information about the factors that determine the level of readiness signaled by the measure. While the ORIC could be used rapidly to inform a "go or no go" decision to implement, further assessment would be needed if the measure signaled low or uneven levels of readiness in order to identify areas in which actions could be taken to increase readiness levels. With both tools publicly available, practitioners interested in readiness assessment can decide which pragmatic measurement quality they value more: actionability (comprehensiveness) versus feasibility (brevity).

There remains much that we need to know about organizational readiness beyond whether it matters and how to increase it. Is organizational readiness equally important for all types of change and likewise is it equally important for all types of organizations? Is organizational readiness necessary, sufficient, both, or neither? Is there a threshold of organizational readiness that should be met prior to initiating implementation? Do all organizational members need to be ready or ready at the same time, or is readiness more important for specific groups of individuals? The answers are out there waiting for social scientists and practitioners to discover and apply them (Tables 5.6 and 5.7).

Table 5.6 Supplemental: descriptive information about organizational readiness for change measures

Measure name	Originating authors	No. of uses	No. of scales	No. of items	Setting type	Level of readiness assessment	Implementation outcomes assessed	Level of outcomes assessment
[not specified]	Acosta et al. (2013)	1	2	NR	O	O	NONE	NA
[not specified]	Al-Somali et al. (2015)	1	2	5	B	O	ADO	O
Organizational Change Recipients' Beliefs Scale	Armenakis et al. (2007)	6	5	24	B (2) CW (1) O (3)	I (6)	ATT (3) NONE (2) OTH	I
Specialty Training's Organizational Readiness for curriculum Change	Bank et al. (2015)	1	10	44	H	O	NONE	NA
Medical Organizational Readiness for Change (MORC)	Bohman et al. (2008)	1	8	45	H	B	NONE	NA
Organizational Change Questionnaire-Process, Context, and Readiness	Bouckenooghe et al. (2009)	2	3	9	O (2)	I (2)	NONE (2)	NA
Readiness to Adopt	Brink et al. (1995)	1	10	41	E	I	NONE	NA
Organizational Readiness	Burnett et al. (2010)	1	3	NR	H	B	OTH	I
Change Readiness	Caldwell et al. (2009)	2	1	7	H (2)	I (2)	OTH (1) NONE (1)	I
Organizational Readiness for Change	Chang et al. (2013)	1	17	58	H	O	ADO	O
Long-Term Care Readiness Tool for EHR Implementation	Cherry (2011)	1	1	21	H	O	NONE	NA
[not specified]	Chilenski et al. (2015)	1	5	13	O	I	ATT	I
Readiness	Chwelos et al. (2001)	2	3	19	B (2)	O (2)	ATT (2)	O (2)
Perceived Organizational Readiness for Change	Cinite et al. (2009)	1	3	11	O	I	OTH	I

(continued)

Table 5.6 (continued)

Measure name	Originating authors	No. of uses	No. of scales	No. of items	Setting type	Level of readiness assessment	Implementation outcomes assessed	Level of outcomes assessment
[not specified]	Claiborne et al. (2013)	1	1	9	CW	I	NONE	NA
Readiness for Use of New Technology	Demiris et al. (2007)	1	0	27	H	O	NONE	NA
Functional Organizational Readiness for Change Evaluation (FORCE)	Devereaux et al. (2006)	1	22	NR	H	I	NONE	NA
Organizational Readiness for Change	Eby et al. (2000)	2	1	9	B (2)	I (2)	NONE OTH	NA
e-Readiness	Fathian et al. (2008)	1	4	13	B	O	NONE	NA
Technology Adoption Readiness Scale	Finch et al. (2012)	1	0	30	H	I	NONE	NA
Training and Resources	Friedmann et al. (2007)	6	6	26	CJ (6)	O (6)	ADO (6)	O (6)
Psychological Climate	Garner and Hunter (2013)	2	5	56	SU (2)	I (2)	OTH (2)	I (2)
E-Commerce Readiness	Ghobakhloo et al. (2014)	1	1	6	B	O	IMP ATT	O
Readiness for Change	Hameed et al. (2013)	1	1	3	B	I	NONE	NA
Readiness for Change	Hanpachern et al. (1998)	1	1	14	B	I	NONE	NA
Organizational Readiness to Change Assessment	Helfrich et al. (2009)	8	19 (3 super-scales)	77	H (8)	B (I = 4) (O = 4)	I (2) NONE (6)	O (2)
Training Resources	Herbeck et al. (2008)	1	1	6	SU	O	IMP	I
Individual Readiness for Organizational Change	Holt et al. (2007)	11	4	25	B (6) H (4) E	I (11)	NONE (7) IMP (2) OTH (2)	I (3) O (1)
Organizational e-Readiness	Hung et al. (2014)	1	6	32	B	O	IMP	O

Scale	Citation							
Organizational Telehealth Readiness Assessment Tool	Jennett et al. (2003)	1	4	28	H	O	NONE	NA
Medical School's Organizational Readiness for Curriculum Change (MORC)	Jippes et al. (2013)	2	3	53	E (2)	B (2)	NONE (2)	NA
Readiness for Change	Jones et al. (2005)	1	1	7	B	I	IMP OTH	I
Readiness for Change-Cognitive Emotional Intentional	Kondakci et al. (2013)	3	3	12	E (3)	I (3)	NONE (3)	NA
Organizational Readiness	Kurnia et al. (2015)	1	2	9	B	O	ADO	O
Readiness for Change	Kwahk and Lee (2008)	2	1	6	B (2)	I (2)	ATT (2)	I (2)
Employee Readiness for e-Business	Lai and Ong (2010)	1	4	18	B	I	OTH	I
e-Business Readiness	Lai et al. (2013)	1	1	6	B	O	OTH	O
TCU Organizational Readiness for Change	Lehman et al. (2002)	63	18 (4 super-scales)	118	H (7)* E (2) CW (4) SU (40) MH (11) CJ (6)	I (27) O (28) B (8)	ADO (4)* IMP (10) ATT (9) OTH (25) NONE (19)	I (24) O (16) B (4) NA (19)
Readiness for Organizational Change	Madsen et al. (2005)	3	1	14	M (1) E (2)	I (3)	NONE (3)	NA
Readiness for Change	McCrae et al. (2014)	1	3	24	CW	I	IMP	O
Change Readiness	Medley and Nickel (1999)	1	0	16	H	O	NONE	NA
Readiness for Change	Ming-Chu and Hsui (2015)	1	1	19	B	I	ATT	I
Health Reform Readiness Index	Molfenter et al. (2012)	2	0	13	SU (2)	O (2)	NONE (2)	NA
Perceived Organizational E-Readiness	Molla and Licker (2005)	1	6	33	B	O	ADO	O

(continued)

Table 5.6 (continued)

Measure name	Originating authors	No. of uses	No. of scales	No. of items	Setting type	Level of readiness assessment	Implementation outcomes assessed	Level of outcomes assessment
Perceived Organizational E-Readiness	Molla et al. (2010)	1	1	6	B	O	ADO	O
Health-Oriented Readiness for Change	Mueller et al. (2012)	2	1	8	B (2)	I (2)	OTH NONE	I
Proactive Organizational Change: Assessing Critical Success Factors	Nelson et al. (1998)	1	6	29	H	I	NONE	NA
Organizational Readiness for Change	Nordin (2012)	1	1	40	E	I	NONE	NA
Readiness for Technological Innovation	Parker Oliver and Demiris (2004)	1	0	17	H	I	NONE	NA
Change Readiness	O'Neill and Downer (2004)	1	1	12	H	O	NONE	NA
Organizational Readiness	Pinto et al. (2011)	2	1	8	H (2)	O (2)	OTH (2)	I (2)
Readiness for Change	Rafferty and Simons (2006)	1	1	9	B	I	NONE	NA
Organizational Readiness	Ram et al. (2013)	3	1	4–6	B (3)	O (3)	ADO OTH (2)	O (3)
Organizational Readiness for Data Warehousing	Sen et al. (2006)	1	1	3	B	O	NONE	NA
Organizational Readiness for Implementing Change	Shea et al. (2014)	1	2	10	H	O	NONE	NA
Organizational Resources	Smith and Manfredo (2011)	1	1	9	SU	O	I	I
Organizational Information Technology Innovation Readiness Scale	Snyder-Halpern (2002)	2	8	41	H (2)	I (2)	NONE (2)	NA

Readiness	Spoth et al. (2015)	1	10 [8]	80 [38]	O	O	NONE	NA
CPOE Readiness Assessment Tool	Stablein et al. (2003)	1	9	25	H	O	NONE	NA
Organizational E-Readiness	Tan et al. (2007)	1	6	33	B	O	ADO	O
Organizational Needs Assessment	Taxman et al. (2008)	2	7	22	CJ (2)	O (2)	ADO IMP	O (2)
Readiness for Change	Taxman et al. (2014)	1	1 (5 subscales)	NR	CJ	I	NONE	NA
Change Readiness	Timmor and Zif (2010)	1	1	6	B	O	OTH	I
e-Health Readiness Measure	Touré et al. (2012)	1	3	57	H	I	NONE	NA
Readiness	Trzcinski and Sobeck (2012)	2	1	15	B (2)	O (2)	OTH (2)	O (2)
Individual Readiness to Change	Vakola (2014)	1	1	6	B	I	NONE	NA
Organizational Readiness	Wang and Ahmed (2009)	1	1	6	B	O	ADO	O
Readiness for Change	Weeks et al. (2004)	1	1	4	B	I	OTH	I
Readiness Implementation Model	Wen et al. (2010)	1	7	41	H	O	OTH	O
Change Readiness	West (1998)	1	0	16	H	O	NONE	NA
Readiness to Utilize Technology	Wittenberg-Lyles et al. (2012)	1	0	31	H	I	NONE	NA
Organizational Readiness	Yan Xin et al. (2014)	1	1	3	B	O	IMP	O
Organizational Readiness	Yang et al. (2015)	1	2	6	B	O	ATT	O
Organizational Readiness	Yusof and Shafiei (2011)	1	1	4	B	O	ATT	O
Organizational Readiness for Change	Zeitlin (2014)	1	1	9	CW	I	OTH	I
Organizational Readiness	Zhu et al. (2010)	1	2	5	B	O	OTH	O

Notes: Number of settings for Lehman exceeds 48 because some studies included two types of settings (e.g., SU and MH)

Numbers in parenthesis indicate study frequencies. Spoth et al. (2015) developed separate readiness scales for university extension services and state agencies (departments of education and health). State agency scales in brackets

Table 5.7 Evidence-based assessment of the psychometric properties of organizational readiness for change measures

Measure name	Originating authors	Inter-item consistency	Structural validity	Known-groups validity	Predictive validity (ADO and IMP only)
[not specified]	Acosta et al. (2013)	Cohesion = 4 Change receptivity = 3	0	Other = 0	0 (NY)
[not specified]	Al-Somali et al. (2015)	IT readiness = 0 Receptivity to change = 0	1	0 (NY)	2
Organizational Change Recipients' Beliefs Scale	Armenakis et al. (2007)	Discrepancy = 4 Appropriateness = 4 Efficacy = 4 Principal support = 3 Valence = 4 OCRBS = 4	4	Demographics = 1	0 (NY)
Specialty Training's Organizational Readiness for curriculum Change	Bank et al. (2015)	0	0	0 (NY)	
Medical Organizational Readiness for Change	Bohman et al. (2008)	Guidance = 4 Pressure = 4 Org. readiness = 3 Ind. readiness = 2 Group functioning = 3 Work environ. = 3 Autonomy = 3 Alcohol/drug focus = 2	0	Organization = 2 Role/profession = 2	0 (NY)
Organizational Change Questionnaire-Process, Context, and Readiness	Bouckenooghe et al. (2009)	Intentional readiness = 4 Cognitive readiness = 2 Emotional readiness = 4	4	Organization = 3 Role/profession = 3	0 (NY)

Readiness to Adopt	Brink et al. (1995)	Relative advantage = 2 Compatibility = 3 Complexity = 3 Innovativeness = 1 Innovation attitudes = 3 Policy attitudes = 2 Self-efficacy = 1 Outcome expectations = 1 Norms and support = 4 Decentralized decision = 3	0	Other = 2	0 (NY)
Organizational Readiness	Burnett et al. (2010)	0	0	Organization = 0	0 (NY)
Change Readiness	Caldwell et al. (2009)	4	0	0 (NY)	0 (NY)
Organizational Readiness for Change	Chang et al. (2013)	Financial insufficiency = 4 Space sufficiency = 4 IT support sufficiency = 3 Provider insufficiency = 2 Champion in clinic = NA Psychiatrist on staff = NA Psychologist on staff = NA Social worker on staff = NA Training retreat = NA Network endorsement = NA Teamwork = NA Comm. and cooperation = 4 Orientation toward QI = 4 Demands and stress = 4 Internal clinic authority = 4 External clinic authority = 4 Resistance = 4	0	Organization = 2	4

(continued)

Table 5.7 (continued)

Measure name	Originating authors	Inter-item consistency	Structural validity	Known-groups validity	Predictive validity (ADO and IMP only)
Long-Term Care Readiness Tool for EHR Implementation	Cherry (2011)	4	0	0 (NY)	0 (NY)
[not specified]	Chilenski et al. (2015)	Openness to change = 3 Leadership openness = NA Morale = NA Communication = 4 Resources = NA	0	0 (NY)	0 (NY)
Readiness	Chwelos et al. (2001)	Financial resources = 3 IT sophistication = 4 Partner readiness = 4	3	0 (NY)	0 (NY)
Perceived Organizational Readiness for Change	Cinite et al. (2009)	Management commitment = 4 Change agent competence = 4 Immediate manager support = 3	4	0 (NY)	0 (NY)
Organizational Readiness for Change	Claiborne et al. (2013)	Readiness = 3	3	Demographics = 2	0 (NY)
Readiness for Use of New Technology	Demiris et al. (2007)	0 (NA)	0	0 (NY)	0 (NY)
Functional Organizational Readiness for Change Evaluation (FORCE)	Devereaux et al. (2006)	11 scales <=1 11 scales >1	0	Demographics = 2 Role/profession = 1	0 (NY)

Organizational Readiness for Change	Eby et al. (2000)	3	0 (NY)	0	0 (NY)
e-Readiness	Fathian et al. (2008)	0	0 (NY)	4	0 (NY)
Technology Adoption Readiness Scale	Finch et al. (2012)	0 (NA)	Other = 3	0	0 (NY)
Training and Resources	Friedmann et al. (2007)	Funding = 3 Physical plant = 3 Staffing = 1 Training = 4 Resources = 2 Internal support = NR	Organization = 0	0	4
Psychological Climate	Garner and Hunter (2013)	Supervisor support = 4 Coworker support = 4 Role overload = 4 Role clarity = 4 Job challenge/autonomy = 2	0 (NY)	4	0 (NY)
E-Commerce Readiness	Ghobakhloo et al. (2014)	4	0 (NY)	4	2
Readiness for Change	Hameed et al. (2013)	4	0 (NY)	3	0 (NY)
Readiness for Change	Hanpachern et al. (1998)	4	Demographics = 2	0	0 (NY)

(continued)

Table 5.7 (continued)

Measure name	Originating authors	Inter-item consistency	Structural validity	Known-groups validity	Predictive validity (ADO and IMP only)
Organizational Readiness to Change Assessment Instrument	Helfrich et al. (2009)	Evidence = 3 Context = 4 Facilitation = 4 Subscales: Research = 2 Clinical experience = 3 Patient preferences = 2 Leader culture = 4 Staff culture = 4 Leadership behavior = 4 Measurement = 4 Opinion leaders = 4 General resources = 4 Leader practices = 4 Clinical champion = 4 Leader implem. roles = 4 Implem. team roles = 4 Implementation plan = 4 Project Comm. = 4 Progress tracking = 4 Project resources = 4 Project evaluation = 4	1	Role/profession = 1 Organization = 0	4
Training Resources	Herbeck et al. (2008)	Training resources = 3	0	0 (NY)	4

Readiness for Organizational Change	Holt et al. (2007)	Appropriateness = 4, Management support = 4, Change efficacy = 3, Personal valence = 2, IROC = 4	4	Demographics = 1 Role/profession = 2, Organization = 1, Other = 4	4
Organizational e-Readiness	Hung et al. (2014)	Aware corporate website = 4, Enterprise resources = 4, Website governance = 4, Sen. exec. commit = 4, Technol. resources = 4, Human resources = 2	3	0 (NY)	3
Organizational Telehealth Readiness Assessment Tool	Jennett et al. (2003)	0	0	0 (NY)	0 (NY)
Medical School's Organizational Readiness for Curriculum Change (MORC)	Jippes et al. (2013)	Motivation = 4, Capability = 4, External pressure = 2	3	0 (NY)	0 (NY)
Readiness for Change	Jones et al. (2005)	4	0	0 (NY)	2
Readiness for Change-Cognitive Emotional Intentional	Kondakci et al. (2013)	Cognitive readiness = 4, Emotional readiness = 4, Intentional readiness = 4	3	Demographics = 0 Organization = 4	0 (NY)
Organizational Readiness	Kurnia et al. (2015)	Perceived benefits = 4, Perceived organizational resources and governance = 4	2	0 (NY)	4
Readiness for Change	Kwahk and Lee (2008)	3	3	0 (NY)	0 (NY)
Employee Readiness for e-Business	Lai and Ong (2010)	Benefit = 4, Security = 4, Collaboration = 4, Certainty = 4	4	0 (NY)	0 (NY)
e-Business Readiness	Lai et al. (2013)	4	4	0 (NY)	0 (NY)

(continued)

Table 5.7 (continued)

Measure name	Originating authors	Inter-item consistency	Structural validity	Known-groups validity	Predictive validity (ADO and IMP only)
TCU Organizational Readiness for Change	Lehman et al. (2002)	Program needs = 4 Training needs = 4 Pressure for change = 3 Offices = 3 Staffing = 2 Training = 2 Computer access = 2 E-communication = 2 Growth = 2 Efficacy = 2 Influence = 3 Adaptability = 2 Mission = 3 Cohesion = 4 Autonomy = 1 Communication = 3 Stress = 3 Change = 2 Organizational climate = 3 Motivation for change = 2 Staff attributes = 3 Adequacy of resources = 3 ORC scale = 4	1	Role/profession = 4 Organization = 1 Other = 1	4
Readiness for Organizational Change	Madsen et al. (2005)	4	4	Demographics = 1	0 (NY)
Readiness for Change	McCrae et al. (2014)	0	0	0 (NY)	0
Readiness for Managed Care	Medley and Nickel (1999)	0 (NA)	0	0	0 (NY)

Readiness for Change	Ming-Chu and Hsui (2015)	Belief = 4 Attitude = 4 Intention = 4	4	0 (NY)	0 (NY)
Health Reform Readiness Index	Molfenter et al. (2012)	0 (NA)	0	Organization = 2	0 (NY)
Perceived Organizational E-Readiness	Molla and Licker (2005)	Awareness = 4 Human resources = 4 Business resources = 4 Technology resources = 4 Commitment = 4 Governance = 4	1	0 (NY)	1
Perceived Organizational E-Readiness	Molla et al. (2010)	3	0	0 (NY)	0
Health-Oriented Readiness for Change	Mueller et al. (2012)	3	4	0 (NY)	0 (NY)
Proactive Organizational Change: Assessing Critical Success Factors	Nelson et al. (1998)	0	0	0 (NY)	0 (NY)
Organizational Readiness for Change	Nordin (2012)	0	0	0 (NY)	0 (NY)
Readiness for Technological Innovation	Oliver and Demiris (2004)	0	0	Organization = 2 Role/profession = 2	0 (NY)
Change Readiness	O'Neill and Downer (2004)	3	1	Organization = 1	0 (NY)
Organizational readiness	Pinto et al. (2011)	4	0	0 (NY)	0 (NY)
Readiness for Change	Rafferty and Simons (2006)	4	0	0 (NY)	0 (NY)
Organizational Readiness	Ram et al. (2013)	4	4	0 (NY)	2
Organizational Readiness for Data Warehousing	Sen et al. (2006)	3	4	Organization = 1	0 (NY)
Organizational Readiness for Implementing Change	Shea et al. (2014)	4	4	Other = 3	0 (NY)
Organizational Resources	Smith and Manfredo (2011)	3	0	0 (NY)	2

(continued)

Table 5.7 (continued)

Measure name	Originating authors	Inter-item consistency	Structural validity	Known-groups validity	Predictive validity (ADO and IMP only)
Organizational Information Technology Innovation Readiness Scale	Snyder-Halpern (2002)	Resources = 4 End-users = 4 Technology = 4 Knowledge = 4 Processes = 4 Values and goals = 4 Manage. structures = 4 Admin. support = 4	3	0 (NY)	0 (NY)
Readiness	Spoth et al. (2015) Extension service scales (state agency scales in parentheses)	State engagement = 4 (2) Prevention support = 4 (NA) Knowledge of EBPs = 3 (2) Evaluation = 4 (NA) EBP collaboration = 4 (4) Organizational capacity = 4 (4) Perceived resources = 3 (2) Collaboration experience 3 (3) Openness to change = 3 (NA) Train and development = 2 (NA)	2	Organization = 1 Other = 1	0 (NY)
CPOE Readiness Assessment Tool	Stablein et al. (2003)	0	0	0 (NY)	0 (NY)
Organizational e-Readiness	Tan et al. (2007)	Awareness = 4 Commitment = 4 Human resources = 1 Technol. resources = 4 Business resources = 3 Governance = 4	0	0 (NY)	1

Instrument	Citation				
Organizational Needs Assessment	Taxman et al. (2008)	Staffing needs = 1 / Retention = 1 / Training emphasis = 3 / Perceived funding for new programs = 2 / Physical facilities = 3 / IT support = 3 / Community support = 1	0	Organization = 0	0
Readiness for Change	Taxman et al. (2014)	0	4	Other = 3	0 (NY)
Change Readiness	Timmor and Zif (2010)	3	0	0 (NY)	0 (NY)
e-Health Readiness Measure	Toure et al. (2007)	Individual = 4 / Organizational = 4 / Technology = 4	0	Demographics = 1 / Role/profession = 1 / Organization = 1	0 (NY)
Readiness	Trzcinski and Sobeck (2012)	4	3	0 (NY)	0 (NY)
Individual Readiness to Change	Vakola (2014)	3	2	0 (NY)	0 (NY)
Organizational Readiness	Wang and Ahmed (2009)	4	1	0 (NY)	0
Readiness for Change	Weeks et al. (2004)	4	3	0 (NY)	0 (NY)
Readiness Implementation Model	Wen et al. (2010)	0	0	0 (NY)	0 (NY)
Change Readiness	West (1998)	0 (NA)	0	0 (NY)	0 (NY)
Readiness to Utilize Technology	Wittenberg-Lyles et al. (2012)	0 (NA)	0	0 (NY)	0 (NY)
Organizational Readiness	Yan Xin et al. (2014)	3	1	0 (NY)	0
Organizational Readiness	Yang et al. (2015)	IT infrastructure = 3 / Top management support = 4	1	0 (NY)	0 (NY)
Organizational Readiness	Yusof and Shafiei (2011)	3	0	0 (NY)	0 (NY)
Organizational Readiness for Change	Zeitlin (2014)	0	4	0 (NY)	0 (NY)
Organizational Readiness	Zhu et al. (2010)	Leadership involve. = 4 / Organizational fit = 4	1	0 (NY)	0 (NY)

ADO adoption, *IMP* implementation, *NY* not yet assessed, *NA* not applicable

References

Ajzen, I. (1991). The theory of planned behavior. *Organizational Behavior and Human Decision Processes, 50*(2), 179–211. https://doi.org/10.1016/0749-5978(91)90020-t

Al-Somali, S. A., Gholami, R., & Clegg, B. (2015). A stage-oriented model (SOM) for e-commerce adoption: A study of Saudi Arabian organisations. *Journal of Manufacturing Technology Management, 26*(1), 2–35. https://doi.org/10.1108/JMTM-03-2013-0019

Anderson, N. R., & West, M. A. (1998). Measuring climate for work group innovation: Development and validation of the team climate inventory. *Journal of Organizational Behavior, 19*(3), 235–258. https://doi.org/10.1002/(sici)1099-1379(199805)19:3<235::aid-job837>3.3.co;2-3

Armenakis, A. A., & Bedeian, A. G. (1999). Organizational change: A review of theory and research in the 1990s. *Journal of Management, 25*(3), 293–315. https://doi.org/10.1177/014920639902500303

Armenakis, A. A., Bernerth, J. B., Pitts, J. P., & Walker, H. J. (2007). Organizational change recipients' beliefs scale: Development of an assessment instrument. *Journal of Applied Behavioral Science, 43*(4), 481–505. https://doi.org/10.1177/0021886307303654

Armenakis, A. A., Harris, S. G., & Mossholder, K. W. (1993). Creating readiness for organizational-change. *Human Relations, 46*(6), 681–703.

Baer, J. S., Wells, E. A., Rosengren, D. B., Hartzler, B., Beadnell, B., & Dunn, C. (2009). Agency context and tailored training in technology transfer: A pilot evaluation of motivational interviewing training for community counselors. *Journal of Substance Abuse Treatment, 37*(2), 191–202. https://doi.org/10.1016/j.jsat.2009.01.003

Bank, L., Jippes, M., Van Luijk, S., Den Rooyen, C., Scherpbier, A., & Scheele, F. (2015). Specialty Training's Organizational Readiness for curriculum Change (STORC): Development of a questionnaire in a Delphi study. *BMC Medical Education, 15*(1), 1–8. https://doi.org/10.1186/s12909-015-0408-0

Becan, J. E., Knight, D. K., & Flynn, P. M. (2012). Innovation adoption as facilitated by a change-oriented workplace. *Journal of Substance Abuse Treatment, 42*(2), 179–190. https://doi.org/10.1016/j.jsat.2011.10.014

Beidas, R. S., Edmunds, J., Ditty, M., Watkins, J., Walsh, L., Marcus, S., & Kendall, P. (2014). Are inner context factors related to implementation outcomes in cognitive-behavioral therapy for youth anxiety? *Administration and Policy in Mental Health, 41*(6), 788–799. https://doi.org/10.1007/s10488-013-0529-x

Beidas, R. S., Mychailyszyn, M. P., Edmunds, J. M., Khanna, M. S., Downey, M. M., & Kendall, P. C. (2012). Training School Mental Health Providers to Deliver Cognitive-Behavioral Therapy. *School Mental Health, 4*(4), 197–206. https://doi.org/10.1007/s12310-012-9074-0

Bohman, T. M., Kulkarni, S., Waters, V., Spence, R. T., Murphy-Smith, M., & McQueen, K. (2008). Assessing health care organizations' ability to implement screening, brief intervention, and referral to treatment. *Journal of Addiction Medicine, 2*(3), 151–157. https://doi.org/10.1097/ADM.0b013e3181800ae5

Bouckenooghe, D. (2010). Positioning change recipients' attitudes toward change in the organizational change literature. *Journal of Applied Behavioral Science, 46*(4), 500–531. https://doi.org/10.1177/0021886310367944

Bouckenooghe, D., Devos, G., & Van Den Broeck, H. (2009). Organizational change questionnaire-climate of change, processes, and readiness: Development of a new instrument. *Journal of Psychology: Interdisciplinary and Applied, 143*(6), 559–599. https://doi.org/10.1080/00223980903218216

Brink, S. G., Basenengquist, K. M., Oharatompkins, N. M., Parcel, G. S., Gottlieb, N. H., & Lovato, C. Y. (1995). Diffusion of an effective tobacco prevention program.1. Evaluation of the dissemination phase. *Health Education Research, 10*(3), 283–295.

Burnett, S., Benn, J., Pinto, A., Parand, A., Iskander, S., & Vincent, C. (2010). Organisational readiness: Exploring the preconditions for success in organisation-wide patient safety improvement programmes. *Quality & Safety in Health Care, 19*(4), 313–317. https://doi.org/10.1136/qshc.2008.030759

Caldwell, S. D., Roby-Williams, C., Rush, K., & Ricke-Kiely, T. (2009). Influences of context, process and individual differences on nurses' readiness for change to Magnet status. *Journal of Advanced Nursing, 65*(7), 1412–1422. https://doi.org/10.1111/j.1365-2648.2009.05012.x

Chang, E. T., Rose, D. E., Yano, E. M., Wells, K. B., Metzger, M. E., Post, E. P., ... Rubenstein, L. V. (2013). Determinants of readiness for primary care-mental health integration (PC-MHI) in the VA health care system. *Journal of General Internal Medicine, 28*(3), 353–362. https://doi.org/10.1007/s11606-012-2217-z

Chaudoir, S. R., Dugan, A. G., & Barr, C. H. I. (2013). Measuring factors affecting implementation of health innovations: A systematic review of structural, organizational, provider, patient, and innovation level measures. *Implementation Science, 8*. https://doi.org/10.1186/1748-5908-8-22

Cherry, B. (2011). Assessing organizational readiness for electronic health record adoption in long-term care facilities. *Journal of Gerontological Nursing, 37*(10), 14–19. https://doi.org/10.3928/00989134-20110831-06

Chilenski, S. M., Olson, J. R., Schulte, J. A., Perkins, D. F., & Spoth, R. (2015). A multi-level examination of how the organizational context relates to readiness to implement prevention and evidence-based programming in community settings. *Evaluation and Program Planning, 48*, 63–74. https://doi.org/10.1016/j.evalprogplan.2014.10.004

Choi, N. G., Lee, A., & Goldstein, M. (2011). Meals on wheels: Exploring potential for and barriers to integrating depression intervention for homebound older adults. *Home Health Care Services Quarterly, 30*(4), 214–230. https://doi.org/10.1080/01621424.2011.622251

Chor, K. H. B., Wisdom, J. P., Olin, S. C. S., Hoagwood, K. E., & Horwitz, S. M. (2015). Measures for predictors of innovation adoption. *Administration and Policy in Mental Health and Mental Health Services Research, 42*(5), 545–573. https://doi.org/10.1007/s10488-014-0551-7

Chwelos, P., Benbasat, I., & Dexter, A. S. (2001). Research report: Empirical test of an EDI adoption model. *Information Systems Research, 12*(3), 304–321. https://doi.org/10.1287/isre.12.3.304.9708

Cinite, I., Duxbury, L. E., & Higgins, C. (2009). Measurement of perceived organizational readiness for change in the public sector. *British Journal of Management, 20*(2), 265–277. https://doi.org/10.1111/j.1467-8551.2008.00582.x

Claiborne, N., Auerbach, C., Lawrence, C., & Schudrich, W. Z. (2013). Organizational change: The role of climate and job satisfaction in child welfare workers' perception of readiness for change. *Children and Youth Services Review, 35*(12), 2013–2019. https://doi.org/10.1016/j.childyouth.2013.09.012

Demiris, G., Courtney, K. L., & Meyer, W. (2007). Current status and perceived needs of information technology in critical access hospitals: A survey study. *Informatics in Primary Care, 15*(1), 45–51. https://doi.org/10.14236/jhi.v15i1.643

Devereaux, M. W., Drynan, A. K., Lowry, S., MacLennan, D., Figdor, M., Fancott, C., & Sinclair, L. (2006). Evaluating organizational readiness for change: A preliminary mixed-model assessment of an interprofessional rehabilitation hospital. *Healthcare Quarterly, 9*(4), 66–74.

Eby, L. T., Adams, D. M., Russell, J. E. A., & Gaby, S. H. (2000). Perceptions of organizational readiness for change: Factors related to employees' reactions to the implementation of team-based selling. *Human Relations, 53*(3), 419–442.

Fathian, M., Akhavan, P., & Hoorali, M. (2008). E-readiness assessment of non-profit ICT SMEs in a developing country: The case of Iran. *Technovation, 28*(9), 578–590. https://doi.org/10.1016/j.technovation.2008.02.002

Finch, T. L., Mair, F. S., Odonnell, C., Murray, E., & May, C. R. (2012). From theory to "measurement" in complex interventions: Methodological lessons from the development of an e-health normalisation instrument. *BMC Medical Research Methodology, 12*, 1–16. https://doi.org/10.1186/1471-2288-12-69

Friedmann, P. D., Taxman, F. S., & Henderson, C. E. (2007). Evidence-based treatment practices for drug-involved adults in the criminal justice system. *Journal of Substance Abuse Treatment, 32*(3), 267–277. https://doi.org/10.1016/j.jsat.2006.12.020

Gagnon, M. P., Attieh, R., Ghandour, E. K., Légaré, F., Ouimet, M., Estabrooks, C. A., & Grimshaw, J. (2014). A systematic review of instruments to assess organizational readiness for knowledge translation in health care. *PLoS One, 9*(12). https://doi.org/10.1371/journal.pone.0114338

Garner, B. R., & Hunter, B. D. (2013). Examining the temporal relationship between psychological climate, work attitude, and staff turnover. *Journal of Substance Abuse Treatment, 44*(2), 193–200. https://doi.org/10.1016/j.jsat.2012.05.002

Ghobakhloo, M., Hong, T. S., & Standing, C. (2014). Business-to-business electronic commerce success: A supply network perspective. *Journal of Organizational Computing and Electronic Commerce, 24*(4), 312–341. https://doi.org/10.1080/10919392.2014.956608

Guerrero, E. G., He, A., Kim, A., & Aarons, G. A. (2014). Organizational implementation of evidence-based substance abuse treatment in racial and ethnic minority communities. *Administration and Policy in Mental Health and Mental Health Services Research, 41*(6), 737–749. https://doi.org/10.1007/s10488-013-0515-3

Guerrero, E. G., & Kim, A. (2013). Organizational structure, leadership and readiness for change and the implementation of organizational cultural competence in addiction health services. *Evaluation and Program Planning, 40*, 74–81. https://doi.org/10.1016/j.evalprogplan.2013.05.002

Haffar, M., Al-Karaghouli, W., & Ghoneim, A. (2013). The mediating effect of individual readiness for change in the relationship between organisational culture and TQM implementation. *Total Quality Management and Business Excellence, 24*(5–6), 693–706. https://doi.org/10.1080/14783363.2013.791112

Haffar, M., Al-Karaghouli, W., & Ghoneim, A. (2014). An empirical investigation of the influence of organizational culture on individual readiness for change in Syrian manufacturing organizations. *Journal of Organizational Change Management, 27*(1), 5–22. https://doi.org/10.1108/JOCM-04-2012-0046

Hameed, I., Roques, O., & Arain, G. A. (2013). Nonlinear moderating effect of tenure on organizational identification (OID) and the subsequent role of OID in fostering readiness for change. *Group & Organization Management, 38*(1), 101–127. https://doi.org/10.1177/1059601112472727

Hanpachern, C., Morgan, G. A., & Griego, O. V. (1998). An extension of the theory of margin: A framework for assessing readiness for change. *Human Resource Development Quarterly, 9*(4), 339–350. https://doi.org/10.1002/hrdq.3920090405

Helfrich, C. D., Li, Y. F., Sharp, N. D., & Sales, A. E. (2009). Organizational readiness to change assessment (ORCA): Development of an instrument based on the Promoting Action on Research in Health Services (PARIHS) framework. *Implementation Science, 4*. https://doi.org/10.1186/1748-5908-4-38

Henderson, C. E., Taxman, F. S., & Young, D. W. (2008). A Rasch model analysis of evidence-based treatment practices used in the criminal justice system. *Drug and Alcohol Dependence, 93*(1–2), 163–175. https://doi.org/10.1016/j.drugalcdep.2007.09.010

Henderson, C. E., Young, D. W., Farrell, J., & Taxman, F. S. (2009). Associations among state and local organizational contexts: Use of evidence-based practices in the criminal justice system. *Drug and Alcohol Dependence, 103*, S23–S32. https://doi.org/10.1016/j.drugalcdep.2008.12.006

Henderson, C. E., Young, D. W., Jainchill, N., Hawke, J., Farkas, S., & Davis, R. M. (2007). Program use of effective drug abuse treatment practices for juvenile offenders. *Journal of Substance Abuse Treatment, 32*(3), 279–290. https://doi.org/10.1016/j.jsat.2006.12.021

Henggeler, S. W., Chapman, J. E., Rowland, M. D., Halliday-Boykins, C. A., Randall, J., Shackelford, J., & Schoenwald, S. K. (2008). Statewide adoption and initial implementation of contingency management for substance-abusing adolescents. *Journal of Consulting and Clinical Psychology, 76*(4), 556–567. https://doi.org/10.1037/0022-006x.76.4.556

Herbeck, D. A., Hser, Y. I., & Teruya, C. (2008). Empirically supported substance abuse treatment approaches: A survey of treatment providers' perspectives and practices. *Addictive Behaviors, 33*(5), 699–712. https://doi.org/10.1016/j.addbeh.2007.12.003

Herscovitch, L., & Meyer, J. P. (2002). Commitment to organizational change: Extension of a three-component model. *Journal of Applied Psychology, 87*(3), 474–487.

Holt, D. T., Armenakis, A. A., Harris, S. G., & Feild, H. S. (2006). *Toward a comprehensive definition of readiness for change: A review of research and instrumentation research in organizational change and development*. Greenwich, CT: JAI Press.

Holt, D. T., Armenakis, A. A., Feild, H. S., & Harris, S. G. (2007). Readiness for organizational change: The systematic development of a scale. *Journal of Applied Behavioral Science, 43*(2), 232–255. https://doi.org/10.1177/0021886306295295

Holt, D. T., Helfrich, C. D., Hall, C. G., & Weiner, B. J. (2010). Are you ready? How health professionals can comprehensively conceptualize readiness for change. *Journal of General Internal Medicine, 25*(Suppl 1), 50–55. https://doi.org/10.1007/s11606-009-1112-8

Hung, W. H., Chang, L. M., Lin, C. P., & Hsiao, C. H. (2014). E-readiness of website acceptance and implementation in SMEs. *Computers in Human Behavior, 40*, 44–55. https://doi.org/10.1016/j.chb.2014.07.046

Jennett, P., Yeo, M., Pauls, M., & Graham, J. (2003). Organizational readiness for telemedicine: implications for success and failure. *Journal of Telemedicine and Telecare, 9*(Suppl 2), 27–30. https://doi.org/10.1258/135763303322596183

Jippes, M., Driessen, E. W., Broers, N. J., Majoor, G. D., Gijselaers, W. H., & Van Der Vleuten, C. P. M. (2013). A medical school's organizational readiness for curriculum change (MORC): Development and validation of a questionnaire. *Academic Medicine, 88*(9), 1346–1356. https://doi.org/10.1097/ACM.0b013e31829f0869

Jippes, M., Driessen, E. W., Broers, N. J., Majoor, G. D., Gijselaers, W. H., & Van Der Vleuten, C. P. M. (2015). Culture matters in successful curriculum change: An international study of the influence of national and organizational culture tested with multilevel structural equation modeling. *Academic Medicine, 90*(7), 921–929. https://doi.org/10.1097/ACM.0000000000000687

Jones, R. A., Jimmieson, N. L., & Griffiths, A. (2005). The impact of organizational culture and reshaping capabilities on change implementation success: The mediating role of readiness for change. *Journal of Management Studies, 42*(2), 361–386.

Kondakçi, Y., Zayim, M., & Çalişkan, O. (2013). Development and validation of readiness for change scale. *Elementary Education Online, 12*(1), 23–35.

Kotter, J. P. (1996). *Leading change*. Boston, MA: Harvard Business Press.

Kurnia, S., Choudrie, J., Mahbubur, R. M., & Alzougool, B. (2015). E-commerce technology adoption: A Malaysian grocery SME retail sector study. *Journal of Business Research, 68*(9), 1906–1918. https://doi.org/10.1016/j.jbusres.2014.12.010

Kwahk, K. Y., & Lee, J. N. (2008). The role of readiness for change in ERP implementation: Theoretical bases and empirical validation. *Information and Management, 45*(7), 474–481. https://doi.org/10.1016/j.im.2008.07.002

Lai, J. Y., & Ong, C. S. (2010). Assessing and managing employees for embracing change: A multiple-item scale to measure employee readiness for e-business. *Technovation, 30*(1), 76–85. https://doi.org/10.1016/j.technovation.2009.05.003

Lai, J. Y., Kan, C. W., & Ulhas, K. R. (2013). Impacts of employee participation and trust on e-business readiness, benefits, and satisfaction. *Information Systems and e-Business Management, 11*(2), 265–285. https://doi.org/10.1007/s10257-012-0193-9

Lehman, W. E. K., Greener, J. M., & Simpson, D. D. (2002). Assessing organizational readiness for change. *Journal of Substance Abuse Treatment, 22*(4), 197–209.

Lewis, C. C., Fischer, S., Weiner, B. J., Stanick, C., Kim, M., & Martinez, R. G. (2015). Outcomes for implementation science: An enhanced systematic review of instruments using evidence-based rating criteria. *Implementation Science, 10*. https://doi.org/10.1186/s13012-015-0342-x

Lewis, C. C., Stanick, C. F., Martinez, R. G., Weiner, B. J., Kim, M., Barwick, M., & Comtois, K. A. (2015). The society for implementation research collaboration instrument review project: A methodology to promote rigorous evaluation. *Implementation Science, 10*. https://doi.org/10.1186/s13012-014-0193-x

Lewis, C. C., Weiner, B. J., Stanick, C., & Fischer, S. M. (2015). Advancing implementation science through measure development and evaluation: A study protocol. *Implementation Science, 10*. https://doi.org/10.1186/s13012-015-0287-0

Lundgren, L., Chassler, D., Amodeo, M., D'Ippolito, M., & Sullivan, L. (2012). Barriers to implementation of evidence-based addiction treatment: A national study. *Journal of Substance Abuse Treatment, 42*(3), 231–238. https://doi.org/10.1016/j.jsat.2011.08.003

Lundgren, L., Amodeo, M., Chassler, D., Krull, I., & Sullivan, L. (2013). Organizational readiness for change in community-based addiction treatment programs and adherence in implementing evidence-based practices: a national study. *Journal of Substance Abuse Treatment, 45*(5), 457–465. https://doi.org/10.1016/j.jsat.2013.06.007

Madsen, S. R., Miller, D., & John, C. R. (2005). Readiness for organizational change: Do organizational commitment and social relationships in the workplace make a difference? *Human Resource Development Quarterly, 16*(2), 213–233.

McCrae, J. S., Scannapieco, M., Leake, R., Potter, C. C., & Menefee, D. (2014). Who's on board? Child welfare worker reports of buy-in and readiness for organizational change. *Children and Youth Services Review, 37*, 28–35. https://doi.org/10.1016/j.childyouth.2013.12.001

Medley, T. W., & Nickel, J. T. (1999). Predictors of home care readiness for managed care: A multivariate analysis. *Home Health Care Services Quarterly, 18*(2), 27–42. https://doi.org/10.1300/j027v18n02_02

Ming-Chu, Y., & Meng-Hsiu, L. (2015). Unlocking the black box: Exploring the link between perceive organizational support and resistance to change. *Asia Pacific Management Review, 20*(3), 177–183. https://doi.org/10.1016/j.apmrv.2014.10.003

Molfenter, T., Capoccia, V. A., Boyle, M. G., & Sherbeck, C. K. (2012). The readiness of addiction treatment agencies for health care reform. *Substance Abuse: Treatment, Prevention, and Policy, 7*, 1–8. https://doi.org/10.1186/1747-597X-7-16

Molla, A., & Licker, P. S. (2005). Perceived e-readiness factors in e-commerce adoption: An empirical investigation in a developing country. *International Journal of Electronic Commerce, 10*(1), 83–110.

Molla, A., Peszynski, K., & Pittayachawan, S. (2010). The use of E-business in agribusiness: Investigating the influence of E-readiness and OTE factors. *Journal of Global Information Technology Management, 13*(1), 56–76.

Mueller, F., Jenny, G. J., & Bauer, G. F. (2012). Individual and organizational health-oriented readiness for change: Conceptualization and validation of a measure within a large-scale comprehensive stress management intervention. *International Journal of Workplace Health Management, 5*(3), 220–236. https://doi.org/10.1108/17538351211268872

Nelson, J. C., Raskind-hood, C., Galvin, V. G., Essien, J. D. K., & Levine, L. M. (1998). Assessing public health agency readiness. *American Journal of Preventive Medicine, 16*(99), 103–117.

Noe, T. D., Kaufman, C. E., Kaufmann, L. J., Brooks, E., & Shore, J. H. (2014). Providing culturally competent services for American Indian and Alaska native veterans to reduce health care disparities. *American Journal of Public Health, 104*(SUPPL. 4), S548–S554. https://doi.org/10.2105/AJPH.2014.302140

Nordin, N. (2012). The influence of leadership behavior and organizational commitment on organizational readiness for change in a higher learning institution. *Asia Pacific Education Review, 13*(2), 239–249. https://doi.org/10.1007/s12564-011-9200-y

O'Neill, M. L., & Downer, P. (2004). Change readiness for SAP in the Canadian Healthcare System. *Healthcare Management Forum, 17*(1), 18–25. https://doi.org/10.1016/S0840-4704(10)60312-2

Oser, C. B., Knudsen, H. K., Staton-Tindall, M., Taxman, F., & Leukefeld, C. (2009). Organizational-level correlates of the provision of detoxification services and medication-based treatments for substance abuse in correctional institutions. *Drug and Alcohol Dependence, 103*, S73–S81. https://doi.org/10.1016/j.drugalcdep.2008.11.005

Oser, C. B., Tindall, M. S., & Leukefeld, C. G. (2007). HIV testing in correctional agencies and community treatment programs: The impact of internal organizational structure. *Journal of Substance Abuse Treatment, 32*(3), 301–310. https://doi.org/10.1016/j.jsat.2006.12.016

Parker Oliver, D. R., & Demiris, G. (2004). An assessment of the readiness of hospice organizations to accept technological innovation. *Journal of Telemedicine and Telecare, 10*(3), 170–174. https://doi.org/10.1258/135763304323070832

Pinto, A., Benn, J., Burnett, S., Parand, A., & Vincent, C. (2011). Predictors of the perceived impact of a patient safety collaborative: An exploratory study. *International Journal for Quality in Health Care, 23*(2), 173–181. https://doi.org/10.1093/intqhc/mzq089

Rafferty, A. E., Jimmieson, N. L., & Armenakis, A. A. (2013). Change readiness: A multilevel review. *Journal of Management, 39*(1), 110–135. https://doi.org/10.1177/0149206312457417

Rafferty, A. E., & Simons, R. H. (2006). An examination of the antecedents of readiness for fine-tuning and corporate transformation changes. *Journal of Business and Psychology, 20*(3), 325–350.

Ram, J., Corkindale, D., & Wu, M. L. (2013). Enterprise resource planning adoption: Structural equation modeling analysis of antecdants. *Journal of Computer Information Systems, 54*(1), 53–65.

Scaccia, J. P., Cook, B. S., Lamont, A., Wandersman, A., Castellow, J., Katz, J., & Beidas, R. S. (2015). A practical implementation science heuristic for organizational readiness: R = MC2. *Journal of Community Psychology, 43*(4), 484–501. https://doi.org/10.1002/jcop.21698

Sen, A., Sinha, A. P., & Ramamurthy, K. (2006). Data warehousing process maturity: An exploratory study of factors influencing user perceptions. *IEEE Transactions on Engineering Management, 53*(3), 440–455.

Shah, N., & Shah, S. G. S. (2010). Relationships between employee readiness for organisational change, supervisor and peer relations and demography. *Journal of Enterprise Information Management, 23*(5), 640–652. https://doi.org/10.1108/17410391011083074

Shea, C. M., Jacobs, S. R., Esserman, D. A., Bruce, K., & Weiner, B. J. (2014). Organizational readiness for implementing change: A psychometric assessment of a new measure. *Implementation Science, 9*. https://doi.org/10.1186/1748-5908-9-7

Simpson, D. D., Joe, G. W., & Rowan-Szal, G. A. (2007). Linking the elements of change: Program and client responses to innovation. *Journal of Substance Abuse Treatment, 33*(2), 201–209. https://doi.org/10.1016/j.jsat.2006.12.022

Smith, B. D., & Manfredo, I. T. (2011). Frontline counselors in organizational contexts: A study of treatment practices in community settings. *Journal of Substance Abuse Treatment, 41*(2), 124–136. https://doi.org/10.1016/j.jsat.2011.03.002

Snyder-Halpern, R. (2002). Development and pilot testing of an Organizational Information Technology/Systems Innovation Readiness Scale (OITIRS). *Proceedings of the AMIA Symposium, 702*–706.

Stablein, D., Welebob, E., Johnson, E., Metzger, J., Burgess, R., & Classen, D. C. (2003). Understanding Hospital Readiness for Computerized Physician Order Entry. *Joint Commission Journal on Quality and Safety, 29*(7), 336–344.

Stevens, G. W. (2013). Toward a process-based approach of conceptualizing change readiness. *Journal of Applied Behavioral Science, 49*(3), 333–360. https://doi.org/10.1177/0021886313475479

Spoth, R., Schainker, L. M., Redmond, C., Ralston, E., Yeh, H. C., & Perkins, D. F. (2015). Mixed picture of readiness for adoption of evidence-based prevention programs in communities: Exploratory surveys of state program delivery systems. *American Journal of Community Psychology, 55*(3–4), 253–265. https://doi.org/10.1007/s10464-015-9707-1

Tan, J., Tyler, K., & Manica, A. (2007). Business-to-business adoption of eCommerce in China. *Information & Management, 44*(3), 332–351.

Taxman, F. S., Cropsey, K. L., Melnick, G., & Perdoni, M. L. (2008). COD services in community correctional settings: An examination of organizational factors that affect service delivery. *Behavioral Sciences & the Law, 26*(4), 435–455. https://doi.org/10.1002/bsl.830

Taxman, F. S., Henderson, C., Young, D., & Farrell, J. (2014). The impact of training interventions on organizational readiness to support innovations in Juvenile justice offices. *Administration and Policy in Mental Health and Mental Health Services Research, 41*(2), 177–188. https://doi.org/10.1007/s10488-012-0445-5

Taxman, F. S., & Kitsantas, P. (2009). Availability and capacity of substance abuse programs in correctional settings: A classification and regression tree analysis. *Drug and Alcohol Dependence, 103*, S43–S53. https://doi.org/10.1016/j.drugalcdep.2009.01.008

Timmor, Y., & Zif, J. (2010). Change readiness: An alternative conceptualization and an exploratory investigation. *EuroMed Journal of Business, 5*(2), 138–165. https://doi.org/10.1108/14502191011065482

Touré, M., Poissant, L., & Swaine, B. R. (2012). Assessment of organizational readiness for e-health in a rehabilitation centre. *Disability and Rehabilitation, 34*(2), 167–173. https://doi.org/10.3109/09638288.2011.591885

Trzcinski, E., & Sobeck, J. L. (2012). Predictors of growth in small and mid-sized nonprofit organizations in the Detroit metropolitan area. *Administration in Social Work, 36*(5), 499–519. https://doi.org/10.1080/03643107.2011.627492

Vakola, M. (2013). Multilevel readiness to organizational change: A conceptual approach. *Journal of Change Management, 13*(1), 96–109. https://doi.org/10.1080/14697017.2013.768436

Vakola, M. (2014). What's in there for me? Individual readiness to change and the perceived impact of organizational change. *Leadership and Organization Development Journal, 35*(3), 195–209. https://doi.org/10.1108/LODJ-05-2012-0064

Wang, Y., & Ahmed, P. K. (2009). The moderating effect of the business strategic orientation on eCommerce adoption: Evidence from UK family run SMEs. *Journal of Strategic Information Systems, 18*(1), 16–30. https://doi.org/10.1016/j.jsis.2008.11.001

Weeks, W. A., Roberts, J., Chonko, L. B., & Jones, E. (2004). Organizational readiness for change, individual fear of change, and sales manager performance: An empirical investigation. *Journal of Personal Selling and Sales Management, 24*(1), 7–17. https://doi.org/10.1080/08853134.2004.10749012

Weiner, B. J. (2009). A theory of organizational readiness for change. *Implementation Science, 4*, 67. https://doi.org/10.1186/1748-5908-4-67

Weiner, B. J., Amick, H., & Lee, S. Y. D. (2008). Review: Conceptualization and measurement of organizational readiness for change. A review of the literature in health services research and other fields. *Medical Care Research and Review, 65*(4), 379–436. https://doi.org/10.1177/1077558708317802

Wen, K. Y., Hawkins, D. H. G., Brennan, P. F., Dinauer, S., Johnson, P. R., & Siegler, T. (2010). Developing and validating a model to predict the success of an IHCS implementation: The Readiness for implementation model. *Journal of the American Medical Informatics Association, 17*(6), 707–713. https://doi.org/10.1136/jamia.2010.005546

West, T. D. (1998). Comparing change readiness, quality improvement, and cost management among Veterans Administration, for-profit, and nonprofit hospitals. *Journal of Health Care Finance, 25*(1), 46–58. Retrieved from: https://www.ncbi.nlm.nih.gov/pubmed/9718511

Wittenberg-Lyles, E., Shaunfield, S., Oliver, D. P., Demiris, G., & Schneider, G. (2012). Assessing the readiness of hospice volunteers to utilize technology. *American Journal of Hospice & Palliative Medicine, 29*(6), 476–482. https://doi.org/10.1177/1049909111429559

Yan Xin, J., Ramayah, T., Soto-Acosta, P., Popa, S., & Ai Ping, T. (2014). Analyzing the use of web 2.0 for brand awareness and competitive advantage: An empirical study in the Malaysian hospitability industry. *Information Systems Management, 31*(2), 96–103. https://doi.org/10.1080/10580530.2014.890425

Yang, Z., Sun, J., Zhang, Y., & Wang, Y. (2015). Understanding SaaS adoption from the perspective of organizational users: A tripod readiness model. *Computers in Human Behavior, 45*, 254–264. https://doi.org/10.1016/j.chb.2014.12.022

Young, D. W., Farrell, J. L., Henderson, C. E., & Taxman, F. S. (2009). Filling service gaps: Providing intensive treatment services for offenders. *Drug and Alcohol Dependence, 103*, S33–S42. https://doi.org/10.1016/j.drugalcdep.2009.01.003

Yusof, N., & Shafiei, M. W. M. (2011). Factors affecting housing developers' readiness to adopt innovative systems. *Housing Studies, 26*(3), 369–384. https://doi.org/10.1080/02673037.2011.542097

Zayim, M., & Kondakci, Y. (2015). An exploration of the relationship between readiness for change and organizational trust in Turkish public schools. *Educational Management Administration & Leadership, 43*(4), 610–625. https://doi.org/10.1177/1741143214523009

Zeitlin, W. (2014). Factors impacting perceptions of organizational cultural competence in voluntary child welfare. *Children and Youth Services Review, 44*, 1–8. https://doi.org/10.1016/j.childyouth.2014.05.006

Zhu, Y., Li, Y., Wang, W., & Chen, J. (2010). What leads to post-implementation success of ERP? An empirical study of the Chinese retail industry. *International Journal of Information Management, 30*(3), 265–276. https://doi.org/10.1016/j.ijinfomgt.2009.09.007

Chapter 6
Changing Organizational Social Context to Support Evidence-Based Practice Implementation: A Conceptual and Empirical Review

Nathaniel J. Williams and Charles Glisson

Introduction

Conceptual models of evidence-based practice (EBP) implementation assert the importance of organizational social context for implementation success. Beginning with Rogers' (Rogers, 2003) well-known diffusion of innovations theory to more recent models such as the Consolidated Framework for Implementation Research (CFIR; Damschroder et al., 2009); the exploration, preparation, implementation, and sustainment (EPIS) model (Aarons, Hurlburt, & Horwitz, 2011); and the PARiHS model (Kitson et al., 2008), many models share the assumption that social characteristics of organizations influence the adoption and use of innovative practices (Mendel, Meredith, Schoenbaum, Sherbourne, & Wells, 2008). These models suggest variation in organizational social context contributes to differences in clinicians' propensity to adopt and implement EBPs and imply that purposeful change of an organization's social context is one mechanism for improving the adoption and integration of EBPs into practice (Williams & Glisson, 2014b).

Empirical research offers preliminary support for this hypothesis. Studies conducted across a range of health service settings in several countries reveal significant variation in the organizational social contexts of settings that deliver health, mental health, substance abuse, and social services (Glisson, Green, & Williams, 2012; Glisson, Landsverk et al., 2008; Helfrich et al., 2010; Henderson et al., 2007), and data from both national and regional studies show this variation is associated with differences in clinical, services, and implementation outcomes (Friedmann, Taxman, & Henderson, 2007; Glisson & Green, 2006; Glisson, Hemmelgarn,

N. J. Williams (✉)
School of Social Work, Boise State University, Boise, ID, USA
e-mail: natewilliams@boisestate.edu

C. Glisson
Center for Behavioral Health Research, University of Tennessee, Knoxville, TN, USA

© Springer Nature Switzerland AG 2020
B. Albers et al. (eds.), *Implementation Science 3.0*,
https://doi.org/10.1007/978-3-030-03874-8_6

Green, & Williams, 2013; Marty, Rapp, McHugo, & Whitley, 2008; Scott, Mannion, Marshall, & Davies, 2003; Williams & Glisson, 2013, 2014a; Zazzali et al., 2008). For example, within mental health services, organizational culture and climate have been linked to clinicians' attitudes toward EBPs, EBP adoption, EBP fidelity, and EBP sustainment (Aarons et al., 2012; Baer et al., 2009; Beidas et al., 2015; Glisson, Schoenwald et al., 2008; Olin et al., 2014; Williams, Glisson, Hemmelgarn, & Green, 2017; Williams, Ehrhart, Aarons, Marcus, & Beidas, 2018). These findings parallel a larger body of research from the organizational sciences which documents strong population-average correlations of $\rho = 0.41$ to $\rho = 0.59$ between features of organizational social context and innovative workplace behavior (Hartnell, Ou, & Kinicki, 2011; Kuenzi & Schminke, 2009).

Despite this growing body of research, critics argue that organizational social context is poorly conceptualized, may not be susceptible to planned change, and could be a consequence of, rather than antecedent to, changes in practitioners' implementation behaviors (Parmelli et al., 2011; Scott et al., 2003). These critiques question the effectiveness of efforts to influence EBP implementation by changing organizational social context and raise four questions which are addressed by the present chapter. First, how can we most usefully conceptualize organizational social context and its relation to EBP implementation? That is, what empirically supported theoretical bases exist for defining and measuring facets of organizational social context and using them to predict EBP implementation? Second, what evidence is there that organizational social context can be purposefully changed by implementation strategies? Third, what evidence is there that implementation strategies that target organizational social context positively influence implementation outcomes such as EBP acceptability, adoption, fidelity, and sustainment (Proctor et al., 2011)? Fourth, what evidence is there that organizational social context mediates the effects of context-focused implementation strategies on implementation outcomes? The purpose of this chapter is to address these questions through a conceptual and empirical review.

The chapter begins with a brief review of empirically supported theories that characterize and link organizational social context with implementation outcomes in health services. The review includes a description of the salient social characteristics of organizations and the levers that can be used to modify those characteristics. Next, the chapter reviews randomized controlled trials (RCTs) that manipulate organizational social context to support EBP implementation. Such studies offer the best evidence for understanding the malleability of organizational social context and for testing its effects on implementation outcomes. The review examines RCTs that tested the effects of organizational social context-focused implementation strategies on implementation outcomes in behavioral health, substance abuse, and social service settings. Special attention is given to RCTs that test organizational social context as a mediating mechanism that explains the effects on implementation outcomes. The chapter concludes with recommendations for advancing research on organizational social context, implementation strategies, and EBP implementation.

The Dimensionality of Organizational Social Context and Its Association with EBP Implementation

Theory and research on the social characteristics of organizations has resulted in a diverse body of scholarly work with at least three distinct streams (Ostroff, Kinicki, & Tamkins, 2003; Verbeke, Volgering, & Hessels, 1998). These streams characterize organizational social context in terms of three dimensions: organizational culture defined as the shared norms and expectations that characterize a workplace (Cooke & Rousseau, 1988; Glisson, Landsverk, et al., 2008; Hofstede, Neuijen, Ohayv, & Sanders, 1990); molar organizational climate defined as shared employee perceptions regarding the psychological impact of the work environment on their own personal well-being (James et al., 2008); and strategic organizational climate defined as employees' shared perceptions regarding the organization's policies and procedures and the behaviors that are expected, rewarded, and supported within the organization (Schneider, Ehrhart, & Macey, 2013). Together, these three constructs encapsulate the majority of empirical research on organizational social context from the last 50 years and offer the theoretical and empirical basis for understanding the influence of organizational social context on individuals' EBP implementation behavior (Ostroff et al., 2003). Our discussion of these three constructs with respect to EBP implementation adopts Novins, Green, Legha, and Aarons' (2013) definition of EBPs as those interventions that are supported by rigorous scientific research, allow for clinical judgment and expertise in their application, and provide for consumer choice. We characterize implementation outcomes in terms of the taxonomy suggested by Proctor et al. (2011) which includes: EBP acceptability, adoption, appropriateness, cost, feasibility, fidelity, penetration, and sustainability.

Our discussion of organizational culture, molar climate, and strategic climate is couched within a broader view of organizational context that includes other constructs identified by implementation frameworks. This broader organizational context, which is often referred to as the inner setting, includes features such as leadership, formal structure, resources, networks and communications, and organizational readiness or tension for change, among others (Aarons, Hurlburt, & Horwitz, 2011; Damschroder et al., 2009). Although all of these constructs have implications for EBP implementation, we focus on the social contextual features of organizational culture, molar climate, and strategic climate. This emphasis reflects the theoretical and empirical bases of these constructs as well as our conclusion that they represent malleable features of an organization's social environment that uniquely influence the implementation of EBPs. It is particularly important that organizations operating within the same external policy and service environments and with the same resource constraints are characterized by different organizational cultures and climates that shape clinical processes (including EBP implementation), service quality, and outcomes for clients (Beidas et al., 2015; Williams, Ehrhart et al., 2018; Glisson et al., 2013; Williams & Glisson, 2013, 2014a; Williams, Glisson et al., 2017; Glisson & Green, 2006, 2011). Moreover, there is evidence that other features of the inner setting, such as leadership, influence behavior through their effects on organizational social context (Aarons & Sommerfeld, 2012).

Organizational Culture

Research on organizational culture is characterized by several different connotations (Verbeke et al., 1998). The most prominent and empirically supported stream of research focuses on the content or substance of various culture *domains* and their relationships to organizational, work unit, small group, and individual outcomes (Hartnell et al., 2011). From this perspective, organizational culture consists of the shared norms and behavioral expectations that guide and direct individuals' role-related behaviors within a work environment (Cooke & Rousseau, 1988; Glisson, Landsverk, et al., 2008; Hofstede et al., 1990). Shared norms and behavioral expectations arise from common work experiences with leadership, organizational design, organizational systems, and reward structures that inform employees of how they ought to behave (Schein, 2004). Cultural norms and expectations can be associated with implicit, shared, and underlying values and assumptions (Cameron & Quinn, 2011; Schein, 2004). However, given the difficulty in measuring implicit beliefs and the possibility that employees comply with norms and expectations without embracing underlying values, the quantitative assessment of organizational culture most often focuses on explicit behaviors that are normative and expected within the work environment (Glisson & James, 2002; Hofstede et al., 1990). There is considerable evidence, summarized by a recent meta-analysis of 84 studies (Hartnell et al., 2011), supporting the predictive validity of a variety of organizational culture domains for a range of outcome criteria. Outcomes associated with organizational culture include employees' job satisfaction and commitment ($\rho = 0.50$), organizational innovation ($\rho = 0.59$), product and service quality ($\rho = 0.38$), and organizational growth ($\rho = 0.18$). The strong theoretical and empirical bases of research on organizational culture suggest it represents a promising area for research on EBP implementation (Grol, Bosch, Hulscher, Eccles, & Wensing, 2007).

Implementation researchers have linked several domains of organizational culture to implementation outcomes in mental health and substance abuse service settings. Analyses of qualitative data from 49 sites across 8 states in the National Evidence-Based Practices Implementation project (McHugo et al., 2007) indicated an *outcome-focused* organizational culture contributed to high implementation fidelity of outcome monitoring in mental health organizations (Marty et al., 2008). Similarly, analyses of key informant interviews from a statewide multi-year implementation of Functional Family Therapy (FFT) in New York indicated an *innovative* organizational culture facilitated the successful adoption and implementation of FFT (Zazzali et al., 2008). Aarons and Sawitzky (2006) showed that clinicians working in public youth mental health agencies with *constructive* cultures characterized by norms that emphasize achievement and motivation had more open and positive attitudes toward EBPs ($r = 0.22$) after controlling for organizational- and clinician-level demographics. Investigators have shown that a *performance-oriented* organizational culture predicts the provision of EBP services to drug-involved adults in the criminal justice system ($\beta = 0.13$) after controlling for a host of organizational characteristics including support for training and resources (Friedmann et al., 2007).

One organizational culture domain that has been the focus of multiple investigations in mental health services is *proficiency*. Proficient organizational cultures are characterized by norms and expectations that clinicians prioritize improving client well-being and maintain competence in up-to-date treatment practices for doing so (Glisson, Landsverk et al., 2008). Proficient organizational cultures are associated with positive clinician attitudes toward EBPs ($r = 0.24$), clinician intentions to adopt EBPs ($r = 0.55$), EBP adoption ($r = 0.25$), and the use of EBPs with clients ($r = 0.40$) among outpatient mental health clinicians serving youth (Aarons et al., 2012; Beidas et al., 2015; Williams, Glisson et al., 2017). Research by Olin et al. (2014) showed that more proficient organizational cultures were associated with higher observer-rated fidelity at both the program level ($r = 0.44$) and the individual clinician level ($r = 0.58$). Finally, organizational culture profiles that were two standard deviations above the national mean on *proficiency* and two standard deviations below the mean on *rigidity* and *resistance* sustained innovative programs almost twice as long (50 months vs. 24 months) as organizations with the opposite culture profiles in a national study of children's mental health agencies in the United States (Glisson, Schoenwald et al., 2008).

Molar Organizational Climate

Research on organizational climate most often examines employees' shared perceptions or meanings regarding the attributes of their work environment with respect to one of two referents—the work environment's impact on the employees' own personal well-being or the specific strategic objectives or processes that are supported, rewarded, and expected within the work environment (Ehrhart, Schneider, & Macey, 2014; Glisson, Landsverk et al., 2008; Ostroff et al., 2003). Employees' shared perceptions regarding the meaning of the work environment for their personal well-being are described as molar organizational climate. Molar climate consists of multiple dimensions (e.g., functionality, engagement, stress) with an overall general factor (PCg) describing employees' shared perceptions of the impact of their work environment on their own personal well-being and functioning (Glisson & James, 2002). In this research paradigm, employees' individual-level perceptions, labeled *psychological climate*, are assessed and aggregated to the organizational unit level to describe *organizational climate* (James et al., 2008).

Although research on the molar climate construct has the longest history among studies of organizational social context, it has been criticized by those who define climate in strategic terms (e.g., Ehrhart, Schneider, & Macey, 2014). Despite this, investigators working in the area of behavioral health and social services have found the molar construct especially powerful in characterizing the social contexts of organizations engaged in the complex, demanding, and emotion-laden work of delivering behavioral health and social services (Glisson & Hemmelgarn, 1998; Glisson & James, 2002; Williams & Glisson, 2014a). Psychometric research has demonstrated that molar climate is a unique factor distinct from both organizational culture and clinicians' work attitudes (Glisson, Green, & Williams, 2012; Glisson, Landsverk et al., 2008). Most importantly, studies have shown molar climate is predictive of work attitudes, clinician turnover, service quality, and outcomes (Glisson & Green, 2011; Glisson & Hemmelgarn, 1998; Glisson & James, 2002; Glisson et al., 2013; Glisson, Schoenwald et al., 2008; Olin et al., 2014; Williams & Glisson, 2014a).

Several studies of EBP implementation in behavioral health and social services have linked molar organizational climate to implementation outcomes. Wang, Saldana, Brown, and Chamberlain (2010) showed that leaders' perceptions of more positive organizational climates, including high functionality, high engagement, and low stress, predicted faster rates of adoption of Multidimensional Treatment Foster Care in county public service systems (hazard ratio = 1.22). In a national study of 100 mental health service organizations in 26 states, Aarons et al. (2012) showed more engaged and more functional climates were associated with more positive clinician attitudes toward EBPs ($r = 0.18$ and $r = 0.14$, respectively), whereas more stressed climates were related to more negative attitudes toward EBPs ($r = 0.14$). More functional organizational climates were also associated with increased clinician use of cognitive behavioral therapy (CBT) with youth in a large public mental health system after controlling for organizational culture, strategic climate for EBP implementation, and other clinician and organizational factors (Beidas et al., 2015).

Schoenwald et al. (2008) found that climates more conducive to therapists' growth and advancement predicted increased therapist adherence to multisystemic therapy. Lundgren, Chassler, Amodeo, D'Ippolito, and Sullivan (2012) found that more cohesive climates were correlated with fewer perceived barriers to EBP adoption among therapists ($r = -0.21$) and more stressful climates were associated with greater perceived barriers ($r = 0.21$). In a multivariate model that controlled for numerous clinician- and organization-level covariates, Lundgren et al.'s study also showed stressful climate was the second strongest predictor of perceived EBP barriers ($\beta = 0.12$) behind only program needs ($\beta = 0.14$). More demoralizing climates (i.e., those that are high in emotional exhaustion, depersonalization, and role conflict) were associated with increased clinician perceptions that EBPs diverge from their preferred method of practice ($r = 0.23$) and increased perceived burden of EBPs ($\beta = 0.55$) (Aarons & Sawitzky, 2006; Brimhall et al., 2016). Demoralizing climate has also been shown to mediate the relationship between low levels of transformational leadership and increased perceived burden of EBP among clinicians (standardized indirect effect = -0.14) (Brimhall et al., 2016).

Strategic Organizational Climate

A second stream of research on organizational climate focuses on employees' shared perceptions of the extent to which specific strategic outcomes (e.g., innovation implementation, safety) or processes (e.g., ethics, diversity) are supported, rewarded, or expected within the work environment (Ostroff et al., 2003; Schneider et al., 2013). These shared perceptions result in the emergence of focused or strategic climates such as a *climate for safety* or a *climate for implementation* (Kuenzi & Schminke, 2009). In behavioral health and social service settings, a strategic *climate for EBP implementation* is defined as employees' shared perceptions of the importance of EBP implementation within the organization and the extent to which EBP use is expected, rewarded, and supported (Ehrhart, Aarons, & Farahnak, 2014).

Similar to the organizational culture domains defined as norms and expectations, strategic climates derive from leadership behaviors and social processes within organizations which cue employees to the underlying logics of action and the normative and expected behaviors in a work environment (Zohar & Hofmann, 2012). Although investigators have sought to differentiate the concept of strategic climate from organizational culture domains (e.g., Ostroff et al., 2003; Zohar & Hofmann, 2012), there is overlap between the two constructs (e.g., the role of expectations), and further research is needed to empirically establish their conceptual boundaries (West, Topakas, & Dawson, 2014).

Strategic climates focused on rewarding and supporting specific EBPs, such as the Triple P parenting program, are correlated with increased program use ($r = 0.26$) and program adherence ($\beta = 0.48$) even after controlling for agency resources and training needs (Asgary-Eden & Lee, 2012). Henderson et al. (2007) showed a strategic climate focused on quality treatment was associated with greater use of EBPs among juvenile justice drug treatment programs in both bivariate ($r = 0.36$) and multivariate models that controlled for organizational characteristics and administrator attitudes ($\beta = 0.31$). Aarons and Sommerfeld (2012) showed a strategic climate for innovation was associated with more positive clinician attitudes toward EBPs during a system-wide EBP implementation effort. Lundgren et al. (2012) showed a strategic climate for change was correlated with fewer perceived barriers to EBP adoption ($r = -0.16$). Finally, increased EBP implementation climate is related to increased use of cognitive behavioral therapy (CBT) among mental health clinicians treating youth ($r = 0.28$) although this relationship is moderated by molar climate such that implementation climate exerts its strongest effects when accompanied by a positive molar climate (Williams, Ehrhart et al., 2018).

Strategies for Changing or Sustaining Organizational Social Contexts for EBP Implementation

Three types of strategies are used to improve and sustain organizational social contexts to support EBP implementation. There is both theoretical and empirical support for the use of each type of strategy in changing social context, and each makes a unique contribution to understanding how the social contexts of organizations can be used to support the implementation of innovations such as EBPs. The three types of strategies focus on different facets of organizational social contexts: (a) organizational principles and priorities, (b) shared meaning and interpretation among coworkers, and (c) organizational infrastructure and processes.

   The first strategy for changing social context promotes guiding principles that determine organizational priorities (Osborne & Gaebler, 1992). This strategy is based on the idea that a variety of strategic goals and operational demands compete for emphasis in organizations and employees are influenced by their perceptions of the goals or demands that organizational leaders prioritize (Quinn & Rohrbaugh, 1983; Schneider & Bowen, 1995). Organizations that do similar work differ in the priorities they place on the competing goals and demands they face (e.g., quality of care versus quantity of billable units). Employees discern which competing priorities are favored in the organization and develop shared perceptions of the organization's norms and expectations (i.e., culture) and beliefs about what actions are most supported or punished (i.e., strategic climate). Shared perceptions regarding the organization's priorities are influenced by (a) the *content* of the enacted priorities (i.e., the specific goal or task demands that are given precedence); (b) the *alignment* between the organization's espoused and enacted priorities, that is, the degree to which an organization does what is says (Argyris & Schon, 1996; Pate-Cornell, 1990; Simons, 2002); and (c) the *internal consistency* of the organization's priorities, that is, the extent to which major organizational priorities complement rather than conflict with one another (Weick, 1979).

   Implementation strategies may target any of these priority issues or all three of them simultaneously as a mechanism for changing organizational culture and climate. The priorities placed on competing demands (that specify what is most important to the organization), the alignment of enacted and espoused priorities (ensuring the organization's actions reflect what it says is most important), and the consistencies in enacted priorities (the extent to which the organization's priorities complement rather than conflict with each other) affect an organization's social context and distinguish effective from ineffective organizations (Zohar & Hofmann, 2012).

   The second strategy alters the shared mental or cognitive models that coworkers use to interpret and provide meaning to their work experiences. Such models influence work behavior by explaining the behavior and predicting the responses from coworkers and superiors that are likely to result from the behavior. One of the best examples is *psychological safety* which describes the extent to which workers feel comfortable in identifying errors among peers and superiors, are quick to make suggestions for improvements in work, and attempt to master new skills and technologies without fear of reprisal and criticism. Edmundson and colleagues found that psychological safety explained why some surgical teams were more successful than others in implementing new cardiac surgery techniques (Edmondson, Bohner & Pisano, 2001). Those teams whose members experienced higher levels of psychological safety were more effective in implementation of the innovation.

   Another mental model that is shared by members of a work environment to interpret and give meaning to their work experience is their orientation toward intrinsic or extrinsic motivation (Ryan & Deci, 2000). Based on self-determination theory, coworkers in social contexts characterized by autonomy, competence, and relatedness promote intrinsic assumptions about the underlying motivation for work behavior that are different from extrinsic models. Intrinsic models assume workers find meaning and value in doing a job well independent of the extrinsic rewards (e.g., money, prestige) associated with the work. The model of motivation that is most used and shared among coworkers in interpreting and giving meaning to their work experience affects work behavior required for implementation. Based on self-determination theory, we argue that service providers in behavioral health and social service systems that share intrinsic models of work motivation are more likely to extend the additional effort to learn new skills and knowledge necessary for innovation. That is, social contexts characterized by autonomy, competence, and relatedness motivate individuals in a way that engenders the commitment, effort, and high-quality performance needed for successful EBP implementation (Ryan & Deci, 2000).

The third strategy for changing or sustaining organizational social contexts creates organizational structures and processes that support implementation in three ways. The first focuses on using leadership and network development to improve *collaboration* (Edmondson et al., 2001; Gustafson et al., 2003). The second uses teamwork and decentralized decision-making to improve *participation* (Baer & Frese, 2003; Denis, Hebert, Langley, Lozeau, & Trottier, 2002; Ensley & Pearce, 2001; Rentsch & Klimoski, 2001). The third uses goal setting and continuous improvement to facilitate *innovation* (Lemieux-Charles et al., 2002: Shortell, Bennett, & Byck, 1998). These three organizational processes (collaboration, participation, and innovation) are interrelated in the roles they play in creating and sustaining the types of organizational social contexts that are necessary for supporting EBP implementation.

Effects of EBP Implementation Strategies on Organizational Social Context and Implementation Outcomes: A Review of RCTs

This section reviews RCTs of implementation strategies in behavioral health and social service settings to address three questions. First, what is the evidence that EBP implementation strategies change organizational social context? If organizational culture, molar climate, and strategic climates cannot be changed, they cannot be activated as potential mechanisms for improving EBP implementation. Second, to what extent do context-focused implementation strategies influence implementation outcomes? This question indirectly addresses the efficacy of context-focused interventions by indicating whether strategies that attempt to change culture and climate have the expected effects on salient implementation outcomes. Third, what evidence is there that improvement in organizational social context mediates the effects of context-focused implementation strategies on implementation outcomes? This question directly addresses the causal influence of organizational social context on EBP implementation and informs its status as a potential mechanism for system change.

The review examines RCTs that tested strategies for implementing behavioral health EBPs in any setting. Studies were identified through electronic database searches of PubMed and PsycINFO and by examination of the reference lists of five earlier reviews of implementation strategies in mental health and social services (Barwick et al., 2012; Landsverk, Brown, Reutz, Palinkas, & Horwitz, 2011; Novins et al., 2013; Powell, Proctor, & Glass, 2014; Williams, 2015). Electronic searches focused on four constructs: (a) dissemination/implementation, (b) evidence-based practice, (c) mental health/substance use, and (d) randomized controlled trials. Given our objectives, we included RCTs in our review if they (a) tested an implementation strategy for an EBP that addressed mental health or substance use disorders; (b) attempted to influence implementation outcomes by targeting some facet of organizational social context including organizational culture, molar climate, or strategic climate; and (c) reported quantitative results from a randomized controlled trial (RCT). In order to include as many studies as possible, the definitional criteria were intentionally broad. This resulted in the inclusion of a few RCTs that targeted organizational social context even if this was not explicitly stated by the investigators.

The initial search resulted in a pool of 1357 unique articles. Screening of titles and abstracts resulted in the identification of 89 articles reporting 88 RCTs that tested an implementation strategy for a substance use or mental health EBP. Ten of these articles, reporting the results of nine separate RCTs, tested an organizational social context-focused implementation strategy and were included in the review. For each study, we describe the study setting and sample, implementation strategy, comparison or control conditions, facet of organizational social context targeted, measurement approach for organizational social context, effects of the strategy on organizational social context, effects of the strategy on implementation outcomes, and tests of mediation linking change in organizational social context to improvement in implementation outcomes. Table 6.1 presents a summary of the included studies.

Characterization of Trials

The RCTs in Table 6.1 reflect the diverse settings in which EBPs have been introduced into services for mental health and substance use disorders. Trials were conducted in juvenile justice settings, outpatient mental health clinics, substance abuse treatment facilities, elementary schools, and community medical practices. The EBPs targeted for implementation included motivational interviewing, collaborative care for bipolar disorder, multisystemic therapy, a range of clinician-selected EBPs, clinical guidelines for depression, and a protocol for evidence-based assessment, referral, and treatment planning. The variety of settings targeted and the range of EBPs implemented attest to the broad-based interest in organizational social context interventions and their relevance to a range of service systems.

Table 6.1 Randomized controlled trials of implementation strategies targeting organizational social context

Study	Setting and sample	EBP(s)	Implementation strategy (IS)	What dimension(s) of OSC was targeted?	What measure of OSC was used?	What effect did IS have on OSC?	What effect did IS have on implementation outcomes?	Results of mediation test (X-M; M-Y adjusted for X)
Rohrbach et al., (1993)	$n = 60$ elementary school teachers $n = 25$ principals	Adol. Alcohol prevention trial curriculum	2×2 design: 1. Training intensity (full day vs. 2 h) 2. Principal encouraged to support implementation (PS) vs. control	Strategic climate for implementation	Study-developed measures of principal encouragement based on (a) teacher report and (b) principal self-report	PS condition did not increase principal encouragement per teacher or self-report	PS condition increased teachers' quantity of implementation; training intensity did not affect implementation	Not tested
Atkins et al. (2008)	$n = 115$ teachers $k = 10$ elementary schools	Best practices for classroom mgmt. of ADHD	1. Trained key opinion leader (KOL) teachers + workshop + mental health professional (MHP) consults 2. Workshop + MHP consults	Organizational culture	Study-developed measure of KOL support	Not reported	KOL increased teachers' self-report adoption of 11 EBP strategies during the preceding month	The effect of the KOL intervention condition was no longer significant when measures of KOL support and MHP support were added to the model; only KOL support was sig.
Baer et al. (2009)	$n = 144$ substance abuse (SA) counselors $k = 6$ SA treatment facilities from NIDA's CTN	Motivational interviewing (MI)	1. Context-tailored training (CTT) 2. Standard 2-day workshop	Strategic climate for (a) autonomy and (b) change	ORC subscales (Lehman et al., 2002): (a) Autonomy (b) Change	Not reported	No effects of CTT on rater-coded MI fidelity indicators of "MI spirit" or reflection to question ratio	Not tested; however, baseline climate for change sig predicted MI fidelity on both indicators

(continued)

Table 6.1 (continued)

Study	Setting and sample	EBP(s)	Implementation strategy (IS)	What dimension(s) of OSC was targeted?	What measure of OSC was used?	What effect did IS have on OSC?	What effect did IS have on implementation outcomes?	Results of mediation test (X-M; M-Y adjusted for X)
Forsner et al. (2010)	$k = 6$ public adult outpatient psychiatric clinics in Sweden	Clinical practice guidelines for treatment of depression and suicidality	1. Tailored org learning IS + receipt of guidelines 2. Receipt of guidelines	Organizational learning culture	Not measured	NA	IS sig improved quality indicators for management of depression and suicide (based on chart review); no improvements observed in control clinics	NA
Glisson et al. (2010)	$k = 7$ MST treatment teams $k = 14$ rural counties	Multisystemic therapy (MST)	1. 36-months Availability, responsiveness, and continuity (ARC) organizational intervention + MST quality assurance (QA) protocol 2. MST QA protocol	Organizational culture and molar climate	Not measured	NA	ACR had no effect on MST therapist or supervisor fidelity ARC influenced therapists' distribution of MST effort	NA

			Strategic climate for learning and molar climate	Factor scores incorporating: Climate for learning, communication, cynicism toward change, supervisor leadership, emphasis on case mgmt. Activities	SN condition increased strategic and molar climate at 12-month follow-up relative to KS and mgmt. Directive No sig differences between KS and mgmt. Directive on social context	Not reported	NA
Taxman et al. (2014)	$n = 231$ case mgmt. Staff $k = 12$ juvenile justice offices	Juvenile assessment, referral, placement, and treatment planning protocol (JARPP)	3 post-training conditions: 1. Social network (SN) focused 2. Knowledge and skill-building (KS) focused 3. Mgmt. directive to use JARPP				
Waxmonsky et al. (2014)	$k = 5$ community-based medical practices	Life goals collaborative care model for treatment of bipolar disorder	1. Standard REP (training + technical assist.) 2. Enhanced REP (+ external and internal facilitation)	Organizational culture	Not measured	NA	Enhanced REP sig improved fidelity (number of sessions and contacts delivered) compared to standard REP
Aarons et al. (2015)	$n = 100$ MH clinicians $n = 12$ MH supervisors	Clinician-selected EBPs	1. 6-month Leadership and organizational change for implementation (LOCI) 2. Two-session general leadership webinar	Strategic climate for EBP implementation	Not measured	NA	LOCI increased EBP acceptability for supervisors as measured by clinician-rated leader EBP support and leader EBP readiness	NA

(continued)

Table 6.1 (continued)

Study	Setting and sample	EBP(s)	Implementation strategy (IS)	What dimension(s) of OSC was targeted?	What measure of OSC was used?	What effect did IS have on OSC?	What effect did IS have on implementation outcomes?	Results of mediation test (X-M; M-Y adjusted for X)
Glisson et al. (2016a)	$n = 475$ MH clinicians $k = 14$ child MH agencies	Clinician-selected EBPs	1. 36-month ARC org. Intervention 2. Control	Proficient culture	OSC proficiency subscale (Glisson et al., 2008)	ARC improved proficiency culture at 12-month follow-up (48 months Post-baseline)	ARC increased clinicians' attendance at voluntary EBP workshops offered in the community over a 3-year period	ARC's effects on EBP workshop attendance were mediated by improved proficiency culture
Williams et al. (2017)	$n = 475$ MH clinicians $k = 14$ child MH agencies	Clinician-selected EBPs	1. 36-month. ARC org. Intervention 2. Control	Proficient culture	OSC proficiency subscale (Glisson et al., 2008)	ARC improved proficiency culture mid-way through the intervention period (24 months. Post-baseline)	At 12-month follow-up, ARC increased clinicians' odds of adopting ≥1 name-brand EBPs and increased clinicians' use of EBPs with clients	ARC's effects on EBP adoption and use at 12-month follow-up were mediated by improved proficiency culture and increased clinician EBP intentions

All three facets of organizational social context (i.e., culture, molar climate, strategic climate) were targeted by at least one trial included in the review. The most frequently targeted facet was organizational culture (five trials) followed by strategic climate (four trials). Molar climate was only targeted by two trials, and in both cases it was paired with either a culture or strategic climate focus as well. The prominence of organizational culture and strategic climate, both of which represent expectation-focused facets of social context, is consistent with some writers' suggestion that these facets may be the most powerful for shaping individuals' EBP implementation behavior (Grol et al., 2007).

Consistent with these diverse foci, investigators used several different instruments to assess organizational social context including the Organizational Social Context (OSC) measure developed by Glisson and colleagues (Glisson, Green, & Williams, 2012; Glisson, Landsverk et al., 2008) and the Organizational Readiness for Change (ORC) measure developed by Lehman, Grenner, and Simpson (2002) among others. Some trials used study-specific measures with minimal information provided about the psychometric characteristics of the measure. Others relied on study-specific factor scores that incorporated information from several different measures that tapped various facets of organizational social context. The wide range of contextual facets targeted and the divergent measurement approaches reflect the need for further research to clarify the specific dimensions of organizational social context that are most relevant to EBP implementation. Four trials did not measure any facet of organizational social context although the implementation strategy clearly targeted a social contextual domain as a mechanism for improving EBP implementation. These studies reflect the emergence of organizational social context as a potential mechanism for influencing EBP implementation as well as the importance of examining unstudied dimensions of OSC.

The Empirical Status of Organizational Social Context as a Mechanism for EBP Implementation

Malleability of Organizational Social Context

This section describes the effects of implementation strategies on organizational social context for those RCTs included in our review. Other RCTs have shown organizational social context can be changed in mental health and social services (e.g., Glisson, Dukes, & Green, 2006; Glisson et al., 2012, 2016b); however, here we focus specifically on RCTs of efforts to implement EBPs. All nine strategies included in our review targeted organizational social context in their effort to implement EBPs; however, only five of the trials measured organizational social context, and only three reported the effects of the strategy on this criterion. Two studies reported positive effects on organizational social context, and one study reported the strategy did not influence organizational social context. Importantly, the one study reporting null results used a low-intensity implementation strategy that involved simply asking school principals to support implementation of a curriculum (Rohrbach, Graham & Hansen, 1993).

Two of the three trials reported positive effects of an implementation strategy on organizational social context. In the first trial (Glisson et al., 2016a; Williams, Glisson et al., 2017), a 3-year organizational intervention labeled ARC (for Availability, Responsiveness, and Continuity) improved organizational proficiency culture 2 years after baseline and maintained these gains at 1-year follow-up to the intervention (4 years post-baseline). These results replicate a preliminary RCT which showed the 36-month ARC intervention improved organizational culture and climate in mental health clinics (Glisson et al., 2012). In the second trial, Taxman, Henderson, Young, and Farrell (2014) showed a briefer and less intensive 12-month post-training strategy focused on developing and reinforcing social networks for EBP implementation improved strategic climate for learning and molar climate more than a strategy that exclusively targeted EBP knowledge and skills and a control condition consisting of management directive to use the EBP. This trial highlighted the importance of specifically targeting organizational social context for change because neither the management directive nor the knowledge and skill-building conditions improved social context. Together, these trials indicate organizational culture, strategic climate, and molar climate are malleable facets of organizational social context that can be influenced by EBP implementation strategies.

Effects of Context-Focused Implementation Strategies on Implementation Outcomes

Eight of the nine trials reported the effects of the implementation strategy on implementation outcomes. In six of these trials (75%), the strategy had a positive effect on implementation outcomes including EBP exploration (Glisson et al., 2016a), EBP acceptability (Aarons, Ehrhart, Farahnak, & Hurlburt, 2015), EBP adoption (Atkins et al., 2008; Rohrbach, Graham, & Hansen, 1993; Williams, Glisson et al., 2017), and EBP fidelity (Forsner et al., 2010; Waxmonsky et al., 2014). In two studies (25%), there were no observed effects of the context-focused strategy on EBP fidelity (Baer et al., 2009; Glisson et al., 2010). However, in one of these trials, the ARC organizational intervention did influence clinicians' distribution of effort in implementing the EBP and significantly improved both the short- and long-term clinical outcomes for youth who received the EBP (Glisson et al., 2010). The other trial (Baer et al., 2009) showed that although the context-tailored training strategy did not influence fidelity to motivational interviewing, a strategic organizational climate for change predicted increased fidelity several months later. Given that strategic climate for change was related to both fidelity measures but was not impacted by the strategy, these findings suggest the strategy may not have influenced implementation outcomes because it did not change organizational social context. Taken together, the evidence suggests implementation strategies that target and activate organizational social context positively influence EBP implementation outcomes.

Organizational Social Context as a Mediator of Strategies' Effects on Implementation Outcomes

Two trials tested organizational social context as a mediator of implementation strategies' effects on implementation outcomes; both trials supported this hypothesis. Atkins et al. (2008) showed support from key opinion leader teachers (but not mental health professionals) mediated the effect of an implementation strategy on teachers' adoption of evidence-based management techniques for students with attention deficit/hyperactivity disorder. The implementation strategy included workshop training, recruitment and training of teacher key opinion leaders (KOL), support and encouragement from KOLs to facilitate teachers' EBP adoption, and consultation from mental health professionals. This trial drew on Rogers' (2003) diffusion of innovations theory to argue that the use of natural opinion leaders in social influence processes (i.e., changing norms and expectations around use of the innovation) supports innovation adoption. We view this emphasis on creating norms and peer-level expectations that support the innovation as an effort to influence organizational culture defined as organizational norms and expectations. Results of the trial indicated the implementation strategy increased teachers' EBP use, and this effect was no longer statistically significant once a variable measuring KOL support was added to the model. Because the investigators did not directly test the effect of the strategy on KOL support, it is impossible to formally assess the mediated effect; however, the pattern of results suggests KOL support may have mediated the strategy's effects on teachers' EBP adoption.

The most robust evidence supporting the mediational role of organizational social context comes from a RCT with 14 mental health organizations of the effects of the ARC organizational intervention on clinicians' EBP exploration and adoption behavior (Glisson et al., 2016a; Williams, Glisson et al., 2017). The 3-year ARC organizational intervention is designed to create proficient organizational cultures that support the use of effective practices (e.g., EBPs) and an organization's capacity to eliminate barriers that hinder service effectiveness. ARC employs all three strategies described above to improve an organization's social context: (a) embed principles of service effectiveness to affect organizational priorities; (b) develop an organizational infrastructure to promote collaboration, participation, and innovation; and (c) generate shared mental models (e.g., psychological safety, intrinsic motivation) among staff and leadership that support innovation and service improvement efforts (Glisson et al., 2010).

Results from the trial indicated ARC increased clinicians' voluntary attendance at a series of community-based EBP workshops offered over a 3-year period (OR = 1.69), increased clinicians' odds of adopting one or more "name brand" EBPs at 12-month follow-up (OR = 3.19), and increased the percentage of clients treated using an EBP at 12-month follow-up (ARC = 81% vs. control = 56%). All three of these effects were shown to be formally mediated by improvement in proficiency culture. In a three-level growth model, Glisson et al. (2016a) showed the ARC clinicians' significant increase in the odds of attending an EBP workshop over the 3-year study period was mediated by improvement in proficiency culture measured at 12-month follow-up. In a serial multiple mediation analysis, Williams, Glisson et al. (2017) showed ARC's effects on EBP adoption and use at 48 months post-baseline were mediated by improvement in proficiency culture at 24 months post-baseline, which subsequently increased clinicians' intentions to adopt EBPs at 36 months post-baseline. This analysis demonstrated the time precedence of change in organizational social context (proficiency culture) relative to the implementation outcomes (EBP adoption, EBP use) and also identified a cross-level mediator of this effect (clinicians' EBP intentions). Results from this trial provide direct evidence that implementation strategies can increase clinicians' EBP exploration, adoption, and use by improving the organizational social contexts in which they work.

Future Directions for Implementation Science and Practice in Organizations

The trials reviewed in this chapter underscore the role of organizational social context in EBP implementation and how social context can be improved to influence EBP implementation. Research on EBP implementation has progressed from an exclusive focus on training, in which organizational social context was largely overlooked (Beidas & Kendall, 2010), to the development of theoretical models that acknowledge the importance of organizational social context (Mendel et al., 2008; Tabak, Khoong, Chambers, & Brownson, 2012), to the development of valid measures to assess organizational social context in behavioral health and social service settings (Ehrhart, Aarons, & Farahnak, 2014; Glisson, Landsverk et al., 2008), to testing whether organizational social context can be used as a causal mechanism for improving EBP implementation (Glisson et al., 2016a; Williams, Glisson et al., 2017). Although much work remains to be done, several facets of organizational social context have been linked to implementation outcomes, RCTs have demonstrated organizational social context can be changed, and implementation strategies that target organizational social context have demonstrated positive effects on EBP implementation through their influence on social context.

A growing number of intervention studies with a variety of organizations show that organizational social context can be changed and that interventions targeting organizational social context have the intended effects on clinician behavior and service outcomes (Glisson et al., 2012, 2013; Glisson et al., 2010; Glisson, Williams, Glisson et al., 2016a; Larson, Early, Cloonan, Sugrue, & Parides, 2000; Zohar & Polachek, 2014). These intervention studies support organizational culture and strategic climate theories which suggest changes in the prevailing norms and behavioral expectations that characterize a workplace influence individual behavior (Schein, 2004; Williams & Glisson, 2014b). They highlight the importance of addressing organizational social context to support EBP implementation as opposed to focusing exclusively on the technical (e.g., training) aspects of implementation.

Advancing Implementation Science

Our review highlights several directions for advancing implementation science in health services organizations. First, the range of constructs and measures used to characterize organizational social context in this review underscores the need for theoretical refinement and clearer operationalization of constructs in research designs, coupled with the careful selection of measurement instruments for assessing organizational social context.

Second, trials should focus on theory-backed hypothesis testing in which specific dimensions of organizational social context are linked to specific implementation strategies and outcomes. Consistent with other reviews of implementation strategies in mental health, our review points toward a need for implementation scientists to articulate how and why an implementation strategy is hypothesized to influence specific domains of organizational social context and what theoretical basis explains how and why organizational social context influences the targeted implementation outcomes (Williams, 2015).

Third, investigators should move beyond simply targeting and testing organizational social context as a mediator toward a comparative effectiveness paradigm in which alternative dimensions of social context are compared to identify which is most effective as a mediator for improving implementation and clinical outcomes in service organizations. For example, trials could test the differential efficacy of organizational proficiency culture and strategic EBP implementation climate for influencing a range of implementation and clinical outcomes (Ehrhart, Aarons, & Farahnak, 2014; Glisson, Landsverk et al., 2008). Proficiency culture and EBP implementation climate overlap in their emphasis on norms and expectations that support the use of effective treatment practices; however, they diverge in their emphasis on promoting clinicians' *aspirations* versus obtaining their *compliance*. Proficiency culture has a broader *aspirational* focus that emphasizes competence in state-of-the-art treatment practices as a means toward the ultimate end of improving client well-being. In contrast, strategic climate for EBP implementation is *compliance-focused* in that it captures work environment characteristics that support clinicians' adherence to particular protocols (i.e., EBP implementation). This difference in focus likely has implications for the type of clinician motivation that is activated (e.g., internally regulated vs. externally regulated), the breadth of implementation outcomes influenced, and the downstream effects on clinical outcomes. Examining the comparative effectiveness of these dimensions of social context is particularly important in light of growing concerns that community-based agencies that adopt EBPs vary in their ability to improve services beyond usual care because of other factors that also play a role in service outcomes (Kazdin, 2015; Weisz, Krumholz, Santucci, Thomassin, & Ng, 2015; Weisz, Ugueto, Cheron, & Herren, 2013).

Fourth, studies are needed to identify effective and efficient levers for creating, changing, and sustaining organizational social contexts that support innovation. Research on interventions to change organizational social context for improved behavioral health and social services is in its infancy. A great deal of work is needed not only to identify effective levers for improving services but also to address questions of cost-effectiveness. The strategies tested in this review ranged from very minimal (i.e., a single contact with an administrator) to very intense (i.e., a 3-year, multilevel internally and externally facilitated change process). Change in organizational social context occurred in as little as 12–24 months with strategies that varied in intensity. Data are lacking, however, on the effects of different strategies on implementation and clinical outcomes. Determining what intervention components represent the minimally necessary and sufficient conditions for leveraging social context to improve EBP implementation is a top priority for future research.

Fifth, studies are needed to identify the cross-level mechanisms that transmit social context's effects on individual clinicians' behavior and patient outcomes. There is evidence to suggest motivation is the primary carrier of organizational culture's effects on EBP implementation (Williams, Glisson et al., 2017); however, additional studies are needed. Identifying these cross-level links may be an important step in increasing the efficiency and effectiveness of implementation strategies in the future.

Sixth, there is a need for experimental studies that examine the effects of organizational social context interventions in countries outside of North America. Only one of the nine RCTs identified by this review occurred outside of the United States (Forsner et al., 2010). Within the larger organizational climate literature, investigators have conducted experimental intervention studies in countries outside the United States (e.g., Zohar & Polachek, 2014); however, to our knowledge this work has not been conducted in health services contexts. Studies are needed to explore how differences in national culture, social and political environments, infrastructure, and health policies shape and interact with organizational social context as well as the generalizability of organizational implementation strategies that target social context as a mechanism for change.

Advancing Implementation Practice

The findings of this review also have important implications for implementation practice in health services organizations. First, results from our review support the idea that organizational social context acts on practitioners' EBP implementation as either a supportive accelerant or a formidable detriment to their implementation success. The implication of this for those who lead health service organizations is that significant attention should be paid to the cultural norms and behavioral expectations that characterize the workplace to ensure that these align in a way that supports EBP implementation. Leaders should use psychometrically valid instruments to assess the organizational culture and climate of their agency from the perspective of frontline staff (Beidas et al., 2016) and should use this information to either (a) affirm the presence of a social context that supports EBP implementation or (b) identify the presence of a social context that is a likely detriment to successful EBP implementation. Findings from this review suggest two empirically supported measures predict effective EBP implementation and may be particularly useful to organizational leaders. These include the proficiency subscale of the Organizational Social Context measure developed by Glisson and colleagues (Glisson, Landsverk et al., 2008) and the EBP implementation climate measure developed by Ehrhart, Aarons, and Farahnak (2014). Organizational leaders can use these measures to assess their social contexts and take action to create supportive cultures and strategic climates based on the results.

Second, findings from this review affirm the idea that organizational social contexts are unlikely to change in ways that support EBP implementation without the implementation of strategies that specifically target social context for change. Two studies are especially supportive of this conclusion. First, in a study by Taxman et al. (2014), molar and strategic climate were only improved in the implementation condition that specifically focused on building social networks and norms to support EBP use. In the two comparison implementation conditions, which involved a leadership mandate to use EBP or a training intervention that provided technical assistance for EBP, organizational social context was not improved. Second, a study of tailored training for motivational interviewing showed that the implementation strategy did not influence strategic climate for MI implementation even though this facet of the agencies' social context was related to MI implementation success (Baer et al., 2009). This study provides further support for the idea that training alone is insufficient to create an organizational social context that supports EBP implementation. Furthermore, these studies' findings can be compared to those of a trial of the ARC organizational intervention in which an implementation strategy that specifically focused on improving organizational social context resulted in improved proficiency culture and increased EBP exploration and adoption behaviors (Glisson et al., 2016a; Williams, Glisson et al., 2017). Together, these studies suggest that merely providing training or a mandate to use EBPs is not enough to create the type of culture or strategic climate that is necessary for implementation success—specific implementation strategies are needed in order to change organizational social context.

Third, although there is still much to learn, it appears that certain types of organizational social contexts are most conducive to EBP implementation. These contexts are characterized by an emphasis on clinician competence in using up-to-date treatments, an expectation for improvement in client well-being, a learning orientation that strives to improve outcomes through the systematic evaluation of practice, and a strategic emphasis on supporting the implementation of EBPs. These foci paint a stark contrast to health service cultures and climates that emphasize the routinization of services, optimization of billable units, and minimization of costs. Consistent with the larger literature on organizational culture and climate (Hartnell et al., 2011; Kuenzi & Schminke, 2009), findings from this review indicate employees in health service organizations shift their behavior to match the expectations and norms of their workplaces. To the extent that these expectations focus on continual learning from local data, clinician competence, use of EBPs, and optimal clinical outcomes, clinicians' EBP implementation is enhanced; to the extent that other expectations are primary, clinicians adjust their behavior accordingly and EBP implementation is not as robust.

The conclusion that specific types of cultures and climates support EBP implementation whereas others hinder implementation leads to questions of resources. Organizations that deliver mental health services are under increasing financial pressure and strain related to diminishing resources for service delivery, increased demands for efficiency, and increased pressure to improve outcomes by implementing EBPs. While these issues are beyond the scope of the present review, we wish to acknowledge these challenges and argue that more information is needed about how organizations address competing priorities in service delivery (Glisson et al., 2016b).

Fourth, contrary to the predictions of some theoretical models (Ehrhart, Aarons, & Farahnak, 2014; Weiner, Belden, Bergmire, & Johnston, 2011), the studies reviewed in this chapter indicate a strategic climate for EBP implementation is neither the only type of organizational social context that supports EBP implementation nor necessarily the optimal type of social context for supporting EBP implementation. To date, the evidence for EBP implementation climate includes only correlational studies which offer mixed results (Beidas et al., 2015) and show that its effects are contingent upon the presence of a positive molar climate that supports clinicians' well-being (Williams, Ehrhart et al., 2018). In comparison, proficient organizational culture, which focuses on clinician competence and improvement in client well-being, as opposed to addressing EBP implementation directly, has been strongly correlated with numerous EBP implementation outcomes (Aarons et al., 2012; Glisson, Schoenwald et al., 2008; Olin et al., 2014; Williams & Glisson, 2014a) and has been shown in RCTs to explain the effects of an organizational implementation strategy on clinicians' EBP exploration, adoption, and implementation behavior (Glisson et al., 2016a; Williams, Glisson et al., 2017). Clearly, there is much more to learn as EBP implementation climate has not been directly tested as a mediator of an implementation strategy. However, these preliminary results have important implications for implementation practice. It appears that program directors need not focus exclusively, or even primarily, on developing a strategic climate for EBP implementation in order to improve implementation outcomes. Instead, increased EBP implementation can result from a proficient culture with an emphasis on clinician competence and improvement in client well-being. Assuming that improved client outcomes are the impetus behind increased EBP implementation and that organizations can accrue additional benefits beyond improved EBP implementation from a proficient culture (e.g., decreased turnover, improved clinical outcomes), organizational leaders may be able to optimize a multitude of outcomes (e.g., fiscal, services, implementation, clinical) by targeting proficiency culture for improvement rather than narrowly targeting EBP implementation climate.

Conclusion

Our review of EBP implementation strategies that focus on organizational social context supports the idea that implementation success depends in part on social context and provides implementation scientists and practitioners with guidelines for improving EBP implementation. However, gaps in our knowledge include the need for a better understanding of the mechanisms that link specific organizational strategies to EBP implementation at the individual level through contextual mediators. Addressing this knowledge gap requires studies that identify the cross-level effects of various implementation strategies to explain how each improves specific dimensions of social context to increase an individual's commitment to acquiring and using EBP knowledge and skills. Studies show that EBP exploration, adoption, and use can be increased by creating proficient organizational cultures and other contextual characteristics, but more work is needed to specify mediation models that link implementation strategies, dimensions of social context, and outcomes. Information from these mediation models will contribute to efficient and transportable implementation strategies that generate supportive organizational cultures and climates to improve clinicians' use of EBPs.

References

Aarons, G. A., Ehrhart, M. G., Farahnak, L. R., & Hurlburt, M. S. (2015). Leadership and organizational change for implementation (LOCI): A randomized mixed method pilot study of a leadership and organization development intervention for evidence-based practice implementation. *Implementation Science, 10*(11), 1–12.

Aarons, G. A., Glisson, C., Green, P. D., Hoagwood, K., Kelleher, K. J., Landsverk, J. A., & The Research Network on Youth Mental Health. (2012). The organizational social context of mental health services and clinician attitudes toward evidence-based practice: A United States national study. *Implementation Science, 7*(56), 1–15.

Aarons, G. A., Hurlburt, M., & Horwitz, S. M. (2011). Advancing a conceptual model of evidence-based practice implementation in public service sectors. *Administration and Policy in Mental Health, 38*, 4–23.

Aarons, G. A., & Sawitzky, A. C. (2006). Organizational culture and climate and mental health provider attitudes toward evidence-based practice. *Psychological Services, 3*, 61–72.

Aarons, G. A., & Sommerfeld, D. H. (2012). Leadership, innovation climate, and attitudes toward evidence-based practice during a statewide implementation. *Journal of the American Academy of Child and Adolescent Psychiatry, 51*, 423–431.

Argyris, C., & Schon, D. A. (1996). *Organizational learning: Theory, method and practice* (2nd ed.). Reading, MA: Addison-Wesley.

Asgary-Eden, V., & Lee, C. M. (2012). Implementing an evidence-based parenting program in community agencies: What helps and what gets in the way? *Administration and Policy in Mental Health, 39*, 478–488.

Atkins, M. S., Frazier, S. L., Leathers, S. J., Graczyk, P. A., Talbott, E., Jakobsons, L., … Bell, C. C. (2008). Teacher key opinion leaders and mental health consultation in low-income urban schools. *Journal of Consulting and Clinical Psychology, 76*, 905–908.

Baer, J. S., Wells, E. A., Rosengren, D. B., Hartzler, B., Beadnell, B., & Dunn, C. (2009). Agency context and tailored training in technology transfer: A pilot evaluation of motivational interviewing training for community counselors. *Journal of Substance Abuse Treatment, 37*, 191–202.

Baer, M., & Frese, M. (2003). Innovation is not enough: Climates for initiatives and psychological safety, process innovations and firm performance. *Journal of Organizational Behavior, 24*, 45–68.

Barwick, M. A., Schachter, H. M., Bennett, L. M., McGowan, J., Ly, M., Wilson, A., ... Manion, I. (2012). Knowledge translation efforts in child and youth mental health: A systematic review. *Journal of Evidence-Based Social Work, 9*, 369–395.

Beidas, R. S., & Kendall, P. C. (2010). Training therapists in evidence-based practice: A critical review of studies from a systems-contextual perspective. *Clinical Psychology: Science & Practice, 17*, 1–30.

Beidas, R. S., Marcus, S., Aarons, G. A., Hoagwood, K. E., Schoenwald, S., Evans, A. C., ... Mandell, D. S. (2015). Predictors of community therapists' use of therapy techniques in a large public mental health system. *JAMA Pediatrics, 169*, 374–382.

Beidas, R. S., Williams, N. J., Green, P. D., Aarons, G. A., Becker-Haimes, E., Evans, A. C., ... Marcus, S. C. (2016). Concordance between administrator and clinician ratings of organizational culture and climate. *Administration and Policy in Mental Health and Mental Health Services Research.* https://doi.org/10.1007/s10488-016-0776-8

Brimhall, K. C., Fenwick, K., Farahnak, L. R., Hurlburt, M. S., Roesch, S. C., & Aarons, G. A. (2016). Leadership, organizational climate, and perceived burden of evidence-based practice in mental health services. *Administration and Policy in Mental Health and Mental Health Services Research, 43*(5), 629–639.

Cameron, K. S., & Quinn, R. E. (2011). *Diagnosing and changing organizational culture: Based on the competing values framework* (3rd ed.). Hoboken, NJ: Jossey-Bass.

Cooke, R. A., & Rousseau, D. M. (1988). Behavioral norms and expectations: A quantitative approach to the assessment of organizational culture. *Group & Organization Studies, 13*, 245–273.

Damschroder, L. J., Aron, D. C., Keith, R. E., Kirsh, S. R., Alexander, J. A., & Lowery, J. C. (2009). Fostering implementation of health services research findings into practice: A consolidated framework for advancing implementation science. *Implementation Science, 4*(50), 1–15.

Denis, J. L., Hebert, Y., Langley, A., Lozeau, D., & Trottier, L. H. (2002). Explaining diffusion patterns for complex health care innovations. *Health Care Management Review, 27*, 60–73.

Edmondson, A. C., Bohmer, R. M., & Pisano, G. P. (2001). Disrupted routines: Team leaning and new technology implementation in hospitals. *Administrative Science Quarterly, 46*(4), 685–716.

Ehrhart, M. G., Aarons, G. A., & Farahnak, L. R. (2014). Assessing the organizational context for EBP implementation: The development and validity testing of the implementation climate scale (ICS). *Implementation Science, 9*, 157.

Ehrhart, M. G., Schneider, B., & Macey, W. H. (2014). *Organizational climate and culture: An introduction to theory, research, and practice.* New York: Routledge.

Ensley, M. D., & Pearce, C. L. (2001). Shared cognition in top management teams: Implications for new venture performance. *Journal of Organizational Behavior, 22*, 145–160.

Forsner, T., Wistedt, A. A., Brommels, M., Janszky, I., de Leon, A. P., & Forsell, Y. (2010). Supported local implementation of clinical guidelines in psychiatry: A two-year follow-up. *Implementation Science, 5*(4), 1–11.

Friedmann, P. D., Taxman, F. S., & Henderson, C. E. (2007). Evidence-based treatment practices for drug-involved adults in the criminal justice system. *Journal of Substance Abuse Treatment, 32*, 267–277.

Glisson, C., Dukes, D., & Green, P. (2006). The effects of the ARC organizational intervention on caseworker turnover, climate, and culture in children's service systems. *Child Abuse and Neglect, 30*, 855–880.

Glisson, C., & Green, P. (2006). The effects of organizational culture and climate on the access to mental health care in child welfare and juvenile justice systems. *Administration and Policy in Mental Health and Mental Health Services Research, 33*, 433–448.

Glisson, C., & Green, P. (2011). Organizational climate, services, and outcomes in child welfare systems. *Child Abuse and Neglect, 35*, 582–591.

Glisson, C., Green, P., & Williams, N. J. (2012). Assessing the organizational social context (OSC) of child welfare systems: Implications for research and practice. *Child Abuse and Neglect, 36*, 621–632.

Glisson, C., & Hemmelgarn, A. (1998). The effects of organizational climate and interorganizational coordination on the quality and outcomes of children's service systems. *Child Abuse & Neglect, 22*, 401–421.

Glisson, C., Hemmelgarn, A., Green, P., Dukes, D., Atkinson, S., & Williams, N. J. (2012). Randomized trial of the availability, responsiveness, and continuity (ARC) organizational intervention with community-based mental health programs and clinicians serving youth. *Journal of the American Academy of Child and Adolescent Psychiatry, 51*, 780–787.

Glisson, C., Hemmelgarn, A., Green, P., & Williams, N. J. (2013). Randomized trial of the availability, responsiveness and continuity (ARC) organizational intervention for improving youth outcomes in community mental health programs. *Journal of the American Academy of Child and Adolescent Psychiatry, 52*, 493–500.

Glisson, C., & James, L. R. (2002). The cross-level effects of culture and climate in human service teams. *Journal of Organizational Behavior, 23*, 767–794.

Glisson, C., Landsverk, J., Schoenwald, S., Kelleher, K., Hoagwood, K. E., Mayberg, S., ... The Research Network on Youth Mental Health. (2008). Assessing the organizational social context (OSC) of mental health services: Implications for research and practice. *Administration and Policy in Mental Health, 35*, 98–113.

Glisson, C., Schoenwald, S. K., Hemmelgarn, A., Green, P., Dukes, D., Armstrong, K. S., & Chapman, J. E. (2010). Randomized trial of MST and ARC in a two-level evidence-based treatment implementation strategy. *Journal of Consulting and Clinical Psychology, 78*, 537–550.

Glisson, C., Schoenwald, S. K., Kelleher, K., Landsverk, J., Hoagwood, K. E., Mayberg, S., ... The Research Network on Youth Mental Health. (2008). Therapist turnover and new program sustainability in mental health clinics as a function of organizational culture, climate, and service structure. *Administration and Policy in Mental Health, 35*, 124–133.

Glisson, C., Williams, N. J., Hemmelgarn, A., Proctor, E., & Green, P. (2016a). Increasing clinicians' EBT exploration and preparation behavior in youth mental health services by changing organizational culture with ARC. *Behaviour Research and Therapy, 76*, 40–46.

Glisson, C., Williams, N. J., Hemmelgarn, A., Proctor, E., & Green, P. (2016b). Aligning organizational priorities with ARC to improve youth mental health service outcomes. *Journal of Consulting and Clinical Psychology, 84*(8), 713–725.

Grol, R., Bosch, M. C., Hulscher, M., Eccles, M. P., & Wensing, M. (2007). Planning and studying improvement in patient care: The use of theoretical perspectives. *Milbank Quarterly, 85*, 93–138.

Gustafson, D. H., Sainfort, F., Eichler, M., Adams, L., Bisognano, M., & Steudel, H. (2003). Developing and testing a model to predict outcomes of organizational change. *Health Services Research, 38*, 751–776.

Hartnell, C. A., Ou, A. Y., & Kinicki, A. (2011). Organizational culture and organizational effectiveness: A meta-analytic investigation of the competing values framework's theoretical suppositions. *Journal of Applied Psychology, 96*, 677–694.

Helfrich, C. D., Damschroder, L. J., Hagedorn, H. J., Daggett, G. S., Sahay, A., Ritchie, M., ... Stetler, C. B. (2010). A critical synthesis of literature on the promoting action on research implementation in health services (PARIHS) framework. *Implementation Science, 5*(82), 1–20.

Henderson, C. E., Young, D. W., Jainchill, N., Hawke, J., Farkas, S., & Davis, M. (2007). Program use of effective drug abuse treatment practices for juvenile offenders. *Journal of Substance Abuse Treatment, 32*, 279–390.

Hofstede, G., Neuijen, B., Ohayv, D. D., & Sanders, G. (1990). Measuring organizational cultures: A qualitative and quantitative study across twenty cases. *Administrative Science Quarterly, 35*, 286–316.

James, L. R., Choi, C. C., Ko, C. E., McNeil, P. K., Minton, M. K., Wright, M. A., & Kim, K. (2008). Organizational and psychological climate: A review of theory and research. *European Journal of Work and Organizational Psychology, 17*, 5–32.

Kazdin, A. E. (2015). Treatment as usual and routine care in research and clinical practice. *Clinical Psychology Review, 42*, 168–178.

Kitson, A. L., Rycroft-Malone, J., Harvey, G., McCormack, B., Seers, K., & Titchen, A. (2008). Evaluating the successful implementation of evidence into practice using the PARiHS framework: Theoretical and practical challenges. *Implementation Science, 3*(1), 1–12.

Kuenzi, M., & Schminke, M. (2009). Assembling the fragments into a lens: A review, critique, and proposed research agenda for the organizational work climate literature. *Journal of Management, 35*, 634–717.

Landsverk, J., Brown, C. H., Reutz, J. R., Palinkas, L., & Horwitz, S. M. (2011). Design elements in implementation research: A structured review of child welfare and mental health studies. *Administration and Policy in Mental Health, 38*, 54–63.

Larson, E. L., Early, E., Cloonan, P., Sugrue, S., & Parides, M. (2000). An organizational climate intervention associated with increased handwashing and decreased nosocomial infections. *Behavioral Medicine, 26*, 14–22.

Lehman, W. E. K., Grenner, J. M., & Simpson, D. D. (2002). Assessing organizational readiness for change. *Journal of Substance Abuse Treatment, 22*, 197–209.

Lemieux-Charles, L., Murray, M., Baker, G. R., Barnsley, J., Tasa, K., & Ibrahim, S. A. (2002). The effects of quality improvement practices on team effectiveness: A meditational model. *Journal of Organizational Behavior, 23*, 533–553.

Lundgren, L., Chassler, D., Amodeo, M., D'Ippolito, M., & Sullivan, L. (2012). Barriers to implementation of evidence-based addiction treatment: A national study. *Journal of Substance Abuse Treatment, 42*, 231–238.

Marty, D., Rapp, C., McHugo, G., & Whitley, R. (2008). Factors influencing consumer outcome monitoring in implementation of evidence-based practices: Results from the national EBP implementation project. *Administration and Policy in Mental Health, 35*, 204–211.

McHugo, G. J., Drake, R. E., Whitley, R., Bond, G. R., Campbell, K., Rapp, C. A., … Finnerty, M. T. (2007). Fidelity outcomes in the National Implementing Evidence-Based Practices project. *Psychiatric Services, 58*, 1279–1284.

Mendel, P., Meredith, L. S., Schoenbaum, M., Sherbourne, C. D., & Wells, K. B. (2008). Interventions in organizational and community context: A framework for building evidence on dissemination and implementation in health services research. *Administration and Policy in Mental Health, 35*, 21–37.

Novins, D. K., Green, A. E., Legha, R. K., & Aarons, G. A. (2013). Dissemination and implementation of evidence-based practices for child and adolescent mental health: A systematic review. *Journal of the American Academy of Child and Adolescent Psychiatry, 52*, 1009–1025.

Olin, S. S., Williams, N. J., Pollock, M., Armusewicz, K., Kutash, K., Glisson, C., & Hoagwood, K. E. (2014). Quality indicators for family support services and their relationship to organizational social context. *Administration and Policy in Mental Health and Mental Health Services Research, 41*, 43–54.

Osborne, D., & Gaebler, T. A. (1992). *Reinventing government*. Reading, MA: Addison-Wesley.

Ostroff, C., Kinicki, A. J., & Tamkins, M. M. (2003). Organizational culture and climate. In W. C. Borman, D. R. Ilgen, R. J. Klimoski, & I. Weiner (Eds.), *Handbook of psychology* (Vol. 12, pp. 565–593). Hoboken, NJ: Wiley.

Parmelli, E., Flodgren, G., Beyer, F., Baillie, N., Schaafsma, M. E., & Eccles, M. P. (2011). The effectiveness of strategies to change organizational culture to improve healthcare performance: A systematic review. *Implementation Science, 6*(33), 1–8.

Pate-Cornell, M. E. (1990). Organizational aspects of engineering system safety: The case of offshore platforms. *Science, 250*, 1210–1217.

Powell, B. J., Proctor, E. K., & Glass, J. E. (2014). A systematic review of strategies for implementing empirically supported mental health interventions. *Research on Social Work Practice, 24*, 192–212.

Proctor, E., Silmere, H., Raghavan, R., Hovmand, P., Aarons, G., Bunger, A., … Hensley, M. (2011). Outcomes for implementation research: Conceptual distinctions, measurement challenges, and research agenda. *Administration and Policy in Mental Health, 38*, 65–76.

Quinn, R. E., & Rohrbaugh, J. (1983). A spatial model of effectiveness criteria: Towards a competing values approach to organizational analysis. *Management Science, 29*, 363–377.

Rentsch, J. R., & Klimoski, R. J. (2001). Why do "great minds" think alike? Antecedents of team member schema agreement. *Journal of Organizational Behavior, 22*, 107–120.

Rogers, E. M. (2003). *Diffusion of innovations* (5th ed.). New York: Free Press.

Rohrbach, L. A., Graham, J. W., & Hansen, W. B. (1993). Diffusion of a school-based substance abuse prevention program: Predictors of program implementation. *Preventive Medicine, 22*, 237–260.

Ryan, R. M., & Deci, E. L. (2000). Self-determination theory and the facilitation of intrinsic motivation, social development, and Well-being. *American Psychologist, 55*, 68–78.

Schein, E. H. (2004). *Organizational culture and leadership*. San Francisco: Jossey-Bass.

Schneider, B., & Bowen, D. (1995). *Winning the service game*. Boston: Harvard Business School Press.

Schneider, B., Ehrhart, M. G., & Macey, W. H. (2013). Organizational climate and culture. *Annual Review of Psychology, 64*, 361–388.

Schoenwald, S. K., Carter, R. E., Chapman, J. E., & Sheidow, A. J. (2008). Therapist adherence and organizational effects on change in youth behavior one year after multisystemic therapy. *Administration and Policy in Mental Health, 35*, 379–394.

Scott, T., Mannion, R., Marshall, M., & Davies, H. (2003). Does organizational culture influence health care performance? A review of the evidence. *Journal of Health Services Research and Policy, 8*, 105–117.

Shortell, S. M., Bennett, C. L., & Byck, G. R. (1998). Assessing the impact of continuous quality improvement on clinical practice: What it will take to accelerate progress. *Milbank Quarterly, 76*, 593–624.

Simons, T. (2002). Behavioral integrity: The perceived alignment between managers' words and deeds as a research focus. *Organization Science, 13*, 18–35.

Tabak, R. G., Khoong, E. C., Chambers, D. A., & Brownson, R. C. (2012). Bridging research and practice: Models for dissemination and implementation research. *American Journal of Preventive Medicine, 43*, 337–350.

Taxman, F. S., Henderson, C., Young, D., & Farrell, J. (2014). The impact of training interventions on organizational readiness to support innovations in juvenile justice offices. *Administration and Policy in Mental Health, 41*, 177–188.

Verbeke, W., Volgering, M., & Hessels, M. (1998). Exploring the conceptual expansion within the field of organizational behavior: Organizational climate and organizational culture. *Journal of Management Studies, 35*, 303–329.

Wang, W., Saldana, L., Brown, C. H., & Chamberlain, P. (2010). Factors that influenced county system leaders to implement an evidence-based program: A baseline survey within a randomized controlled trial. *Implementation Science, 5*(72), 1–8.

Waxmonsky, J., Kilbourne, A. M., Goodrich, D. E., Nord, K. M., Lai, Z., Laird, C., ... Bauer, M. S. (2014). Enhanced fidelity to treatment for bipolar disorder: Results from a randomized controlled implementation trial. *Psychiatric Services, 65*, 81–90.

Weick, K. E. (1979). *The social psychology of organizing*. Reading, MA: Addison-Wesley.

Weiner, B. J., Belden, C. M., Bergmire, D. M., & Johnston, M. (2011). The meaning and measurement of implementation climate. *Implementation Science, 6*(78). https://doi.org/10.1186/1748-5908-6-78

Weisz, J. R., Krumholz, L. S., Santucci, L., Thomassin, K., & Ng, M. Y. (2015). Shrinking the gap between research and practice: Tailoring and testing youth psychotherapies in clinical care contexts. *Annual Review of Clinical Psychology, 11*, 139–163.

Weisz, J. R., Ugueto, A. M., Cheron, D. M., & Herren, J. (2013). Evidence-based youth psychotherapy in the mental health ecosystem. *Journal of Clinical Child & Adolescent Psychology, 42*(2), 274–286.

West, M. A., Topakas, A., & Dawson, J. F. (2014). Climate and culture for health care performance. In B. Schneider & K. M. Barbera (Eds.), *The Oxford handbook of organizational climate and culture* (pp. 335–359). New York: Oxford University Press.

Williams, N. J. (2015). Multilevel mechanisms of implementation strategies in mental health: Integrating theory, research, and practice. *Administration and Policy in Mental Health, 43,* 783–798.

Williams, N. J., & Glisson, C. (2013). Reducing turnover is not enough: The need for proficient organizational cultures to support positive youth outcomes in child welfare. *Children and Youth Services Review, 35,* 1871–1877.

Williams, N. J., & Glisson, C. (2014a). Testing a theory of organizational culture, climate, and youth outcomes in child welfare systems: A United States national study. *Child Abuse & Neglect, 38,* 757–767.

Williams, N. J., & Glisson, C. (2014b). The role of organizational culture and climate in the dissemination and implementation of empirically-supported treatments for youth. In R. S. Beidas & P. C. Kendall (Eds.), *Dissemination and implementation of evidence based practices in child and adolescent mental health* (pp. 61–81). New York: Oxford University Press.

Williams, N. J., Glisson, C., Hemmelgarn, A., & Green, P. (2017). Mechanisms of change in the ARC organizational strategy: Increasing mental health clinicians' EBP adoption through improved organizational culture and capacity. *Administration and Policy in Mental Health and Mental Health Services Research, 44,* 269–283. https://doi.org/10.1007/s10488-016-0742-5

Williams, N. J., Ehrhart, M. G., Aarons, G. A., Marcus, S. C., & Beidas, R. S. (2018). Linking molar organizational climate and strategic implementation climate to clinicians' use of evidence-based psychotherapy techniques: cross-sectional and lagged analyses from a 2-year observational study. *Implementation Science, 13*(85). https://doi.org/10.1186/s13012-018-0781-2.

Zazzali, J. L., Sherbourne, C., Hoagwood, K. E., Greene, D., Bigley, M. F., & Sexton, T. L. (2008). The adoption and implementation of an evidence based practice in child and family mental health services organizations: A pilot study of functional family therapy in New York state. *Administration and Policy in Mental Health, 35,* 38–49.

Zohar, D., & Hofmann, D. A. (2012). Organizational culture and climate. In S. W. J. Kozlowki (Ed.), *The Oxford handbook of organizational psychology* (Vol. 1, pp. 643–666). New York: Oxford University Press.

Zohar, D., & Polachek, T. (2014). Discourse-based intervention for modifying supervisory communication as leverage for safety climate and performance improvement: A randomized field study. *Journal of Applied Psychology, 99,* 113–124.

Chapter 7
Implementation of Effective Services in Community Settings

Luke Wolfenden, Melanie Kingsland, Rachel L. Sutherland, Meghan Finch, Nicole K. Nathan, Christopher M. Williams, John H. Wiggers, and Serene Yoong

Introduction

Chronic diseases are a leading cause of death and disability worldwide. They present a major public policy challenge, threatening the health of individuals and communities and future economic prosperity (McNamara et al., 2015; WHO, 2016). Many chronic diseases are, however, preventable (WHO). The primary modifiable risk factors for chronic diseases such as cancer and cardiovascular disease include tobacco smoking, risky alcohol use, physical inactivity, dietary behaviours and obesity (AIHW, 2012). One approach recommended by the World Health Organization to address the primary modifiable risk factors for chronic disease is through the implementation of evidence based-interventions in community settings. A community setting is a social and culturally defined area of social interaction, where people learn, work or play such as a school, recreation centre or workplace. (Keleher & MacDougall, 2006) Community settings often offer access to large numbers of individuals in the population, often for prolonged periods.

While there are cost-effective interventions in community settings, which address chronic disease risk factors, (Youl, Baade, & Meng, 2012) the implementation of such evidence-based interventions is often poor. For example, childcare services frequently fail to provide food to children that is in line with sector nutrition guidelines, (Yoong, Skelton, Jones, & Wolfenden, 2014) and sporting venues serve alcohol to patrons in a manner that is inconsistent with liquor licensing legislation (Lenk et al., 2010). Impediments to implementation are, however, complex and dynamic. They can include social, cultural, political, organisational, financial and individual

L. Wolfenden (✉) · M. Kingsland · R. L. Sutherland · N. K. Nathan ·
C. M. Williams · J. H. Wiggers · S. Yoong
The University of Newcastle, Callaghan, NSW, Australia
e-mail: luke.wolfenden@health.nsw.gov.au

M. Finch
Centre for Evidence and Implementation, Pyrmont, NSW, Australia

© Springer Nature Switzerland AG 2020
B. Albers et al. (eds.), *Implementation Science 3.0*,
https://doi.org/10.1007/978-3-030-03874-8_7

factors. Implementation science provides a means of understanding these barriers, and can help to identify strategies that can best be employed to overcome them to improve implementation, and in doing so, the health and well-being of the community.

In this chapter, we will discuss the role of implementation science in reducing the burden of chronic disease through interventions delivered in community settings. Specifically, we will describe the following:

(a) The current evidence-base regarding the effectiveness of strategies to improve implementation of chronic disease risk reduction policies, programmes or practices in community settings
(b) The role of formative evaluation and theoretical frameworks in the development of implementation strategies
(c) Three case studies of strategies undertaken in Australia, which aim to improve implementation of evidence-based policies or programmes addressing chronic disease risks in community settings

The Current Evidence-Base Regarding the Effectiveness of Strategies to Improve Implementation of Chronic Disease Risk Reduction Policies, Programmes or Practices in Community Settings

Just as chronic disease prevention interventions should be evidence-based, so too should strategies to improve their implementation. However, to date, there has been limited investment in implementation research, and so little evidence is available for policy-makers and practitioners to guide efforts to implement chronic disease prevention programmes in community settings. For example, implementation and dissemination research represents just 2.5% of all health and medical systematic reviews (Yoong, Clinton-McHarg, & Wolfenden, 2015) and implementation trials comprise just 2% of public health research output (Wolfenden, Milat, et al., 2016).

Systematic reviews across a range of community settings (Williams et al., 2015; Wolfenden et al., 2015) suggest that the effectiveness of strategies to improve implementation of chronic disease prevention programmes is variable and overall improvements in implementation appear modest (Rabin, Glasgow, Kerner, Klump, & Brownson, 2010). A systematic review of strategies by the Agency for Health Research and Quality to support implementation of cancer prevention programmes in community settings identified just 25 trials of any study design. The review concluded that evidence of effectiveness was equivocal, and that the methodological quality of included studies was poor (Rabin et al., 2010). Such findings are corroborated by more recent Cochrane reviews in schools, and childcare services that found a small number of trials of considerable heterogeneity and overall very low quality of evidence (Wolfenden et al., 2015; Wolfenden et al., 2017). Nonetheless, in all reviews, the included studies trialled varying multi-strategic approaches involving combinations of educational outreach, audit and feedback, educational meetings, reminders, printed educational materials and local opinion leaders. The effects of such strategies, either on their own or in combination, have been shown to produce modest yet highly variable improvements to professional practice in primary care(Lau et al., 2015), where a more substantial evidence base exists (See Fig. 7.1). While it is not possible to isolate the effects of individual strategies from reviews of implementation strategies in community settings, the multi-strategic approaches that have been examined typically improved the proportion of childcare services, schools, or staff that implement a targeted policy or programme by 9% in childcare services (Wolfenden et al., 2015) and 19% in schools (Wolfenden et al., 2017).

Previous reviews of implementation strategies for chronic disease prevention initiatives in community settings, and similar reviews in other settings, have consistently found considerable variability in effects of implementation strategies (Wolfenden et al., 2015; Wolfenden et al., 2017). These reviews also show that multifaceted strategies are not necessarily more effective than single faceted implementation strategies (Lau et al., 2015). Such findings might suggest that there is no single reliably effective implementation strategy or approach. Rather, the success of

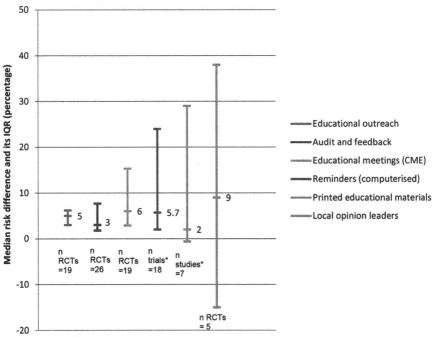

Fig. 7.1 Reviews describing improvements to professional practice in primary care for implementation strategies. Reprinted from Lau et al. (2015), licensed under the terms of the Creative Commons Attribution 4.0 International License (https://creativecommons.org/licenses/by/4.0/)

implementation strategies is highly dependent on the context in which they are delivered and the degree to which they address barriers present within their local context. Enhancing the effects of implementation initiatives in community settings, therefore, requires careful selection of strategies that address the primary barriers to implementation in a way that is suitable to the context in which implementation is occurring.

The Role of Formative Evaluation and Theoretical Frameworks in the Development of Implementation Strategies

Formative Evaluation

A comprehensive understanding of the setting, context and barriers to implementation of a targeted policy or practice will provide a strong grounding for the development of an effective implementation strategy. There are a variety of methods in which this can be achieved. A particularly important source of information is obtained through ongoing engagement with organisations and staff required to implement chronic disease prevention programmes (such as school principals, staff and managers) and observations of their operational environment (Seward et al., 2016). Such processes enable an understanding of the environment in which implementation is required to take place, the available time, resource and infrastructure to support it and other competing demands, priorities and processes that may hinder initiatives that facilitate required practice change. Engagement and observation also enable an appraisal of the suitability of the implementation strategies to the setting, opportunities to integrate support and the feasibility of specific strategies.

A number of formal research methods can improve understanding of the setting, context and implementation barriers. Qualitative research such as interviews or focus groups provide rich contextual information. It is particularly useful to gain an understanding of the perceived importance of implementation issues, and provide an opportunity for researchers to explore in more detail factors that may be pertinent to the likely success or failure of implementation approaches (Peters, Adam, Alonge, Agyepong, & Tran, 2013). Quantitative studies such as the administration of surveys and questionnaires can quantify contextual factors and barriers that may impact on implementation efforts within a setting or organisation. (Peters et al., 2013) A variety of validated tools exist to measure a host of such factors including organisational climate, organisational readiness to change, as well as the confidence and self-efficacy of organisation staff to implement the targeted policy or practice (Clinton-McHarg et al., 2016; Lewis et al., 2015). Quantitative studies provide a measure of the frequency of implementation barriers, and can move beyond the staff perception of barriers or contexts that reportedly influence implementation to empirically examining whether such an association exists (Grady et al., 2017). Qualitative and quantitative research provide different but complementary information to guide implementation efforts and together overcome limitations described in previous research which report that reliance on one form of evidence may overlook potentially importance determinants of implementation in community settings.

Finally, systematic reviews of both qualitative and quantitative research provide a comprehensive assessment of factors that may modify the effects of implementation strategies. By virtue of their intent to capture all relevant research on a particular implementation issue, systematic reviews provide strong evidence to support decisions regarding the development of implementation strategies. Nonetheless, the barriers and operational contexts in which implementation is occurring in community settings of studies included in the review may not generalise to local contexts. As such, assessment to verify local factors influencing implementation is also recommended prior to local intervention.

Theoretical Frameworks

The application of implementation theoretical frameworks is recommended to maximise the benefit of formative evaluation. Implementation theory and theoretical frameworks can help articulate mechanisms by which implementation strategies can exert their effects. The use of implementation theory can ensure that implementation strategies do not overlook important implementation determinants (Seward et al., 2017). Furthermore, without the application of theory, how implementation strategies work can be difficult to discern, providing little guidance for how their effects can be improved. Despite its importance, few strategies to improve implementation of chronic disease prevention interventions in community settings have utilised implementation theories or frameworks (Wolfenden et al., 2015; Wolfenden et al., 2017). The lack of application of theory may, in part, explain the disappointing effects of previous implementation strategies in community settings.

There are now a large number of implementation-relevant theories, frameworks and conceptual models that can be used to understand implementation contexts and barriers (Milat & Li, 2017). The Implementation frameworks such as the Consolidated Framework for Implementation in Health Research (Damschroder et al., 2009) or the Theoretical Domains Framework (French et al., 2012) (TDF) are among the most comprehensive and widely used frameworks in the field of implementation science (Skolarus et al., 2017). The frameworks consolidate a range of implementation-relevant theories and importantly consider multi-level (e.g. individual, organisational and broader environmental factors) determinants. The use of such frameworks can improve the value of formative evaluation to better develop effective implementation initiatives.

For example, guidance documents for the application of the TDF recommend that empirical observations and qualitative studies be undertaken in the setting to identify factors that may influence local improvements in implementation (Atkins et al., 2017). Further, quantitative TDF surveys have been developed to assess a broad range of potential implementation determinants based on TDF theoretical constructs allowing for a range of barriers to be identified to inform implementation strategy development (French et al., 2012; Squires et al., 2013; Taylor, Lawton, Slater, & Foy, 2013). The use of theoretical frameworks such as the TDF in formative evaluations has also been found to provide more comprehensive assessments of implementation contexts and identify important barriers to implementation often overlooked by studies that have not applied them (Grady et al., 2017).

Perhaps most importantly, theoretical frameworks provide a basis for appropriate selection of implementation strategies. Appropriate strategies are those that target the primary impediments to implementation and are congruent with the operational and social context of the organisations in which they are to be introduced. Selection of implementation strategies is guided by a process of theoretical framework mapping whereby barriers identified through theoretically grounded formative evaluations are matched with evidence-based implementation strategies and behaviour change techniques designed to overcome them. Documents supporting the application of frameworks such as the TDF guide this process and help to avoid the use of strategies that do not contribute to addressing barriers to implementation. For example, providing staff skills training to implement a risk reduction policy may not be effective if staff of an organisation already have sufficient skills but do not have management support to do so. Similarly, soliciting organisational leadership to support policy implementation may not be effective if staff do not have the necessary skills for implementation. Further, the application of theory and/or theoretical frameworks in selection of implementation strategies provides a basis for undertaking statistical examination of causal pathways to better understand how the selected implementation strategy exerts its effects on the hypothesised determinants of implementation.

The application of theory and/or theoretical frameworks to the process of implementation strategy selections provides a robust means of maximising the potential impact of an implementation strategy. Regardless of the methods for collecting such information, the more contextual information regarding the setting context that is available, the more likely it is that an appropriate selection of implementation strategies occurs. The triangulation of methods and measures described above is therefore recommended to provide a comprehensive evidence base.

Three Case Studies of Strategies Undertaken in Australia, which Aim to Improve Implementation of Evidence-Based Policies or Programmes Addressing Chronic Disease Risks in Community Settings

Even where theoretically informed approaches are undertaken, the effectiveness of an implementation strategy is not guaranteed. Evaluation of the impact of implementation strategies is recommended to determine if they produce the desired outcome and to provide evidence to identify opportunities for further improvement.

The use of hybrid research designs (Wolfenden, Williams, Wiggers, Nathan, & Yoong, 2016), through which information about the impact of implementation strategies on implementation outcomes (e.g. fidelity of implementation, acceptability) and individual-level health outcomes (e.g. tobacco or alcohol use, or the presence of illness or disease) are measured, provides an informative evidence base to achieve this. For implementation strategies that have been developed on the basis of theory or frameworks, the inclusion of measures in implementation trials that assess these theoretical constructs is particularly valuable, as it provides a means to test theoretical mechanism by which developers hypothesise the strategy will work. Understanding 'how' implementation strategies work provides a basis by which the impact of implementation strategies can be enhanced. A number of tools and statistical techniques (such as causal mediation analyses) are available to assess theoretical constructs in community settings (Clinton-McHarg et al., 2016) and allow assessment of the mechanism by which such strategies exert their effects.

The rest of the chapter discusses three Australian case studies that provide three different approaches to supporting implementation in community-based settings. The approaches differ in the setting which they have been implemented, and in the extent to which formative evaluation and theory informed the selection of implementation strategies was used.

Case Study 1: Implementation of Physical Activity-Promoting Practices in the Childcare Setting

What Was the Evidence–Practice Gap?

Improving physical activity levels in young children is associated with better short- and long-term health outcomes (Timmons et al., 2012). As such, in Australia, as is the case internationally (McWilliams et al., 2009), guidelines for the sector recommend that childcare services have physical activity policies; support active play opportunities including development of movement skills; provide information to parents about active play; and limit small screen recreation (Australian Government Department of Health and Ageing, 2013). Despite the availability of such evidence and guidelines, Australian childcare centres do not routinely implement these recommended practices (Wolfenden et al., 2010).

What Was Known About the Local Context and Implementation Barriers?

Published research literature suggests that childcare staff report a lack of knowledge, resources, confidence and support by parents and staff as barriers to implementing such practices (Froehlich Chow & Humbert, 2011; Tremblay, Boudreau-Larivière, & Cimon-Lambert, 2012). The existence of these or other barriers locally, however, is unknown.

> **Box 7.1: Practices to promote physical activity in childcare**
> - Service has a written physical activity policy
> - Staff programme fundamental movement skills programmes for children every day
> - Service increases time spent on structured physical activities
> - All staff participate in active child play
> - Service has all staff providing verbal prompts for physical activity
> - Service limits small screen recreation opportunities for children to less than once per week
> - Service ensures that children spend no more than 30 min in seated activities at a time (with the exception of eating and sleeping)
> - Service has staff trained in physical activity

How Was the Strategy to Support Implementation Developed?

To address the evidence–practice gap, an implementation support strategy was developed to improve the implementation of the eight physical activity-promoting practices shown to be effective, as outlined in Box 7.1 (Finch et al., 2012).

No local formative qualitative or quantitative research was undertaken, and no explicit theoretical framework was used to guide the selection of the implementation strategies or to specifically match implementation support strategies to identified implementation barriers. A literature review was undertaken to identify implementation strategies that had been found to be effective in other settings, particularly the healthcare sector, as there was little evidence of effective implementation strategies in the childcare setting at the time.

Based on the findings of the literature review, a suite of implementation strategies was then selected by health promotion practitioners in consultation with a regional community advisory group with representation from local childcare service managers, early childhood researchers and physical activity experts. Strategies which had evidence of effectiveness for improving implementation in other settings were then refined by the group according to feasibility, relevance and acceptability to the setting.

What Were the Implementation Support Strategies?

The implementation support package was delivered to childcare centres and included the following five implementation strategies:

1.	*Offer of staff training* (Fees, Trost, Bopp, & Dzewaltowski, 2009; Trost, Ward, & Senso, 2010): Two staff from each service were invited to a 6-hour face-to-face training workshop. Training was conducted by a respected early childhood training organisation, and a local service manager and academic with expertise in child physical activity. The training provided basic information, skill development and guidance regarding service physical activity policies and practices and how they could be modified to better support child activity in care. All services were also provided access to an online web-based training module covering similar content to that provided in the workshop (~40 min in length). Service managers were encouraged to ensure that all service staff who had not attended the workshop completed the online module.
2.	*Offer of information, Programme resources and instructional materials* (McCullum et al., 2004; Schofield, Edwards, & Pearce, 1997): Programme resources and instructional materials included a manual covering topics related to key physical activity-promoting practices, three age-appropriate structured activity handbooks, two DVDs demonstrating fundamental movement skills, laminated game cards and staff lanyards with pictorial and descriptive explanations of fundamental movement skills
3.	*Offer of follow-up support* (Abraham & Michie, 2008; Soumerai & Avorn, 1990): Service managers were offered two 15-min telephone support calls to reinforce key programme messages, identify barriers to practice change and provide additional advice and support. All services were provided with a free contact number direct to a member of the project team for any further queries or support
4.	*Provision of performance monitoring and feedback regarding practice adoption* (Abraham & Michie, 2008; Jamtvedt, Young, Kristoffersen, O'Brien, & Oxman, 2010): Information collected during the telephone support contacts with the service was used to monitor adoption of intervention components and provide performance feedback regarding individual service implementation during telephone contacts
5.	*Offer of incentives* (Grol & Wensing, 2004; Stone et al., 2002): Services that adopted a physical activity policy and/or which had staff who completed online training went in a draw to win vouchers for educational toys and resources. Staff who completed online training also went in a draw to win holiday accommodation

Was the Implementation Support Strategy Effective?

In order to determine if the intervention was successful, childcare service managers in both groups were telephoned and asked to report information on their service's implementation of the eight targeted practices before and after the intervention 18 months later. The evaluation found that improvements in implementation were limited to two of the eight practices. Among services that received the programme, there was a 28% increase in the number of services implementing a physical activity policy, which also included restrictions on small screen recreation (compared to a 4% increase in control services), and an increase of 47% in staff trained in physical activity (compared to an increase of 6% in control services) (Finch et al., 2012). There were no differences observed between the two groups for the other six implementation outcomes (Finch et al., 2012). The trial did not examine differences in child-level physical activity.

Learnings from the Research

- Although the implementation strategies were feasible to deliver and developed in partnership with the setting, they were only effective in improving two of the eight targeted practices to promote physical activity.
- There were no initial formative (qualitative or quantitative) evaluations or observations of the local context in which the intervention was to be delivered. Consequently, important barriers to implementation may have been overlooked.
- Selection of implementation support strategies was based on evidence from outside the childcare sector. The implementation support therefore may not be generalisable to this setting.
- The evaluation of the initiative was limited and did not assess why implementation outcomes were equivocal or the impact of the strategy on child physical activity levels. Accordingly, the evaluation provided limited evidence to identify future opportunities for improvement.

Case Study 2: An Intervention to Improve Sports Club Implementation of Recommended Alcohol Management Practices (the Good Sports Programme)

What Was the Evidence-To-Practice Gap?

Harm caused by excessive alcohol consumption contributes to more than 200 diseases, injuries and other health conditions (World Health Organisation, 1992) and is responsible for around 3.3 million deaths each year (World Health Organisation, 2014). Sporting clubs are one environment in which players and fans of sport are exposed to increased risk of alcohol-related harm. Evidence from systematic reviews indicates that alcohol-related harm can be reduced if controls are placed on the sale and supply of alcohol and if environments in which alcohol is consumed (e.g. sports clubs) are well managed (Babor et al., 2010; Loxley et al., 2005; National Drug Research Institute, 2007). Despite this evidence, sports clubs and venues across the globe, including in Europe (Drygas et al., 2013), the United States (Lenk et al., 2010) and New Zealand (Lyne & Galloway, 2012), have failed to implement alcohol management practices comprehensively and consistently (Drygas et al., 2013).

What Was Known about the Local Context and Implementation Barriers?

The Australian Drug Foundation, a non-government organisation, has conducted formative qualitative and quantitative research and worked with sports clubs and sporting associations to create environments supportive of responsible management of alcohol for over a decade (Australian Drug Foundation, 2013). Through meetings with sports club presidents and committees, players and spectators, as well as visits and observations of sports clubs during competition games and training, the organisation developed an understanding of club alcohol management practices, culture and the operational environment of sports clubs. Consistent with this understanding, empirical research indicated that the capacity of sports clubs to implement best practice initiatives, such as responsible service of alcohol practices, was limited by the volunteer nature of the workforce, resource limitations (Crisp & Swerissen, 2003; Duff & Munro, 2007; Eime, Payne, & Harvey, 2008; Wolfenden et al., 2012), other priorities (Crisp & Swerissen, 2003), structural impediments (e.g. contractual obligations or limited facility access) (Crisp & Swerissen, 2003) and limited support from peak sporting groups (Eime et al., 2008).

How Were Strategies to Support Implementation Developed?

In New South Wales (NSW), Australia, a project was undertaken to improve sports club implementation of recommended alcohol management practices (the *Good Sports* programme). (Australian Drug Foundation, 2013) The programme was undertaken with community-level, non-elite football clubs and specifically aimed to improve the implementation of the 16 alcohol management practices listed in Box 7.2. The development of the implementation support strategy followed the quantita-

---

Box 7.2: Alcohol management practices
- A club management representative is always present when alcohol is served.
- All bar servers have undertaken an accredited responsible service of alcohol training course.
- An up-to-date register of alcohol-related incidents is maintained.
- Bar servers do not consume alcohol while on duty.
- Substantial food is provided when alcohol is served.
- Non-alcoholic drink options are available.
- Low-alcoholic drink options are available.
- Low-alcoholic drink options are cheaper than full strength alcoholic drinks.
- Club has a written alcohol management policy.
- Club has a written safe transport policy.
- Club does not permit or conduct: happy hour, cheap or discounted alcoholic drinks, drinking games, 'all you can drink' promotions, free drink vouchers or alcohol-only awards and prizes.

tive and qualitative research of the Alcohol and Drug Foundation undertaken in the setting.

The NSW Health Framework for Building Capacity to Improve Health (New South Wales Health, 2001) was used as a theoretical basis to develop strategies to support sports clubs to implement the best-practice alcohol management practices. A small group of relevant experts, including Australian Drug Foundation staff, health promotion practitioners and sports club policy and practice experts, developed the implementation support strategies by:

1. Developing a deep understanding of barriers to alcohol management practice implementation based on practical experience and formative research of the sporting club context;
2. Developing implementation support strategies that mapped to all components of the NSW Health Framework for Building Capacity to Improve Health (New South Wales Health, 2001), addressing specific barriers, and based on empirical evidence for effectiveness in other settings.

What Were the Implementation Support Strategies?

The implementation support strategies used to support clubs to undertake best-practice alcohol management practices are outlined Table 7.1, as is the mapping of these strategies to the underlying areas and elements of the NSW Health Framework for Building Capacity to Improve Health.

Was the Implementation Support Strategy Effective?

A randomised controlled trial was undertaken with 87 community football clubs in urban and rural areas of NSW to assess whether the implementation support strategies listed in Table 7.1 were effective in supporting clubs to undertake best-practice alcohol management practices (Kingsland, Wolfenden, Tindall, Rowland, Sidey, et al., 2015). The trial involved half of the clubs being randomly allocated to receive the implementation support strategies for 2 years with the other clubs receiving no support during this time. Telephone Interviews were undertaken with club representatives (e.g. club presidents) from all participating clubs (those that received the support and those that did not) before and after this two-year period to assess club implementation of the 16 alcohol management practices listed in Box 7.2. Implementation of 80% (13 out of 16) of these practices was considered 'adequate implementation'.

At the start of the trial, 40–50% of clubs reported that they implemented 80% of the alcohol management practices. Following the intervention, a significantly greater proportion of clubs that received the implementation support strategies (88%) reported this level of implementation compared to clubs that did not receive any support (65%) (OR: 3.7 [95% CI: 1.1–13.2]; $P = 0.04$). As shown in Table 7.2,

Table 7.1 Implementation support strategies used to support clubs to undertake best-practice alcohol management practices (Kingsland, Wolfenden, Tindall, Rowland, Sidey, et al., 2015)

Strategy	Strategy mapped to action areas and elements in the NSW health framework for building capacity to improve health (New South Wales Health, 2001)
Project officer support (Rohrbach, Grana, Sussman, & Valente, 2006) Each club was allocated a project officer as a resource to enable the club to put in place required alcohol management practice. Assistance was provided in the form of face-to-face meetings and phone/email contact	Resource allocation: 　Human resources Organisational development: 　Management support
Implementation cost recovery (Greenhalgh, Robert, & MacFarlane, 2004) Clubs were provided with \$AU1000 to support the cost of implementing the responsible alcohol strategies	Resource allocation: 　Financial resources
Accreditation merchandise (Greenfield & Braithwaite, 2008; Pomey et al., 2010) Implementation of best-practice alcohol management practices was recognised and rewarded through a three-tier accreditation framework, with incentives including a certificate of accreditation and merchandise (e.g. bar mats, posters) provided at each level of accreditation	Organisational development: 　Recognition and reward systems
Printed resources (Bero et al., 1998; Rohrbach et al., 2006) Clubs received a comprehensive hardcopy of resource kit and electronic versions of resources which included evidence base and external legislative/policy background for responsible alcohol management practices; decision-making tools, case models and simple steps to implement each practice	Resource allocation: 　Physical resources 　Decision-making tools and 　models
Observational audit and feedback (Alvero, Bucklin, & Austin, 2001; Ivers et al., 2012) Observational performance audits of clubs were conducted during football matches before clubs were awarded each level of accreditation. A formal written audit feedback report reflecting on audit results and suggesting strategies to improve practices was provided to clubs following each audit	Workforce development: 　Performance management 　systems
Newsletters (Bero et al., 1998; Rohrbach et al., 2006) Promotion of accreditation status was undertaken via a regular newsletter that was distributed to all participating clubs. Newsletter content also included a ladder comparing club accreditation status; messages of support from peers and champions; evidence base and policy base for key responsible alcohol management practices	Organisational development: 　Recognition and rewards 　systems Partnerships: 　Relationships Resource allocation: 　Physical resources
Training (Bero et al., 1998; Read & Kleiner, 1996) Club staff were engaged and provided with skills to implement responsible alcohol management practices through accredited responsible service of alcohol training.	Workforce development: 　Workforce learning

(continued)

Table 7.1 (continued)

Strategy	Strategy mapped to action areas and elements in the NSW health framework for building capacity to improve health (New South Wales Health, 2001)

Sporting organisation letters of support (Greenhalgh et al., 2004)
Key state sporting associations representing the clubs participating in the study were engaged. Letters of recognition and encouragement were sent from these associations to clubs as they progressed through the accreditation levels
	Partnerships:
	  Relationships
	Organisational development:
	  Recognition and rewards systems

Adapted from Kingsland, Wolfenden, Tindall, Rowland, Sidey, et al. (2015), p. 450, ©2015 Australasian Professional Society on Alcohol and other Drugs, with permission from John Wiley and Sons

Table 7.2 Usefulness and adequacy of each implementation support strategy (Kingsland, Wolfenden, Tindall, Rowland, Sidey, et al., 2015)

Implementation support strategy (n = 34)	Clubs that rated strategy 'very' or 'somewhat' useful	Clubs that rated amount of support as		
		Too little	Just right	Too much
Project officer support	94.1%	2.9%	85.3%	2.9%
Implementation cost recovery	91.2%	26.5%	58.8%	0%
Accreditation merchandise	91.2%	17.7%	73.5%	0%
Printed resources	88.2%	5.9%	85.3%	2.9%
Observational audit feedback	84.9%	11.8%	73.5%	5.9%
Newsletters	81.8%	2.9%	76.5%	0%
Training	79.4%	11.8%	55.9%	0%
State sporting organisation letters of support	68.8%	23.5%	58.8%	0%

Adapted from Kingsland, Wolfenden, Tindall, Rowland, Sidey, et al. (2015), p. 454, ©2015 Australasian Professional Society on Alcohol and other Drugs, with permission from John Wiley and Sons

all implementation support strategies were rated by the majority of club representatives (69–94%) to be either 'very' or 'somewhat' useful. Project officer support was rated as the most useful and letters of support from state sporting organisations was rated as least useful. The amount of support that was provided by each strategy was rated by the majority of club representatives (59–85%) to be 'just right' (Kingsland, Wolfenden, Tindall, Rowland, Sidey, et al., 2015).

Additionally, the trial assessed the impact of the implementation support strategy on the alcohol use of club members. The initiative was found to be effective in reducing episodes of harmful drinking and overall alcohol intake (Kingsland, Wolfenden, Tindall, Rowland, Lecathelinais, et al., 2015).

Learnings from the Research

- A number of improvements in the implementation of best practice alcohol management practices of sports clubs can be achieved through the use of multiple implementation support strategies.
- Prior experience and formative evaluation provided strong grounding for the development of the implementation support package. Formal observations of the environment, however, were not undertaken.
- The use of a capacity-building framework provided a useful basis for implementation support strategy selection. The lack of application of an implementation framework in formative evaluation may have increased the risk that important implementation barriers were undetected.
- The evaluation adopted a hybrid design assessing the impact of the strategy on implementation outcomes, acceptability / usability, and individual health behaviour (alcohol use). Such findings provide data some basis for strategy improvement.

Case Study 3: An Intervention to Facilitate the Implementation of a Statewide Healthy School Canteen Policy in Primary Schools

What Was the Evidence–Practice Gap?

Encouraging healthy eating among children can prevent excessive weight gain and protect against future chronic disease (Jaaskelainen et al., 2012; Kaikkonen et al., 2013; World Cancer Research Fund / American Institute for Cancer Research, 2007). Systematic reviews have reported that interventions that reduce the relative availability of unhealthy foods in schools improve child dietary behaviours (Jaime & Lock, 2009; Kubik, Lytle, & Story, 2005). As such, governments across the globe have released policies restricting the sale of unhealthy foods at school (Ontario Ministry of Education, 2010; Finkelstein, Hill, & Whitaker, 2008; United Kingdom (UK) Department of Education, 2014).

In Australia, a number of states and territories have released mandatory policies requiring government schools to ban the regular sale of unhealthy foods and beverages from canteens (Woods, Bressan, Langelaan, Mallon, & Palermo, 2014). The policy utilises a traffic light system to classify foods as 'red', 'amber' or 'green' based on their nutritional content (i.e. saturated fat, added sugar and/or salt). 'Red' foods are nutrient-poor, high-energy foods such as confectionary and deep-fried foods. 'Amber' foods are considered to have some nutritional value; however, if consumed in large amounts can contribute to excess energy intake (e.g. full fat milk, processed meats). 'Green' foods are considered to provide good sources of nutrients such as fruit, vegetables and lean meats.

The policy was adopted as part of Department of Education policy in NSW and mandated all government schools to remove items classified as 'red' or from regular sale and to comprise their menu with at least 50% of products classified as 'green'. However, research suggests that less than 30% of NSW school canteens complied with the mandatory healthy canteen policy (Woods et al., 2014).

What Was Known About the Local Context and Implementation Barriers?

The local health service had worked with schools to promote healthy eating among children for almost a decade and had developed strong networks with local schools. Limited support, however, had been provided to the canteen managers to comply with the canteen policy. Local audits of school canteen menus found that policy implementation rates were similar to those reported across NSW (Hills, Nathan, Robinson, Fox, & Wolfenden, 2015; Yoong et al., 2015). A number of studies had been published reporting barriers to healthy canteen policy implementation in Australia, suggesting that the primary barriers were the following: perceived complexity of classifying foods according to the guidelines (Ardzejewska, Tadros, & Baxter, 2012), perceived lack of support from school executive, parents or children (Ardzejewska et al., 2012; Pettigrew, Donovan, Jalleh, Pescud, & Cowie, 2009; Woods et al., 2014), concerns regarding the profitability of the canteen and inadequate canteen facilities (Pettigrew et al., 2009; Woods et al., 2014).

How Were the Strategies to Support Implementation Developed?

A project was undertaken to improve the implementation of the governments' healthy canteen policy. To help guide the selection of implementation support strategies, the Theoretical Domains Framework (TDF) (Michie et al., 2013; Michie, Johnston, Francis, Hardeman, & Eccles, 2008) was used. The Theoretical Domains Framework is an integrative framework of organisational change theory that draws on 33 theories relevant to improving implementation across disciplines. Whilst its application in community settings such as schools was, at the time, limited, the framework had been widely used in the development of effective implementation interventions in clinical settings. The procedures recommended by the Theoretical Domains Framework (Michie et al., 2008) were applied to develop the implementation strategy to improve primary schools' implementation of the healthy canteen policy. Specifically, a three-step process was undertaken based on considerable formative evaluation which included the following:

1. Literature reviews to identify studies reporting barriers to the implementation of nutrition policies in schools, with emphasis on the Australian canteen context;
2. Surveys with canteen managers in the study region using a modified Theoretical Domains Framework questionnaire (Huijg et al., 2014) that examined perceived impediments to policy implementation;

Table 7.3 Key impediments to policy implementation identified by literature review, Theoretical Domains Framework survey with canteen managers and observations of canteen practices

Barrier	Literature review	TDF survey	Observation
Perceived lack of support from school community, i.e. principal, students and parents	✓	✓	–
Principal and canteen managers' knowledge of and attitudes to policy.	✓	✓	✓
Canteen manager's knowledge and skills to classify foods according to the policy	✓	✓	✓
Concerns regarding the profitability of the canteen	✓	✓	X
Inadequate canteen facilities.	✓	✓	✓
Lack of volunteers	✓	X	✓
Access to suitable products	X	X	✓

✓ Indicates the presence of a known barrier to implementation

3. On-site observations of canteen management and operational practices to understand canteen processes and qualitative research to better understand implementation context.

Such processes identified a number of factors that impeded the implementation of the healthy canteen policy (see Table 7.3). Information from the various data collection methods was triangulated to identify the key implementation barriers. Observations were particularly useful to understanding implementation context and identified local barriers including, for example, lack of canteen facilitates and access to suitable products that would have been overlooked had the implementation support relied on literature reviews or the TDF quantitative survey alone. The quantitative analyses of the TDF survey, however, provided evidence of strength of an association between a number of barriers and implementation of the policy, aiding in an assessment of the relative importance of such factors in achieving implementation.

Based upon these findings, barriers were mapped to Theoretical Domains Framework constructs, from which implementation strategies to address each key barrier were selected using a matrix and strategy selection process described by Michie et al. (2008). The proposed suite of possible implementation strategies was then reviewed by an advisory group consisting of health promotion practitioners, psychologists, dietitians, teachers, canteen managers and researchers with expertise in child obesity prevention, school-based interventions and implementation science. The advisory group refined the implementation support strategy on the basis that they were feasible and acceptable to school communities. Additionally, given the lack of trials assessing the potential effectiveness of implementation strategies in schools, the advisory group also considered evidence of the effectiveness of implementation strategies delivered in other contexts, such as healthcare settings (Cheung et al., 2012; Grimshaw et al., 2001; Grimshaw et al., 2004; Squires, Sullivan, Eccles, Worswick, & Grimshaw, 2014).

What Were the Implementation Support Strategies?

The implementation support strategies used to facilitate schools' implementation of the healthy canteen policy are outlined Table 7.4. This table also shows the mapping of these strategies to the underlying barriers being addressed and the relevant domains of the Theoretical Domains Framework.

Was the Implementation Support Strategy Effective?

In order to determine if the strategy was successful in supporting school canteens to become 'compliant' with the mandatory canteen policy, a randomised controlled trial was embedded into a routine service delivery programme to primary schools (those catering for children aged 5–12 years) across the Hunter New England Local Health District of NSW Australia with 70 primary schools. Schools were randomly allocated to receive the implementation support strategy or a waitlist control group (who received implementation support following completion of the trial, approximately 12 months later). The evaluation used a hybrid design and assessed a range of implementation and student-level outcomes. Process evaluation with canteen mangers showed that 45% found each implementation support strategy was very helpful or extremely helpful (on a Likert scale) and 94% received six or more of the nine implementation support strategies. Menus were audited at baseline and 12 months after baseline by trained dietitians who were unaware of whether the school had received the intervention or not. The results showed that at follow-up, 70.4% of schools that received the intervention did NOT have any RED items on their menu and 81.5% had mostly items rated as healthy (i.e. green items represented more than 50% of items listed) compared to 3.3% and 26.7%, respectively, in schools that did not receive the intervention. Students at schools that received implementation support also purchased healthier foods from the school canteen. A mediation analysis was undertaken using data from surveys with canteen managers assessing TDF theoretical constructs on which the implementation strategy was based to explore 'how' the implementation strategy achieved its effect (unpublished data).

Learnings from the Research

- Large improvements in policy implementation can be achieved in community settings with well-planned implementation strategies.
- The effectiveness of an implementation support strategy was enhanced through the use of:
- Comprehensive formative evaluation (observation, quantitative and qualitative research as well as systematic review) that was theoretically informed.
- The use of a theoretical frameworks that map implementation strategy selection to implementation barriers and account for local contexts.

Table 7.4 Implementation support strategies mapped to barriers and key domains of the Theoretical Domains Framework (Wolfenden et al., 2014)

Implementation support strategies	Barriers being addressed	Theoretical domain barrier related to	Technique for behaviour change
Schools were allocated a support officer with qualifications in nutrition and dietetics and experience in supporting schools to implement the policy. The support officer was responsible for delivering the intervention strategies below to schools			
Executive support: School principals were asked to communicate support for implementation of the policy to teachers, parents, students and canteen managers during staff meetings, in newsletters, assemblies and through the development of a local school policy	Perceived lack of support from principal	Social influences	Social processes of encouragement, pressure and support
Canteen action plan: Meetings with canteen staff were held to discuss and reach consensus regarding the policy, how best to implement it and to develop local canteen action plans to co-ordinate implementation tasks	Knowledge of and attitudes to policy	Knowledge; beliefs about consequences; motivation and goals	Contract; persuasive communication; feedback
Canteen managers workshop: A one-day training workshop (5 hours) was provided to canteen managers, canteen staff and parent representatives, with the aim of providing education and skill development in the policy, nutrition and food label reading, canteen stock and financial management, pricing and promotion, and change management	Perceived complexity of classifying foods according to the guidelines; concerns regarding the profitability of the canteen; food classification skills; canteen profitability; lack of volunteers; lack of canteen resources	Knowledge; skills; beliefs about capabilities; motivation and goals; memory, attention and decision processes	Information provision; graded tasks; increasing skills; rehearsal of relevant skills
Tools and resources: Canteen managers were provided with a 'canteen resource kit' containing printed instructional materials, sample policies and menus, planning templates, stock management forms, pricing guides, and recipe cards, along with a USB containing relevant templates and kitchen equipment (to the value of AUD$100)	Knowledge of and attitude to policy; food classification skills; canteen profitability; lack of volunteers; lack of canteen resources	Environmental context and resources; knowledge	Information provision; environmental changes (e.g. objects to facilitate behaviour)

(continued)

Table 7.4 (continued)

Implementation support strategies	Barriers being addressed	Theoretical domain barrier related to	Technique for behaviour change
Ongoing support: School canteen visits were conducted one- and three-months post canteen manager training to observe the operational canteen environment, provide feedback and assist with problem-solving	Knowledge of and attitude to policy; food classification skills; canteen profitability; lack of volunteers; lack of canteen resources	Environmental context and resources; knowledge; skills	Information provision; environmental changes (e.g. objects to facilitate behaviour);
Menu feedback: Menu reviews were conducted quarterly with written feedback reports forwarded to the canteen manager and school principal and verbal discussion visits and support calls.	Knowledge of and attitude to policy; food classification skills;	Beliefs about consequences;	Feedback; monitoring
Recognition: Schools with a menu assessed as adhering to the policy received a congratulatory letter, phone call from the research team, and were publically acknowledged via marketing strategies	Perceived lack of support from school community i.e. principal, students, parents; knowledge of and attitude to policy	Beliefs about consequences; social professional role and identity	Persuasive communication, information regarding behaviour, rewards
Marketing strategies: Quarterly project newsletters communicated key messages, provided information and case study successful implementation approaches to common barriers	Perceived lack of support from school community i.e. principal, students, parents; lack of volunteers	Social professional role and identity.	Social processes of encouragement, modelling/ demonstration of behaviour by others

Adapted from Wolfenden et al. (2014), p. 147, licensed under the terms of the Creative Commons Attribution License (https://creativecommons.org/licenses/by/4.0/)

- Programme evaluation is most useful when it provides a comprehensive assessment on the impacts of the implementation strategy on both implementation and individual-level outcomes.
- The effectiveness of implementation strategies is context-specific. Even though some of the research used a comprehensive evidence-based to inform the development to strategies, what works in one setting may not work in another. As a consequence, it is important to understand how the implementation strategy works (or does not) in a setting to generate opportunities for future improvement.

Summary and Conclusion

Despite being preventable, chronic disease continues to be a major source of mortality and morbidity globally. Cost-effective interventions currently exist to address many of these risk factors. The effective implementation of such evidence-based interventions is therefore required to realise their potential to make substantial improvements to reducing the chronic disease burden.

Given the current lack of evidence regarding the effectiveness of implementation strategies in community settings, maximising their potential impact requires a systematic theoretically informed process. This chapter describes three Australian case studies to illustrate the impact of implementation strategies outlining approaches of increasing rigor. Best practice approaches to implementation, as illustrated in case study 3, involved considerable investment in formative evaluation, using multiple data collection methods (e.g. qualitative research, quantitative research and local observation and systematic reviews) that were guided by multi-level theoretical frameworks. Such formative work provided an understanding of the local context and barriers to the implementation of a particular policy, practice or intervention. The mapping of implementation barriers to theory or theoretical frameworks and implementation strategies can then be applied to guide final strategy selection decisions. Evaluation is a recommended part of implementation practice, as it is the basis of continuous quality improvement. Best-practice evaluation identifies whether implementation strategies have their desired impact on both implementation and individual outcomes, providing evidence of how they work, and identifies opportunities for further improvement.

References

Abraham, C., & Michie, S. (2008). A taxonomy of behavior change techniques used in interventions. *Health Psychology, 27*(3), 379–387.

AIHW. (2012). *Risk factors contributing to chronic disease.* Canberra, Australia: AIHW.

Alvero, A. M., Bucklin, B. R., & Austin, J. (2001). An objective review of the effectiveness and essential characteristics of performance feedback in organizational settings (1985-1998). *Journal of Organizational Behavior Management, 21*(1), 3–29.

Ardzejewska, K., Tadros, R., & Baxter, D. (2012). A descriptive study on the barriers and facilitators to implementation of the NSW (Australia) healthy school canteen strategy. *Health Education Journal, 72*, 136–145.

Atkins, L., Francis, J., Islam, R., O'Connor, D., Patey, A., Ivers, N., ... Michie, S. (2017). A guide to using the theoretical domains framework of behaviour change to investigate implementation problems. *Implementation Science, 12*(1), 77.

Australian Drug Foundation. (2013). *Good sports program: Healthy clubs, strong communities.* Available from: http://goodsports.com.au/

Australian Government Department of Health and Ageing. (2013). *Get up and grow: healthy eating and physical activity for early childhood.* [cited 2015 4 Dec]; Available from: http://www.health.gov.au/internet/main/publishing.nsf/Content/phd-early-childhood-nutrition-resources

Babor, T., Caetano, R., Casswell, S., Edwards, G., Giesbrecht, N., Graham, K., ... Rossow, I. (2010). *Alcohol: No ordinary commodity – research and public policy.* Oxford: Oxford University Press.

Bero, L. A., Grilli, R., Grimshaw, J. M., Harvey, E., Oxman, A. D., & Thomson, M. A. (1998). Closing the gap between research and practice: An overview of systematic reviews of interventions to promote the implementation of research findings. *BMJ, 317*(7156), 465–468.

Cheung, A., Weir, M., Mayhew, A., Kozloff, N., Brown, K., & Grimshaw, J. (2012). Overview of systematic reviews of the effectiveness of reminders in improving healthcare professional behavior. *System Review, 1*, 36.

Clinton-McHarg, T., Yoong, S. L., Tzelepis, F., Regan, T., Fielding, A., Skelton, E., ... Wolfenden, L. (2016). Psychometric properties of implementation measures for public health and community settings and mapping of constructs against the consolidated framework for implementation research: A systematic review. *Implementation Science, 11*(1), 148.

Crisp, B. R., & Swerissen, H. (2003). Critical processes for creating health-promoting sporting environments in Australia. *Health Promotion International, 18*(2), 145–152.

Damschroder, L. J., Aron, D. C., Keith, R. E., Kirsh, S. R., Alexander, J. A., & Lowery, J. C. (2009). Fostering implementation of health services research findings into practice: A consolidated framework for advancing implementation science. *Implementation Science, 4*, 50.

Drygas, W., Ruszkowska, J., Philpott, M., BjOrkstrOm, O., Parker, M., Ireland, R., ... Tenconi, M. (2013). Good practices and health policy analysis in European sports stadia: Results from the 'healthy stadia' project. *Health Promotion International, 28*(2), 157–165.

Duff, C., & Munro, G. (2007). Preventing alcohol-related problems in community sports clubs: The good sports program. *Substance Use & Misuse, 42*(12/13), 1991–2001.

Eime, R. M., Payne, W. R., & Harvey, J. T. (2008). Making sporting clubs healthy and welcoming environments: A strategy to increase participation. *Journal of Science and Medicine in Sport, 11*(2), 146–154.

Fees, B., Trost, S., Bopp, M., & Dzewaltowski, D. A. (2009). Physical activity programming in family child care homes: Providers' perceptions of practices and barriers. *Journal of Nutrition Education and Behavior, 41*(4), 268–273.

Finch, M., Wolfenden, L., Falkiner, M., Edenden, D., Pond, N., Hardy, L. L., ... Wiggers, J. (2012). Impact of a population based intervention to increase the adoption of multiple physical activity practices in Centre based childcare services: A quasi experimental, effectiveness study. *International Journal of Behavioral Nutrition and Physical Activity, 9*(1), 101.

Finkelstein, D. M., Hill, E. L., & Whitaker, R. C. (2008). School food environments and policies in US public schools. *Pediatrics, 122*(1), e251–e259.

French, S., Green, S. E., O'Connor, D. A., McKenzie, J. E., Francis, J. J., Michie, S., ... Grimshaw, J. M. (2012). Developing theory-informed behaviour change interventions to implement evidence into practice: A systematic approach using the theoretical domains framework. *Implementation Science, 7*(1), 38.

Froehlich Chow, A., & Humbert, L. (2011). Physical activity and nutrition in early years care Centres: Barriers and facilitators. *Canadian Children, 36*(1), 26–31.

Grady, A., K Seward; M Finch; A Fielding; F Stacey; J Jones ... SL Yoong (2017). Barriers and enablers to implementation of dietary guidelines in early childhood education centers in Australia: Application of the Theoretical Domains Framework. *Journal of Nutrition Education and Behavior*, (in press).

Greenfield, D., & Braithwaite, J. (2008). Health sector accreditation research: A systematic review. *International Journal for Quality in Health Care, 20*(3), 172–183.

Greenhalgh, T., Robert, G., & MacFarlane, F. (2004). Diffusion of innovations in service organizations: Systematic review and recommendations. *The Milbank Quarterly, 82*(4), 581–629.

Grimshaw, J. M., Shirran, L., Thomas, R., Mowatt, G., Fraser, C., Bero, L., ... O'Brien, M. A. (2001). Changing provider behavior: An overview of systematic reviews of interventions. *Medical Care, 39*(8 Suppl 2), Ii2–I45.

Grimshaw, J. M., Thomas, R. E., MacLennan, G., Fraser, C., Ramsay, C. R., Vale, L., ... Donaldson, C. (2004). Effectiveness and efficiency of guideline dissemination and implementation strategies. *Health Technology Assessment, 8*(6), iii–iiv, 1-72.

Grol, R., & Wensing, M. (2004). What drives change? Barriers to and incentives for achieving evidence-based practice. *Medical Journal of Australia, 180*(Supplement 6), 57–60.

Hills, A., Nathan, N., Robinson, K., Fox, D., & Wolfenden, L. (2015). Improvement in primary school adherence to the NSW Healthy School Canteen Strategy in 2007 and 2010. *Health Promotion Journal of Australia, 26*(2), 89–92.

Huijg, J. M., Gebhardt, W. A., Dusseldorp, E., Verheijden, M. W., van der Zouwe, N., Middelkoop, B. J. C., ... Crone, M. R. (2014). Measuring determinants of implementation behavior:

Psychometric properties of a questionnaire based on the theoretical domains framework. *Implementation Science, 9*, 33.

Ivers, N., Jamtvedt, G., Flottorp, S., Young, J. M., Odgaard-Jensen, J., French, S. D., … Oxman, A. D. (2012). Audit and feedback: Effects on professional practice and healthcare outcomes. *Cochrane Database of Systematic Reviews, 6*, CD000259. https://doi.org/10.1002/14651858. CD000259.pub3

Jaaskelainen, P., Magnussen, C. G., Pahkala, K., Mikkila, V., Kahonen, M., Sabin, M. A., … Juonala, M. (2012). Childhood nutrition in predicting metabolic syndrome in adults: The cardiovascular risk in Young Finns Study. *Diabetes Care, 35*(9), 1937–1943.

Jaime, P. C., & Lock, K. (2009). Do school based food and nutrition policies improve diet and reduce obesity? *Preventive Medicine, 48*(1), 45–53.

Jamtvedt G., Young J. M.. Kristoffersen D. T., O'Brien M. A., & Oxman A. D. (2010). Audit and feedback: Effects on professional practice and health care outcomes (review). The Cochrane Collaboration. *The Cochrane Library* (7).

Kaikkonen, J. E., Mikkilä, V., Magnussen, C. G., Juonala, M., Viikari, J. S. A., & Raitakari, O. T. (2013). Does childhood nutrition influence adult cardiovascular disease risk?--insights from the Young Finns Study. *Annals of Medicine, 45*(2), 120–128.

Keleher, H., & MacDougall, C. (2006). In H. Keleher & C. MacDougall (Eds.), *Understanding health: A determinants approach*. South Melbourne, Australia: Oxford University Press.

Kingsland, M., Wolfenden, L., Tindall, J., Rowland Bosco, C., Lecathelinais, C., Gillham, K. E., … John, H. (2015). Tackling risky alcohol consumption in sport: A cluster randomised controlled trial of an alcohol management intervention with community football clubs. *Journal of Epidemiology and Community Health, 69*(10), 993.

Kingsland, M., Wolfenden, L., Tindall, J., Rowland, B., Sidey, M., McElduff, P., … Wiggers, J. H. (2015). Improving the implementation of responsible alcohol management practices by community sporting clubs: A randomised controlled trial. *Drug and Alcohol Review, 34*(4), 447–457.

Kubik, M. Y., Lytle, L. A., & Story, M. (2005). Schoolwide food practices are associated with body mass index in middle school students. *Archives of Pediatrics & Adolescent Medicine, 159*(12), 1111–1114.

Lau, R., Stevenson, F., Ong, B. N., Dziedzic, K., Treweek, S., Eldridge, S., … Murray, E. (2015). Achieving change in primary care-effectiveness of strategies for improving implementation of complex interventions: Systematic review of reviews. *BMJ Open, 5*(12), e009993.

Lenk, K. M., Toomey Traci, L., Erickson Darin, J., Kilian Gunna, R., Nelson Toben, F., & Fabian Lindsey, E. A. (2010). Alcohol control policies and practices at professional sports stadiums. *Public Health Reports, 125*(5), 665–673.

Lewis, C. C., Fischer, S., Weiner, B. J., Stanick, C., Kim, M., & Martinez, R. G. (2015). Outcomes for implementation science: An enhanced systematic review of instruments using evidence-based rating criteria. *Implementation Science, 10*(1), 155.

Loxley, W., Gray, D., Wilkinson, C., Chikritzhs, T., Midford, R., & Moore, D. (2005). Alcohol policy and harm reduction in Australia. *Drug and Alcohol Review, 24*(6), 559–568.

Lyne, M., & Galloway, A. (2012). Implementation of effective alcohol control strategies is needed at large sports and entertainment events. *Australian and New Zealand Journal of Public Health, 36*(1), 55–60.

McCullum, C., Hoelscher, D. M., Eagan, J. M., Ward, J. L., Kelder, S. H., & Barroso, C. S. (2004). Evaluation of the dissemination and implementation of the CATCH eat smart school nutrition program in Texas. *Journal of Child Nutrition and Management, 28*(1).

McNamara, K., Knight, A., Livingston, M., Kypri, K., Malo, J., Roberts, L., … De Courten, M. (2015). *Targets and indicators for chronic disease prevention in Australia*. Melbourne: AHPC, Australian Health Policy Collaboration technical paper No. 2015-08.

McWilliams, C., Ball, S. C., Benjamin, S. E., Hales, D., Vaughn, A., & Ward, D. S. (2009). Best-practice guidelines for physical activity at child care. *Pediatrics, 124*(6), 1650–1659.

Michie, S., Johnston, M., Francis, J., Hardeman, W., & Eccles, M. (2008). From theory to intervention: Mapping theoretically derived Behavioural determinants to behaviour change techniques. *Applied Psychology, 57*(4), 660–680.

Michie, S., Richardson, M., Johnston, M., Abraham, C., Francis, J., Hardeman, W., ... Wood, C. E. (2013). The behavior change technique taxonomy (v1) of 93 hierarchically clustered techniques: Building an international consensus for the reporting of behavior change interventions. *Annals of Behavioral Medicine, 46*(1), 81–95.

Milat, A., & Li, B. (2017). Narrative review of frameworks for translating research evidence into policy and practice. *Public Health Research & Practice, 27*(1), e2711704.

National Drug Research Institute. (2007). *Restrictions on the sale and supply of alcohol: Evidence and outcomes.* Perth, Australia: National Drug Research Institute, Curtin University of Technology.

New South Wales Health. (2001). *A framework for building capacity to improve health.* Gladsville, Australia: Better Health Centre.

Ontario Ministry of Education. (2010). *School food and beverage policy.* [Internet] [cited 2016 23 Mar]; Available from: http://www.edu.gov.on.ca/extra/eng/ppm/150.html

Peters, D. H., Adam, T., Alonge, O., Agyepong, I. A., & Tran, N. (2013). Implementation research: What it is and how to do it. *BMJ: British Medical Journal, 347*, f6753.

Pettigrew S, Donovan R. J., Jalleh G, Pescud M, Cowie S. (2009). *Addressing childhood obesity through school canteens. Report to the WA Department of Education and Training.* In The University of Western Australia and the Centre for Behavioural Research in Cancer Control, (Ed.), Curtin University: Perth, Western Australia.

Pomey, M.-P., Lemieux-Charles, L., Champagne, F., Angus, D., Shabah, A., & Contandriopoulos, A.-P. (2010). Does accreditation stimulate change? A study of the impact of the accreditation process on Canadian healthcare organizations. *Implementation Science, 5*(1), 31. https://doi.org/10.1186/1748-5908-5-31

Rabin, B. A., Glasgow, R. E., Kerner, J. F., Klump, M. P., & Brownson, R. C. (2010). Dissemination and implementation research on community-based cancer prevention: A systematic review. *American Journal of Preventive Medicine, 38*(4), 443–456.

Read, C. W., & Kleiner, B. H. (1996). Which training methods are effective. *Management Development Review, 9*(2), 24–29.

Rohrbach, L. A., Grana, R., Sussman, S., & Valente, T. W. (2006). Type II translation: Transporting prevention interventions from research to real-world settings. *Evaluation & the Health Professions, 29*(3), 302–333.

Schofield, M., Edwards, K., & Pearce, R. (1997). Effectiveness of two strategies for dissemination of sun-protection policy in New South Wales primary and secondary schools. *Australian and New Zealand Journal of Public Health, 21*(7), 743–750.

Seward, K., Finch, M., Yoong, S. L., Wyse, R., Jones, J., Grady, A., ... Wolfenden, L. (2017). Factors that influence the implementation of dietary guidelines regarding food provision in centre based childcare services: A systematic review. *Preventive Medicine, 105*(Supplement C), 197–205.

Seward, K., Wolfenden, L., Finch, M., Wiggers, J., Wyse, R., Jones, J., ... Yoong, S. L. (2016). Multistrategy childcare-based intervention to improve compliance with nutrition guidelines versus usual care in long day care services: A study protocol for a randomised controlled trial. *BMJ Open, 6*(6), e010786.

Skolarus, T. A., Lehmann, T., Tabak, R. G., Harris, J., Lecy, J., & Sales, A. E. (2017). Assessing citation networks for dissemination and implementation research frameworks. *Implementation Science, 12*(1), 97.

Soumerai, S. B., & Avorn, J. (1990). Principles of educational outreach ('academic detailing') to improve clinical decision making. *JAMA, 263*(4), 549–556.

Squires, J. E., Suh Kathryn, N., Stefanie, L., Natalie, B., Kathleen, G., Graham Ian, D., ... Jeremy, M. (2013). Improving physician hand hygiene compliance using behavioural theories: A study protocol. *Implementation Science, 8*, 16.

Squires, J. E., Sullivan, K., Eccles, M. P., Worswick, J., & Grimshaw, J. M. (2014). Are multifaceted interventions more effective than single-component interventions in changing health-care professionals' behaviours? An overview of systematic reviews. *Implementation Science, 9*, 152.

Stone, E. G., Morton, S. C., Hulscher, M. E., Maglione, M. A., Roth, E. A., Grimshaw, J. M., ... Shekelle, P. G. (2002). Interventions that increase use of adult immunization and cancer screening services: A meta-analysis. *Annals of Internal Medicine, 136*(9), 641–651. [Summary for patients in Ann Intern Med. May 7;136(9):I16; PMID: 11992319].

Taylor, N., Lawton, R., Slater, B., & Foy, R. (2013). The demonstration of a theory-based approach to the design of localized patient safety interventions. *Implementation Science, 8*, 123.

Timmons, B., LeBlanc, A. G., Carson, V., Gorber, S. C., Dillman, C., Janssen, I., ... Tremblay, M. S. (2012). Systematic review of physical activity and health in the early years (aged 0-4 years). *Applied Physiology, Nutrition, and Metabolism, 37*, 773–792.

Tremblay, L., Boudreau-Larivière, C., & Cimon-Lambert, K. (2012). Promoting physical activity in preschoolers: A review of the guidelines, barriers, and facilitators for implementation of policies and practices. *Canadian Psychology/Psychologie Canadienne, 53*(4), 280.

Trost, S. G., Ward, D. S., & Senso, M. (2010). Effects of child care policy and environment on physical activity. *Medicine & Science in Sports & Exercise, 42*(3), 520–525.

United Kingdom (UK) Department of Education. (2014). *Press release: new school food standards.* [2014 7th April 2016]. Available from: http://www.gov.uk/government/news/new-school-food-standards

WHO. (2016). Chronic diseases and health promotion. [cited 2016 04/05/2016]. Available from: http://www.who.int/chp/about/integrated_cd/en/.

Williams, C. M., Nathan, N. K., Wyse, R. J., Yoong, S. L., Delaney, T., Wiggers, J., ... Wolfenden, L. (2015). Strategies for enhancing the implementation of school-based policies or practices targeting risk factors for chronic disease. *Cochrane Database of Systematic Reviews, 5.*

Wolfenden, L., Jones, J., Williams, C. M., Finch, M., Wyse, R. J., Kingsland, M., ... Yoong, S. L. (2015). Strategies to improve the implementation of healthy eating, physical activity and obesity prevention policies, practices or programmes within childcare services. *Cochrane Database of Systematic Reviews, 7.*

Wolfenden, L., Kingsland, M., Rowland, B., Kennedy, V., Gillham, K., & Wiggers, J. (2012). Addressing alcohol use in community sports clubs: Attitudes of club representatives. *Australian and New Zealand Journal of Public Health, 36*(1), 93–94.

Wolfenden, L., Milat, A. J., Lecathelinais, C., Sanson-Fisher, R. W., Carey, M. L., Bryant, J., ... Yoong, S. (2016). What is generated and what is used: A description of public health research output and citation. *European Journal of Public Health, 26*(3), 523–525.

Wolfenden, L., Nathan, N., CM Williams, T. D., Reilly, K. L., Freund, M., ... Wiggers, J. (2014). A randomised controlled trial of an intervention to increase the implementation of a heathy canteen policy in Australian primary schools: Study protocol. *Implementation Science, 9*, 147.

Wolfenden, L., Nathan, N. K., Sutherland, R., Yoong, S. L., Hodder, R. K., Wyse, R. J., ... Clinton-McHarg, T. (2017). Strategies for enhancing the implementation of school-based policies or practices targeting risk factors for chronic disease (in press). *Cochrane Database of Systematic Reviews.*

Wolfenden, L., Neve, M., Farrell, L., Lecathelinais, C., Bell, C., Milat, A., ... Sutherland, R. (2010). Physical activity policies and practices of childcare centres in Australia. *Journal of Paediatrics and Child Health, 47*(3), 73–76.

Wolfenden, L., Williams, C. M., Wiggers, J., Nathan, N., & Yoong, S. L. (2016). Improving the translation of health promotion interventions using effectiveness–implementation hybrid designs in program evaluations. *Health Promotion Journal of Australia, 27*(3), 204–207.

Woods, J., Bressan, A., Langelaan, C., Mallon, A., & Palermo, C. (2014). Australian school canteens: Menu guideline adherence or avoidance? *Health Promotion Journal of Australia, 25*(2), 110–115.

World Cancer Research Fund/American Institute for Cancer Research. (2007). *Food, nutrition, physical activity, and the prevention of cancer: A global perspective.* Washington, DC: American Institute for Cancer Research.

World Health Organisation. (1992). *WHO statistical classification of diseases and related health problems (ICD)* (10th revision ed.). Geneva, Switzerland: World Health Organisation.

World Health Organisation. (2014). *Global status report on alcohol and health 2014*. Geneva, Switzerland: World Health Organisation.

Yoong, S. L., Clinton-McHarg, T., & Wolfenden, L. (2015). Systematic reviews examining implementation of research into practice and impact on population health are needed. *Journal of Clinical Epidemiology, 68*(7), 788–791.

Yoong, S. L., Nathan, N. K., Wyse, R. J., Preece, S. J., Williams, C. M., Sutherland, R. L., … Wolfenden, L. (2015). Assessment of the school nutrition environment: A study in Australian primary school canteens. *American Journal of Preventive Medicine, 49*(2), 215–222.

Yoong, S. L., Skelton, E., Jones, J., & Wolfenden, L. (2014). Do childcare services provide foods in line with the 2013 Australian dietary guidelines? A cross-sectional study. *Australian and New Zealand Journal of Public Health, 38*(6), 595–596.

Youl, P., Baade, P., & Meng, X. (2012). Impact of prevention on future cancer incidence in Australia [online]. *Cancer Forum, 36*(1), 37–41.

Chapter 8
Implementation Teams: A Stakeholder View of Leading and Sustaining Change

Allison Metz and Leah Bartley

Introduction

Successful implementation is a collaborative act, requiring more than the efforts of a single charismatic leader. There is growing evidence that "implementation relies on multiple actors, is a process that is multi-faceted, iterative, and often unpredictable" (Rycroft-Malone et al., 2013, p. 14). Implementation researchers and practitioners are promoting a stakeholder view of leadership, where traditional leadership must engage with community members and diverse stakeholder groups to develop a shared understanding of problems and potential solutions, develop strategies with a strong contextual fit in complicated systems, and create a sense of mutual accountability for building the infrastructure needed to sustain change and improve outcomes. Collaboration and teamwork, and specifically the creation of implementation teams, are strategies for stakeholder leadership. Implementation teams are the foundation of effective implementation, collectively leveraging members' diverse skills and perspectives to build an enabling context for interventions. Implementation teams ensure the inclusion of multiple actors and perspectives in activities such as communication, problem-solving, and data-driven decision-making. This shift in focus from solo leaders to implementation teams requires new thinking in how to build teams, identify team functions, facilitate effective team meetings, support individual learning of team members, and develop team members into leaders of implementation.

The growing attention on implementation teams is timely and important for supporting the sustainable use of evidence to improve outcomes. This chapter will provide a state-of-the-field as it relates to use of implementation teams to support, scale, and sustain change efforts to produce population impacts. Specifically, this chapter seeks to:

A. Metz (✉) · L. Bartley
University of North Carolina, Chapel Hill, NC, USA
e-mail: allison.metz@unc.edu

© Springer Nature Switzerland AG 2020
B. Albers et al. (eds.), *Implementation Science 3.0*,
https://doi.org/10.1007/978-3-030-03874-8_8

- Define implementation teams, describing what teams are and what they are not.
- Provide a state-of-the-field regarding the practice and research evidence for the role of teams in supporting and sustaining implementation of evidence-based practices and innovations.
- Describe effective team meeting processes and structures.
- Identify the core functions of implementation teams in building organizational and systems capacity.
- Define the core competencies needed to support the development and facilitation of implementation teams.

Implementation Teams Defined

An implementation team is a group of stakeholders that oversees, attends to, and is accountable for facilitating key activities in the selection, implementation, and continuous improvement of an intervention. They are a group with a common goal, cumulatively responsible for ensuring completion of necessary tasks that involve high interdependence and autonomy (Sprigg, Jackson, & Parker, 2000). While teams serve as an accountable structure for supporting implementation, team members may not be doing all of the activities associated with this work, that is, the selection, implementation, and continuous improvement of interventions. Rather, implementation team members may facilitate the completion of such activities by identifying other qualified individuals to complete implementation tasks or secure resources needed. For example, team members may identify and ensure qualified trainers, but not conduct training themselves, or they may secure available data from the quality assurance and improvement divisions at their organization, but not collect data or analyze the data themselves.

As the formal implementation structure, teams systematically move an intervention through stages of implementation by ensuring stakeholders and community members are engaged, the practice is well defined and a good fit with the context and setting, implementation supports are in place, implementation integrity is measured and improved, and outcomes are achieved and sustained. Without teams, an implementation effort ends up relying on individual leaders who, without a team, are often unable to influence multiple stakeholders. This "solo hero" model of implementation has been demonstrated to fall short on key issues related to successful implementation such as stakeholder buy-in, integration and alignment of the new practice within the system, and sustainability to achieve population outcomes (Higgins, Weiner, & Young, 2012).

Teams include key personnel (e.g., program administrators and practitioners) and key stakeholders who offer diverse perspectives on what is needed to effectively integrate innovations and evidence-based practices into systems and organizations. For example, program developers can provide information related to fidelity requirements for evidence-based programs, funders can offer strategies for fiscal sustainability, and service users and community members can provide input on the likelihood that specific interventions and practices will be accepted by local communities and meet service needs. Ideally, teams should be established at every level of a program or system, or to target different aspects of an initiative. For example, for a complex initiative such as a statewide implementation of a new child assessment, separate implementation teams may be established at the state, local, and service provider levels to monitor and support the initiative. Furthermore, there may be separate implementation teams, perhaps made up of individuals from across the levels of the system, monitoring distinct aspects of the initiative, such as the training of practitioners or the administration of assessments.

The "core" implementation team is responsible for the day-to-day implementation of the initiative and is often limited in the number of people included, so that it can be agile and productive in its day-to-day activities. Teams play an important role in facilitating change within an organization (Lessard et al., 2016). Members of implementation teams should represent different perspectives, including practice, supervision, administrative leadership, and policy perspectives. These different perspectives can be present within a single implementation team or be represented through a linked teaming structure across levels of a program or system. A linked teaming structure supports connections among practice and leadership levels in a system. For example, core implementation teams responsible for overseeing day-to-day activities associated with implementation may report to a leadership team with decision-making authority.

It is important to draw a distinction between what an implementation team is, and what it is not. Implementation teams are different from advisory groups or technical workgroups. Whereas advisory groups or technical workgroups are often relied upon for expert advice or recommendations for time-limited periods, implementation teams are active and committed facilitators of new ways of work and organizational and systems change during a much longer period of time, often up to two to 4 years (Metz & Bartley, 2012). Implementation teams are also different from learning collaboratives or other collective groups that provide more passive learning opportunities. Compared to conventional workgroups, implementation teams have been shown to take more initiative, ensure ongoing improvement, elevate accountability for decision-making within the team, and engage in more innovative problem-solving (Joiner, 2007; Neilsen, Randall, & Christensen, 2017). Shifts in practice, organizational change, and new ways of work require the involvement of multiple perspectives and a range of expertise (Higgins et al., 2012). Implementation teams are the organized and committed capacity that ensures different viewpoints and champions are dedicated to promoting shifts in practice and organizational changes. Implementation team members often take on specific responsibilities for ensuring the success of a new way of work or organizational change. For example, specific team members may facilitate efforts for routinely gathering feedback from frontline practitioners or, when turnover occurs, the collective team capacity can mitigate staffing changes within the team or within the organization.

Evidence for Implementation Teams

Implementation research has identified teams as a key ingredient for facilitating change efforts. For example, in a review of implementation frameworks, 68% ($n = 17$) of 25 frameworks identified the creation and use of an implementation team as a critical component of the implementation infrastructure to ensure quality implementation (Durlak & DuPre, 2008; Meyers, Durlak, & Wandersman, 2012). The Quality Implementation Framework (QIF) proposes implementation teams as a major structural feature for implementation (Meyers et al., 2012). Similarly, the Active Implementation Frameworks (AIF) (Fixsen, Naoom, Blase, Friedman, & Wallace, 2005; Metz, Bartley, et al., 2015; Metz & Bartley, 2012) posit that a key feature for active implementation involves building implementation teams, which – based on their collective knowledge, skills, and abilities – shepherd an innovation through the phases of implementation. Powell et al. (2015) have identified a list of discrete strategies that can serve as "building blocks" for supporting implementation efforts. Several of these strategies refer to teaming, collaboration, and inclusion of key stakeholders, including creating clinical teams, organizing clinical team meetings, creating a learning collaborative, using advisory boards and workgroups, and involving patients/consumers and family members in implementation efforts.

Research has shown that using implementation teams to actively and intentionally support change can produce higher rates of success more quickly than traditional methods of implementation that did not take such an active teaming approach. For example, a randomized controlled trial study testing the community development team (CDT) model – one model of implementation teams – across 60 sites in California and Ohio (randomized to CDT or no implementation team) found that CDT sites had more effective and efficient implementation compared to sites without implementation teams. Specifically, sites with CDTs improved rates of placements for children in foster care, the quality of implementation, and the rigor of implementation as indicated by youth more appropriately placed within care and more completion of implementation activities (Brown et al., 2014).

Chaffin et al. (2015) found that implementation teams produced sustained, high-fidelity implementation of an evidence-based practice (Safe Care) in child welfare. The study used the Interdisciplinary Collaborative Team (ICT) model to test whether seed teams designed to provide ongoing support, quality improvement, and sustainability of Safe Care could build the capacity of later cohorts to implement Safe Care with fidelity. This was confirmed through the study results. ICTs consisted of diverse membership with practice, coaching, and policy expertise. Aarons et al. (2014) also examined the role of ICTs in supporting systemwide scale-up of an evidence-based program, with a particular focus on interagency collaboration. The study identified key constructs that influence collaboration among team members including organizational culture, priorities across levels of leadership, power struggles, communication effectiveness, success in surmounting implementation challenges, and role clarity. In a recent overview of systematic reviews (Lau et al., 2015), active practice facilitation conducted by individuals or teams to support education, consensus building, goal setting, quality improvement, and problem-solving processes in healthcare organizations showed to have positive significant effects on the uptake of guidelines across multiple clinical areas. This trend was present in five included reviews, one of which found the odds of adopting clinical guidelines in primary care practice to be 2.76 times higher (95% confidence interval (CI) 2.18–3.43) for clinics that received active practice facilitation. Finally, in a systematic review of teams in health care, 72.7% of 88 studies reported significant results in positive impacts on patient or practitioner outcomes and changes in practice, knowledge, and economic outcomes attributed to the use of professional interventions, such as educational meetings, local consensus processes, or audit and feedback, embedded within teams (Medves et al., 2010).

Taken together, this recent literature reflects that the field of implementation science is beginning to recognize teams as an important lever for successful implementation. Simultaneously, there is growing interest in also testing the role of implementation teams empirically. However, the number of research studies examining the effectiveness of different types of implementation teams in facilitating implementation and high-fidelity use of evidence-based programs and practices is limited. That said, the research evidence that is available is promising, and with a growing emphasis on the operationalization of implementation strategies, such as the use of teams, there are more opportunities for conducting comparative effectiveness studies on the role of teams and specific team functions in supporting implementation.

The remaining sections of this chapter will be informed by both research and practice evidence. The authors have extensive experience in developing implementation teams, convening team meetings, and supporting team processes and functions. We will use this practice knowledge and combine it with best current evidence when sharing our learning and providing recommendations in the following.

Team Functions

As the "instrument for change" (Higgins et al., 2012) and the central body accountable for advancing implementation of an intervention, implementation teams serve a number of important core functions. Through our experience developing and using implementation teams to support implementation in organizations as well as larger systems (e.g., statewide child welfare and education systems), four core team functions have been identified. These include Core Practice, Improvement Cycles, Infrastructure, and Systems Connection (see Fig. 8.1). Below, we provide more details on each of these.

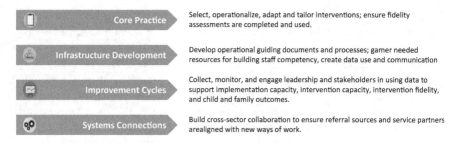

Fig. 8.1 Implementation team core functions

Core Practice

At the outset of an implementation, implementation teams provide support and direction for selecting interventions, operationalizing services or practice to be delivered, and considering potential adaptations of interventions for local contexts and populations. These activities will vary depending on whether teams have a role in selecting the intervention or whether they are charged with supporting a funder's or policymaker's selection of an intervention, which is often the case.

When teams have the ability to support the selection of interventions, teams engage in fit and feasibility assessments that examine the needs of the target population, the level of evidence of potential interventions to meet those needs, the resources that are required to implement the intervention with fidelity (e.g., training and coaching protocols), and the current capacity of the agency to do "what it takes" for effective implementation (e.g., workforce, technology, budget). Teams will often rely on staff throughout the agency to gather the information they need from administrative data systems and other evaluation activities such as community focus groups and interviews with model developers. Teams will also seek to engage stakeholders in an education and selection process (Hurlburt et al., 2014; Saldana & Chamberlain, 2012) to determine the level of buy-in and readiness among them.

In our experience working in larger systems (e.g., states, countries), localized teams (i.e., teams at the provider or agency level) often do not play a role in selecting the interventions. For example, funders or policymakers may select or mandate the use of specific interventions. In such cases, teams can still play a critical role in "preparing" relevant stakeholders and their agency by supporting capacity development, ensuring that selected interventions are well operationalized and core services identified and measurable, and by supporting the assessment of fidelity to continuously improve the intervention and its supports (Saldana & Chamberlain, 2012). Implementation teams also make data-informed decisions about productive adaptations to evidence-based interventions including culturally specific adaptations or modifications to aspects of the model that will not compromise fidelity. This process can include engaging model developers for support in using data for continuous improvement and optimization of practices.

Infrastructure Development

Implementation teams help to identify, build, and improve the implementation supports needed to build practitioner, organization, and systems capacity. Often called "implementation drivers," (Metz, Bartley, et al., 2015) implementation supports include the following:

- Competency drivers, the factors that build staff competency in the intervention – staffing, coaching, training, and fidelity assessment
- Organizational drivers, the factors that build organizational capacity to support the intervention – decision supports, data systems, facilitative administration, and systems connections

As team members seek to build the competency of practitioners to implement new practices, they work with human resources and leadership divisions to recruit and hire staff or redeploy current staff, write job descriptions, and secure training and supervision for practitioners that will support new ways of work. Implementation teams also work with agency staff and division leads to ensure that organizational supports are in place. This type of work might take the form of cowriting procedures and policies to support implementation of practices, identifying data reports that will support continuous quality improvement (CQI) activities, and communicating with collaborative partners such as referral sources on implementation progress.

Team members may have the time and expertise to conduct some of these activities themselves and in other circumstances may rely on organizational staff and leadership and systems partners to develop the infrastructure. Regardless, the implementation team attends to what is needed, looks for gaps, and tries to secure resources where possible to aid implementation efforts (Hurlburt et al., 2014). Once infrastructure is in place, the team continues to use data to ensure sustainability and create efficiencies.

Improvement Cycles

Implementation teams are responsible for supporting processes for the regular use of data for decision-making and continuous improvement. This includes working with evaluation partners, monitoring and performance divisions, and quality assurance and improvement colleagues to systematize the ongoing use of data to inform decision-making. The diverse perspectives present on an implementation team ensure that team members will have different types of questions related to implementation. For example, fiscal staff may have questions related to the cost-effectiveness of the new ways of work. Leadership may ask if child outcomes are being achieved. Supervisors may ask if additional resources are available for training and coaching practitioners and if practitioners are implementing the intervention as intended. Practitioners may focus more on day-to-day implementation activities. Are assessments completed on time? Are treatment slots available for families?

Different types of data are needed to answer these different types of questions. Implementation teams identify the questions and the data sources that can help address these questions. For example, programmatic data provide information on administrative and fiscal information (e.g., enrollment, referrals, service costs, staffing, case closures); fidelity data provide information on whether the intervention is being implemented as intended (e.g., dosage, compliance to content delivery such as a curriculum, competency indicators that demonstrate staff performance); and outcome data provide information on short-term and interim family outcomes (e.g., engagement in services, improved family cohesion, improved family functioning, decreases in risk factors), and long-term impact (e.g., well-being, improved health).

Operational learning (i.e., learning based on day-to-day activities of the organization to support service delivery) should be a core value of the implementation setting (Chambers, Glasgow, & Stange, 2014). Teams should dedicate time for reflecting or debriefing before, during, and after implementation to promote shared learning and improvements along the way (Damschroder et al., 2009). An example of how teams can support the use of data is the following five-step process:

1. *Determine Your Question:* Prioritization of improvement processes requires Implementation Teams to work together to rank key questions that guide the improvement process.
2. *Determine What Data Will Help Answer Questions:* Secondary to determining the improvement questions is the identification of data indicators and sources that will assist in answering the questions. If not already established, teams should consider developing consistent methods for gathering and sharing information with key systems stakeholders and families.
3. *Determine the Simplest Way to Gather the Data:* For improvement efforts to be useful and sustainable, they need to be feasible. Teams should consider and prioritize data sources that are available and feasible to collect.
4. *Put Systems and Structures in Place to Collect Data:* Ideally, implementation teams can facilitate the development of structures (e.g., communication processes) to support improvement processes. A learning culture is facilitated by the inclusion and participation of multiple perspectives in the CQI process (Chovil, 2009), which is why implementation teams with diverse perspectives can have major benefits at the center of improvement efforts.
5. *Analyze Data to Answer Questions:* The final step is the analysis of data. This requires that the data are synthesized and assessed through multiple perspectives. One of the essential aspects of analyzing data for improvement is to look for trends and variation in the data. It is important to note that improvements are not always focused on the intervention itself; rather the competency, organizational, or systems supports necessary to ensure effective practice and improved outcomes for children and families must also be considered.

Systems Connections

Implementation teams support the development of connections across the system with multiple relevant stakeholder groups, including government agencies, model developers, community partners, beneficiaries, and potentially with other systems. By supporting effective, bidirectional feedback loops with key partners, teams can help to improve referral systems, coordinate use of resources – particularly model-specific resources such as training – and promote learning across service providers (Saldana & Chamberlain, 2012).

Implementation teams can support these feedback loops in a few different ways such as convening meetings with various stakeholder groups on a regular basis, collecting information from stakeholders, and responding to challenges via electronic communication, or individual team members who represent different constituent groups can serve as liaisons between the team and the stakeholder groups.

Teams will need to find the least burdensome strategy for supporting effective communication, as many strategies (e.g., in-person meetings) can be time consuming for team members. Our experience in using teams to support communication points to the need for using a range of strategies such as limited in-person meetings coupled with more frequent virtual meetings.

In their role supporting systemwide communication, teams can support a practice-to-policy communication loop, which seems to be a key aspect of successful efforts to implement evidence-based programs and innovations on a scale significant to impact outcomes. In successful system change efforts, leadership teams frequently receive information about what is helping or hindering the efforts to make full and effective use of evidence at the practice level (Supplee & Metz, 2015). The information may consist of descriptions of practitioner experiences or more precise data (e.g., administrative, fidelity, survey, or focus group data). Regardless of the form of the data, based on regular feedback from the practice level, implementation teams have data that can drive their decision-making to change the service system to accommodate for new ways of work. Based on the information from practitioners, leadership can reduce systems barriers to implementation and strengthen the facilitators to achieve the desired outcomes for children and families (Fixsen, Blase, Metz, & Van Dyke, 2013). Teams can also play an important role in liaising with model developers, cocreating adaptations (Hurlburt et al., 2014), and with researchers to support translation research (Aarons, Sommerfeld, Hecht, Silovsky, & Chaffin, 2009).

Implementation Team Structures

There are several key characteristics of successful implementation teams. This section outlines the structural aspects to consider in developing and using implementation teams to support new ways of work and promote organizational and systems change in service to improved outcomes.

- *Size:* At base, an implementation team should "be as small as possible, given the work to be accomplished" (Wageman, Hackman, & Lehman, 2005, p. 4), typically including a limited number of members (e.g., between six and ten members). This promotes the availability and connectivity of the team to support the new ways of work. Members should collectively bring expertise in the intervention or practice, implementation supports such as training, supervision, and coaching, continuous quality improvement and strategies, and collaboration and systems change priorities such as regulatory, policy, and funding environments (Metz, Naoom, Halle, & Bartley, 2015). Implementation team members must have adequate full time staff effort (FTE) dedicated to actively participate as full members. This is often accomplished by including team participation in job descriptions and identifying team meetings as part of everyday duties.
- *Composition:* Teams should have a diversity of perspectives, including members from all organizational levels (Saldana & Chamberlain, 2012), such as administrative and fiscal representation, practitioners, policy staff, supervisors, and community members (Metz, Bartley, et al., 2015). Purposefully including a diversity of representation on teams has several important benefits. Diversity in perspective helps to produce a full range of complementary skills and knowledge enhancing the team's capability to effectively plan implementation activities, to anticipate and diagnose problems that emerge, and to enhance implementation over time. Moreover, inclusion of a diversity of staff roles has been found to strengthen learning among team members (Singer, Benzer, & Hamdan, 2015). Learning has been found to be a critical characteristic for retaining team members in rapidly changing systems environments (Wageman et al., 2005). Finally, change in complex systems requires buy-in from diverse stakeholders. Without diverse team membership, gaining this buy-in will be an ongoing challenge.
- *Terms of Reference:* Once formed, teams need clear guidelines establishing their scope of work and how they will achieve it (Durlak & DuPre, 2008). These guidelines are best established through the development of "terms of reference," a documented memorandum of understanding that carefully outlines the vision and purpose of the group, the scope of work and deliverables for which the group will be held accountable, roles and responsibilities for all members, communication protocols, operational processes, and decision-making authority (Metz, Bartley, et al., 2015). Terms of reference not only provide clarity on ways of work but also help to cultivate basic norms for member behavior that helps to facilitate the work (Wageman et al., 2005). Terms of reference clarify team processes such as decision-making, accountability to leadership, and specify how the implementation team relates to other groups supporting implementation (e.g., Advisory Boards and Leadership Teams). It is our experience that without such clarity, implementation teams often derail early on in the process.
- *Leadership:* In addition to terms of reference, teams need leadership, which includes a number of different elements. First, implementation teams need the support of organizational leadership, which has been identified as a key variable influencing implementation of evidence-based practices (Aarons, 2006; Li, Jeffs, Barwick, & Stevens, 2018; Moullin, Ehrhart, & Aarons, 2017). Installation of

new interventions, or improvement of those already being utilized, requires new ways of working. Implementation teams therefore need the support of leadership to make changes in context to support the intervention – such as the allocation of resources or policy changes. This implies that implementation teams depend on the participation of, or direct access to, departmental or organizational leaders who have the formal authority to initiate required context changes.

Second, the team itself needs coleadership among members. In the context of complex systems change efforts, single leaders who function as "charismatic saviors" (Higgins, Young, Weiner, & Wlodaczyk, 2009) are proving less and less effective. Instead, scholars and practitioners are focusing on models of leadership that utilize collaboration and coleadership of a team to drive organizational and systems change (Higgins et al., 2009). Leadership that is empowering of teams led to higher levels of team learning, coordination, team efficacy, and mental model development over time compared to directive leaders (Lorinkova, Pearsall, & Sims, 2013).

Case Example: Developing Implementation Teams to Support Intervention Development and Implementation

An implementation team structure was developed within a state public child welfare agency in the USA, interested in fully operationalizing its primary prevention community-based efforts to reduce child maltreatment. The agency's prevention model situates community-based centers within neighborhoods or easily accessible locations for families to access and receive needed supports. Even with over 50 community-based centers across the state, the core components and activities of the approach remained unclear. The state public agency embarked on an effort to better define the model in order to organize and ensure effective implementation supports and increase the likelihood of positive outcomes for children and families within the state. As a first step in this process, the state organized an implementation team with a range of expertise and perspectives including representatives from the state agency's program, strategic development, and data and evaluation divisions, as well as local university partners, and frontline community center staff and leadership. The team developed terms of reference that identified responsibilities, communication, expectations, and decision-making processes and authority. In addition to the implementation team, the state decided it was important for leadership to be involved and supportive; however, formal leaders from the agency were not available to participate as intensively on the implementation team as other representatives. Therefore, the state agency created a leadership team that consisted of state-level leadership who oversaw and supported the implementation team's efforts. At one point in the process of defining the model, the implementation team uncovered discrepancies in the understanding of the approach among team members. These included differing understandings of the target population, and the intended outcomes for families served through the community-based centers. The implementation team decided that these questions should be addressed by leadership. Using their bidirectional communication connections, the implementation team shared these questions with the leadership team, and the leadership team spent time developing responses to share with the center community network. This is just one example of how the teaming structure functioned. Throughout the process to better define the prevention model, the implementation team provided intensive support in coordinating efforts, giving feedback on the model definition process, and communicating with the larger community network. Feedback data gathered during this process suggest that the community-based centers were well informed and brought into the new approach because of these formal communication structures and their inclusion in the process.

Team Processes

Effective work processes are critical to the success of implementation teams and implementation research has identified specific best practices. This section describes strategies to support implementation teams in using data and information to support effective and efficient communication and feedback loops within a service system.

- *Meeting Processes:* Implementation teams should have regular, consistent meeting times and follow collaboratively developed meeting procedures that enable members to utilize meetings effectively and achieve planned objectives (Permanency Innovations Initiative Training and Technical Assistance Project, 2016).
- *Communication Processes:* A key task of an implementation team is to communicate at every phase of implementation about what is working, what is not working, and how those conclusions were drawn. Implementation teams should therefore have clear protocols for stakeholder communications that specify the various stakeholders with which the team should communicate (including other linked teams), in what circumstances the team should communicate, the type of information that should be shared, and the specific method (Metz, Bartley, et al., 2015). Communication protocols should support effective communication and feedback loops among practice, supervision, management, and leadership levels of the system (i.e., vertical feedback loops that support communication up and down a system), as well as among service partners, advocacy groups, training networks, and other collaborators (i.e., horizontal feedback loops that support communication across system sectors). Furthermore, teams should consider ways to support bidirectional communication, enabling partners and stakeholders to provide feedback on the information communicated to them and creating broad engagement in the implementation.

WHO should be communicating?	ABOUT WHAT should we be communicating?	HOW OFTEN should we communicate?
• Your team • Vertical team connections • Horizontal team connections 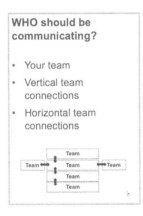	• What is working • What is not working • What we know and what we don't • And how we know that	• Regularly • Using formal process • Opportunities for change 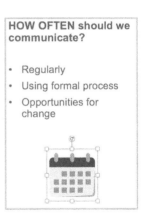

Fig. 8.2 Communication processes

Figure 8.2 provides an overview of key communication processes of teams.

Communication has been demonstrated to be crucial to successful implementation, and frequent and inclusive communication established as a key factor of successful implementation, while limited and exclusive communication has been shown to negatively impact implementation efforts (Hurlburt et al., 2014). For example, frequent communication can help to diminish power imbalances that can occur through informal discussions and sidebar conversations not transparent or inclusive of all stakeholders. Further, stakeholders are more likely to persevere in the face of implementation challenges (Aarons et al., 2014), when early implementation successes are shared, making communication about the achievement of implementation milestones especially important with cross-sector partners.

- *Data Reflection Processes:* Because a core function of an implementation team is using data to make decisions and improve implementation elements and processes (outlined in detail in the core functions section below), teams should also have clearly defined continuous quality improvement processes, such as "plan, do, study, act," explored in detail in the data use section (Metz, Bartley, et al., 2015).
- *Member Engagement Processes:* Research suggests that team members are more likely to stay committed to team participation if they experience opportunities of growth and learning. These findings suggest that for teams to produce the greatest learning and growth for members, teams should provide opportunities for coleadership and peer-to-peer coaching, as well as task-related learning (Higgins et al., 2009). In a study of stakeholder engagement to support the use of evidence-based practices in a public child welfare system, Metz and Bartley (2016) confirm and extend these results by demonstrating that implementation team members were more likely to feel committed and engaged in the change process when they were provided with opportunities to participate in joint prototyping of tools and resources with other team members.

Implementation Team Member Competencies

The development of effective implementation teams requires implementation specialists and technical assistance providers who have the skills and abilities to support team development and improvement in typical service settings. *Technical assistance providers* build the capacity for the service and system changes needed to enable the use of evidence-based approaches. *Implementation specialist* is a term often used to denote technical assistance providers who integrate a range of implementation conceptual models, frameworks, and strategies as part of their technical assistance activities.

There is increasing attention in the literature to specific competencies needed to facilitate implementation and broker knowledge (Berta et al., 2015; Bornbaum, Kornas, Peirson, & Rosella, 2015). Table 8.1 outlines the three major areas and competencies needed for implementation specialists – professionals working to facilitate practice, organizational, and systems change to enhance the use of evidence and of innovations aimed at improving outcomes (Metz, Louison, Ward, & Burk, 2017). While it is probably not realistic that all team members will possess all the skills and competencies described, it is beneficial to have team members who can contribute to the range of skills and competencies needed to support implementation.

These skills and competencies are described as essential functions that detail a range of activities implementation specialists conduct as they provide implementation support to develop teams and facilitate change efforts. Skills and competencies were identified through a multistep methodology including a targeted literature review on relevant team building skills and competencies, an additional document review, interviews with implementation specialists and team members, and a vetting and consensus building process (see Metz, 2016 for a more detailed description of the methodology used to develop practice profiles).

The targeted literature review was conducted to identify skills and abilities required for professionals supporting change efforts. Literature was reviewed across a range of areas where professionals working within these areas would typically support implementation. These areas included technical assistance, team science, community organizing, network development, the role of intermediaries, and cocreation/coproduction. Literature included peer-reviewed publications and gray literature (e.g., white papers, evaluations, working papers, conference proceedings). Materials were initially coded for whether they identified activities, skills, or abilities related to professionals supporting change. References to skill and abilities were limited; however, references to specific activities were more common. Materials were then inductively coded for themes by three reviewers. The three reviewers convened to build consensus on the codes, reduce the number of codes, and categorize the codes by domains. Additional documents were then reviewed deductively to provide additional information for identified themes by domain. Additional documents included a task analysis of intermediary organizations that support implementation of evidence-based practices, as well as logic models and

Table 8.1 Implementation specialist practice profile

Cocreation: Implementation specialists support the active involvement of stakeholders in all stages of the production and implementation process, resulting in service models, approaches, and practices that are contextualized and tailored to settings (Metz & Bartley, 2015; Vargo & Lusch, 2004).

The goal of contextualization is to ensure there is a match between the program or practice and the values, needs, skills, and resources of those delivering interventions, systems stakeholders, and service beneficiaries (Horner et al., 2014)

Essential functions that support cocreation include colearning, brokering, addressing power differentials, codesign, and tailored support

Essential function	Core activities
Colearning – Work collaboratively with systems stakeholders to learn how applied knowledge on how implementation science can be effectively used in the local context. Implementation specialists are open to learning about the history and current priorities in the local context in order to assess the most feasible and relevant uses of implementation science	Understand the system and organizational context and culture
	Create spaces for new ideas to emerge (space can be created through asking questions and structured facilitation processes; and physically created through meeting places and room setup)
	Negotiate, build trust and respect for all perspectives
	Communicate and listen for the purpose of mutual understanding and for collaborative integration of different knowledge perspectives
	Seek ways to introduce and get buy-in for an implementation science approach that fits with existing programs, practices, and processes
	Synthesize diverse perspectives of thought, and check for understanding
	Seek opportunities to reflect on the problem, the implementation specialist's personal experience, and the intention and interaction with others
	Support collaborative implementation planning
Brokering – Enable knowledge exchange and sharing among stakeholders to increase the understanding of diverse perspectives and increase the application of implementation science to improve outcomes	Connect otherwise disconnected individuals or groups in the system by providing advice and serving as a relational resource...
	Position themselves "in between" people or groups in a system network who are disconnected but whose connections are vital for the success of the change effort
	Share evidence and data and promote opportunities for stakeholders and team members to engage with others in the use of data

(continued)

Table 8.1 (continued)

Address power differentials – Address power imbalances between community members, stakeholders in the wider system, technical assistance providers, and researchers, by building trust, supporting two-way communication, cultivating opportunities for mutual consultation, and identifying many accountabilities.	Include diverse expertise in team discussions
	Position the range of service beneficiary experiences at the center of decision-making and implementation activities..
	Recognize and acknowledge loss of status and authority that can impede buy-in and engagement
	Develop an evolving "collective view" or "shared understanding," rather than pushing for consensus which is often artificial and perpetuates power structures
Codesign – Codesign tools, resources, and models through iterative processes and consensus building.	Codesign tools, products, processes, governance structures, service models, and policy
	Facilitate design-centered activities that use collective sense-making and negotiation
	Conduct cyclical tests of change to iteratively improve prototypes of tools, products, and processes to support implementation efforts.
	Ongoing testing and improving of tools, products, processes, governance structures, service models, and policy to support implementation efforts
Tailored support – Frequency, duration, and intensity of implementation supports depend on the needs, goals, and context of the implementation team and systems stakeholders. Implementation specialists refrain from assumptions that a certain level and type of support is always needed.	Assess and agree to the implementation support to be made available to each individual site and/or collectively to a number of sites
	Schedule virtual and onsite meetings based on the goals of the team and stakeholders
	Tailor support based on "just in time" needs of the team and systems stakeholders
	Assess the effectiveness of the level of support in meeting needs, goals, and context of the implementation effort
Ongoing improvement: Implementation specialists support the use of quantitative and qualitative feedback at each stage of implementation accompanied with regular personal, team, and stakeholder debriefings to support improvement (Damschroder et al., 2009). Ongoing improvement includes dedicating time for reflecting or debriefing to promote shared learning and improvements along the way. Ongoing feedback on interventions and approaches should use practical, relevant measures of progress and relevance, and organizational learning should be a core value of the implementation setting	
Essential functions that support ongoing improvement include assessing need and context, applying and integrating implementation science approaches, and conducting improvement cycles	

Essential function	Core activities
Assess need and context – Work with stakeholders to understand population and community needs and the extent to which potential interventions meet identified needs for particular target populations. Support assessments of contextual fit between proposed interventions/approaches and the local service settings before moving forward with implementation. Value the perspectives of multiple stakeholders when identifying the problem space and considering alternatives for addressing problems and improving outcomes.	Clarify stakeholder needs and expectations to help stakeholders understand each other's perspectives regarding the problem to be addressed
	Use data-driven inquiry methods to support "discovery" processes (e.g., needs assessment data, stakeholder analysis, mapping of existing services, initiative inventory)
	Use and/or conduct evidence reviews to determine the relevance and fit of identified interventions and approaches with identified needs
	Assess the contextual fit of the proposed intervention(s)/approach(es) with the values, needs, skills, and resources available in the service setting
	Identify and respond to other changes in the system which could affect implementation
	Identify and support mitigating actions to manage risks and assumptions for the change effort (e.g., assumptions regarding resources, commitments, or buy-in; risks or loss for different stakeholders)
	Involve stakeholders in identifying and understanding the implications and consequences of change efforts
	Work with stakeholders to build strong contextual fit before moving forward with implementation efforts
	Assess the contextual fit of the proposed intervention(s)/approach(es) with the current political, funding and systems and organizational landscape

(continued)

Table 8.1 (continued)

Apply and integrate implementation science approaches – Apply and integrate appropriate implementation science approaches by using systems thinking, participatory methods, and knowledge management and exchange (Bammer, 2005). Systems thinking involves examining how implementation efforts fit within a whole system and choosing appropriate implementation approaches that will address these whole systems issues. Participatory methods recognize that key stakeholders should contribute to choosing implementation approaches. Knowledge management and exchange includes summarizing and synthesizing how a range of implementation approaches address critical issues in order to make informed choices about the approach that will be most suitable for a particular context or setting.	Remain up to date on implementation science concepts, frameworks, and research
	Assess and make judgments about appropriate implementation approaches for different contexts and settings
	Include stakeholders in decision-making regarding the selection of the implementation approach by sharing knowledge and resources
	Apply and integrate implementation approaches, tools, and resources in different service and policy settings
Conduct improvement cycles – Use data throughout implementation to purposefully reexamine implementation processes and continuously improve practice, organization, and systems changes. Through the ongoing use of data, implementation specialists conduct cyclical tests of change to ensure iterative improvements in implementation processes.	Gather and use quantitative and qualitative feedback about the progress and quality of implementation accompanied with regular personal and team debriefings to support improvement (Damschroder et al., 2009)
	Embed processes for data to be collected, analyzed, and reported frequently as a way to monitor progress and to make decisions about the ongoing planning, implementation, and outcomes of an intervention/approach (Chinman, Imm, & Wandersman, 2004)
	Ensure that implementation teams have access to valid and reliable data on how the intervention/approach and implementation infrastructure supports are functioning to guide decision-making along the way
	Develop capacity to assess and use data for decision-making through modeling, instruction, and coaching
	Dedicate time for reflecting or debriefing throughout implementation as a strategy to promote shared learning and improvements along the way
	Use feedback loops that connect policy and practice, identify and address implementation barriers, and ensure that improvements made during implementation are communicated to all stakeholders
	Support implementation teams to prioritize needs, challenges, or problems to be addressed through the use of data

Sustaining change: Implementation specialists support the sustainability of interventions and approaches by developing a shared vision and mutual accountability, building on existing relationships, problem-solving and resource sharing, and maintaining collaboration over time (Green et al., 2016). Implementation specialists seek to understand and address the dynamic changes that occur over time in the use of interventions/approaches, the characteristics of the practice settings, and broader system that establishes how services are delivered (Chambers, Glasgow, & Stange 2014). Sustainability has evolved from being considered as the endgame of a translational process to a suggested "adaptation phase" that integrates and institutionalizes interventions within local organizational and cultural contexts.

Interventions and approaches are classified as sustained when the core elements are maintained or delivered with integrity after initial implementation support has been withdrawn, and adequate capacity exists to continue maintaining these core elements (Stirman et al., 2012).

Essential functions that support sustaining change include growing and sustaining relationships, building capacity, cultivating leadership, and facilitation

Essential function	Core activities
Grow and sustain relationships – Grow and sustain diverse, authentic, respectful, and trusting relationships with stakeholders to guide and support implementation and systems change efforts	Build trust with others by modeling transparent action and accountability
	Engage in ongoing self-assessment and diagnostic assessment of relationship strengths and weaknesses
	Encourage and make use of feedback to strengthen relationships
	Regulate distress in relationships by creating space for stakeholders to discuss challenges and dispute assumptions when conflict emerges
	Work with stakeholders to assess capacity strengths and needs related to mission and goals
Build capacity	Provide or secure training needed for partners to gain capacity and connect with others who can provide training, modeling, and coaching
Increase the knowledge, skills, motivation, and attitudes to achieve their mission and goals	
Successful capacity building includes attention to all types of capacity (psychological, behavioral, and structural), all levels of the system (individual, organization, network, and system). This includes the following:	Model the use of knowledge, skills, behaviors, attitudes, and practices for stakeholders to demonstrate application in a real-world setting
Intervention/approach-specific capacity: The knowledge, skills, motivation, and attitudes about a specific intervention or challenge, such as an understanding of successful evidence-based program (Flaspohler, Duffy, Wandersman, Stillman, & Maras, 2008)..	Coach stakeholders' use of knowledge, skills, behaviors, attitudes, and practices in their daily work, so that partners can gain confidence and competency

(continued)

Table 8.1 (continued)

General capacity: The knowledge, skills, motivation, and attitudes required for overall functioning and achievement, such as bookkeeping (Flaspohler et al., 2008)	Build individual, organizational, and network capacity to respond to future external and internal changes
Analytic capacity: The knowledge, skills, motivation, and attitudes to gather information about a problem, analyze patterns and dynamics, and reflect critically on root causes and potential solutions (Sorgenfrei & Wrigley, 2005)	Identify and implement organizational processes and structures to develop implementation capacity (e.g., human resources, technology)
Adaptive capacity: The knowledge, skills, motivation, and attitudes to adjust actions and strategy in response to analysis (Sorgenfrei & Wrigley, 2005)	Identify and exploit opportunities to build systemwide capacity which will support implementation
Cultivate leadership	Identify emerging and existing leaders in community and/or system through the use of power analysis or systems mapping tools for this purpose
Identify and strengthen leaders to be systems leaders who work across organization and system boundaries and silos	Use appreciative inquiry and reflection techniques to help leaders assess their roles and capacity within the system
Successful leadership cultivation intentionally fosters space for new and emerging leaders, particularly those without historic or current access to power	Support emerging or growing leaders to share responsibilities, such as cofacilitating meetings, so that leaders can gain confidence and competency
	When leadership transitions occur, implementation specialists work with stakeholders to provide planning, continuity, analysis, and support as needed to ease the transition
Facilitation – Enable a process of participatory problem-solving and support that occurs in the context of a recognized need for improvement and supportive interpersonal relationships. Successful facilitation promotes cycles of "mutual consultations" among stakeholders to ensure that different forms of knowledge and ways of knowing are integrated into planning and solutions (Powell et al., 2015). Implementation specialists are guided by four core values for participant engagement (Kaner, 2014):	Serve as formal and informal facilitators as determined by analysis of context and strategy
Full participation where all stakeholders are encouraged to share their perspectives,	Support a balance of divergent and convergent thinking among team members, depending on the type of challenge faced

Mutual understanding where stakeholders accept the legitimacy of one another's needs and goals,	For easily named and easily solved challenges (technical challenges), support stakeholders to evaluate alternatives, summarize key points, sort ideas into categories, and exercise judgment
Inclusive solutions that emerge from the integration of everybody's perspectives and needs	For complex challenges with no easy solution (adaptive challenges), support stakeholders to generate alternatives, free flow open discussion, gather diverse points of view, and suspend judgment
Shared responsibility of stakeholders to implement proposals they endorse and to give and receive input before final decisions are made	Create welcoming spaces for all participants in meetings
	Select and use structured facilitation method ahead of group discussion, depending on the type of challenge, to ensure that appropriate strategies are used to address different types of problems
	Support a communication protocol and process that facilitates interactions among stakeholders

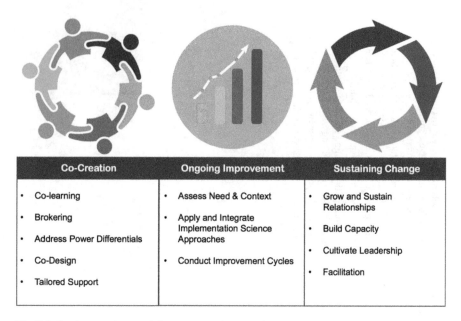

Co-Creation	Ongoing Improvement	Sustaining Change
• Co-learning • Brokering • Address Power Differentials • Co-Design • Tailored Support	• Assess Need & Context • Apply and Integrate Implementation Science Approaches • Conduct Improvement Cycles	• Grow and Sustain Relationships • Build Capacity • Cultivate Leadership • Facilitation

Fig. 8.3 Implementation specialist competencies overview

theories of change for projects within the reviewers' research center. Following the literature and document reviews, an interview protocol was developed to assess the validity of the identified themes and to gather more detailed information. Group interviews and vetting and consensus building were conducted with staff from two nongovernmental agencies (US-based and European-based) that support implementation of evidence and innovations at scale to achieve outcomes. Usability testing will be conducted with up to nine international nongovernmental organizations reflecting on these skills and competencies to validate the content.

The findings from our literature and document review and interviews demonstrate that implementation specialists conduct a range of activities to provide implementation support; three major areas of support emerged, including cocreation, ongoing improvement, and sustaining change (Fig. 8.3).

Within each of these areas, essential functions and activities are operationalized.

- *Cocreation:* Implementation specialists support the active involvement of stakeholders in all stages of the production and implementation process resulting in service models, approaches, and practices that are contextualized and tailored to settings (Metz & Bartley, 2016; Vargo & Lusch, 2004). The goal of contextualization is to ensure there is a match between programs and practices and the values, needs, skills, and resources of those delivering interventions/approaches, systems stakeholders, and service beneficiaries (Horner, Blitz, & Ross, 2014).

Essential functions that support cocreation include colearning, brokering, realigning power structures, codesign, and tailored support.

- *Ongoing Improvement:* Implementation specialists support the use of quantitative and qualitative feedback at each stage of implementation, through regular individual, team, and stakeholder debriefings to support improvement (Damschroder et al., 2009). Ongoing improvement includes dedicating time for reflecting or debriefing to promote shared learning and improvements along the way. Ongoing feedback on interventions and approaches should use practical, relevant measures of progress and relevance, and organizational learning should be a core value of the implementation setting. Essential functions that support ongoing improvement include assessing need and context, applying and integrating implementation science approaches, and conducting improvement cycles.

- *Sustaining Change:* Implementation specialists support the sustainability of interventions and approaches by developing a shared vision and mutual accountability, building on existing relationships, problem-solving, and resource sharing, and maintaining collaboration over time (Green et al., 2016). Implementation specialists seek to understand and address the dynamic changes that occur over time in the use of interventions/approaches, the characteristics of the practice settings, and broader system that establishes how services are delivered (Chambers et al., 2014). Sustainability has evolved from being considered as the endgame of a translational process to a suggested "adaptation phase" that integrates and institutionalizes interventions within local organizational and cultural contexts. Interventions and approaches are classified as sustained when the core elements are maintained or delivered with integrity after initial implementation support has been withdrawn, and adequate capacity exists to continue maintaining these core elements (Stirman, et al., 2012). Essential functions that support sustaining change include growing and sustaining relationships, building capacity, cultivating leadership, and facilitation.

Individual team member learning has been found to be an important dimension of team effectiveness. Implementation specialists can use the identified skills and competencies to support team learning and task completion. Concurrently, implementation specialists can seek to develop these same skills and competencies with team members, so that implementation teams can continue to support change efforts beyond a team's initial formation and development.

Conclusion

This chapter provided suggestions for how to form, utilize, and develop implementation teams, so that they can add value to the implementation of evidence-based approaches in real-world service settings. Implementation in usual care and typical service settings is complex and dynamic, and many factors can hinder and halter meaningful change efforts. Implementation teams can assist in mitigating some of these pervasive challenges and increase an organization's absorptive capacity for the use of research evidence in practice.

Implementation teams differ from workgroups in a variety of distinct ways, most related to their direct role and accountability for supporting new ways of work and engaging with system partners to promote transformation. The size, composition, organization, and connection to leadership are important structural considerations in team development. Teams lead essential communication and facilitation processes that support the alignment and coordination between multiple actors and staff within an organization and system. Without the coordination leveraged by implementation teams, leaders and staff are often isolated and reactive in their communication and engagement efforts.

Individual team members may not be doing all of the activities associated with implementation themselves, however team members are responsible for identifying and securing resources when needed. This means that the role of implementation team members often involves facilitation, relationship development, and brokering skills. Many of these skills are used by teams as they carry out the core components of team functioning. Implementation teams include a diverse array of stakeholder perspectives. The involvement of multiple systems partners is best achieved using high functioning implementation teams.

While the research evidence for implementation teams is still limited, the review of current literature points to how implementation teams are part of conceptual frameworks, indicating that the field of implementation science is beginning to recognize teams as an important lever for implementation success. Further opportunities exist for conducting comparative effectiveness research on the role and contributions of teams and their specific functions in supporting implementation. To conduct this applied research on the use and benefits of implementation, teams will be necessary to better understand how we can scale and sustain evidence to improve population outcomes.

References

Aarons, G. A. (2006). Transformational and transactional leadership: Association with attitudes toward evidence-based practice. *Psychiatric Services, 57*(8), 1162–1169.

Aarons, G. A., Sommerfeld, D. H., Hecht, D. B., Silovsky, J. F., & Chaffin, M. J. (2009). The impact of evidence-based practice implementation and fidelity monitoring on staff turnover: Evidence for a protective effect. *Journal of Consulting and Clinical Psychology, 77*(2), 270–280.

Aarons, G. A., Fettes, D., Hurlburt, M., Palinkas, L., Gunderson, L., Willging, C., & Chaffin, M. (2014). Collaboration, negotiation, and coalescence for interagency-collaborative teams to scale-up evidence-based practice. *Journal of Clinical Child and Adolescent Psychology, 43*(6), 915–928.

Bammer, G. (2005). Integration and implementation sciences: Building a new specialization. *Ecology and Society, 10*(2), 6.

Berta, W., Cranley, L., Dearing, J.W., Dogherty, E.J., Squires, J.E., & Estabrooks, C.A. (2015). Why (we think) facilitation works: Insights from organizational learning theory.

Implementation Science, 10. Retrieved online: https://implementationscience.biomedcentral.com/articles/10.1186/s13012-015-0323-0.

Bornbaum, C.C., Kornas, K., Peirson, L., & Rosella, L.C. (2015). Exploring the function and effectiveness of knowledge brokers as facilitators of knowledge translation in health-related settings: A systematic review and thematic analysis. Implementation Science, 10. Retrieved online: https://implementationscience.biomedcentral.com/articles/10.1186/s13012-015-0351-9.

Brown, C.H., Chamberlain, P., Saldana, L., Padgett, C, Wang, W., & Cruden G. (2014). Evaluation of two implementation strategies in 51 child county public service systems in two states: Results of a cluster randomized head-to-head implementation trial. Implementation Science, 9. Retrieved online: https://www.springermedizin.de/evaluation-of-two-implementation-strategies-in-51-child-county-p/9772796.

Chaffin, M., Hecht, D., Aarons, G., Fettes, D., Hurlburt, M., & Ledesma, K. (2015). EBT fidelity trajectories across training cohorts using the interagency collaborative team strategy. Administration and Policy in Mental Health, 144–156.

Chambers, D. A., Glasgow, R. E., & Stange, K. C. (2014). The dynamic sustainability framework: Addressing the paradox of sustainment amid ongoing change. Implementation Science 8(1), 117. Retrieved online: https://implementationscience.biomedcentral.com/articles/10.1186/1748-5908-8-117.

Chinman, M., Imm, P., & Wandersman, A. (2004). Getting to outcomes 2004: Promoting accountability through methods and tools for planning, implementation, and evaluation (technical report). Santa Monica, CA: RAND Corporation.

Chovil, N. (2009). One small step at a time: Implementing continuous quality improvement in child and youth mental health services. Child and Youth Services, 31, 21–34.

Damschroder, L. J., Aron, D. C., Keith, R. E., Kirsh, S. R., Alexander, J. A., & Lowery, J. C. (2009). Fostering implementation of health services research findings into practice: A consolidated framework for advancing implementation science. Implementation Science, 4, 1–15. https://doi.org/10.1186/1748-5908-4-50

Durlak, J. A., & DuPre, E. P. (2008). Implementation matters: A review of research on the influence of implementation on program outcomes and the factors affecting implementation. American Journal of Community Psychology, 41, 327–350.

Fixsen, D. L., Naoom, S. F., Blase, K. A., Friedman, R. M., & Wallace, F. (2005). Implementation research: A synthesis of the literature (FMHI publication no. 231). Tampa, FL: University of South Florida, Louis de la Parte Florida Mental Health Institute, National Implementation Network.

Fixsen, D., Blase, K., Metz, A., & Van Dyke, M. (2013). Statewide implementation of evidence-based programs. Exceptional Children, 79, 213–230.

Flaspohler, P., Duffy, J., Wandersman, A., Stillman, L., & Maras, M. A. (2008). Unpacking prevention capacity: An intersection of research-to-practice models and community-centered models. American Journal of Community Psychology, 41, 182–196. https://doi.org/10.1007/s10464-008-9162-3

Green, A. E., Trott, E., Willging, C. E., Finn, N. K., Ehrhart, M. G., & Aarons, G. A. (2016). The role of collaborations in sustaining and evidence-based intervention to reduce child neglect. Child Abuse and Neglect, 53, 4–16.

Higgins, M. C., Young, L., Weiner, J., & Wlodaczyk, S. (2009). Leading teams of leaders: What helps team member learning? The Phi Delta Kappan, 91, 41–45.

Higgins, M. C., Weiner, J., & Young, L. (2012). Implementation teams: A new lever for organizational change. Journal of Organizational Behavior, 33, 366–388.

Horner, R., Blitz, C., & Ross, S. W. (2014). Investing in what works issue brief: The role of contextual fit when implementing evidence-based interventions. Washington, DC: American Institutes for Research. Retrieved from https://www.cde.state.co.us/cdesped/eec2015_day01_breakoutc_ebp_issuebrief

Hurlburt, M., Aarons, G. A., Fettes, D., Willging, C., Gunderson, L., & Chaffin, M. J. (2014). Interagency collaborative team model for capacity building to scale-up evidence-based practice. *Children and Youth Services Review, 39*, 160–168.

Joiner, T. A. (2007). Total quality management and performance: The role of organization support and coworker support. *International Journal of Quality & Reliability Management, 24*, 617–627.

Kaner, S. (2014). *Facilitator's guide to participatory decision-making* (3rd ed.). San Francisco: Jossey Bass.

Lau, R., Stevenson, F., Ong, B. N., Dziedzic, K., Treweek, S., Eldridge, S., … Peacock, R. (2015). Achieving change in primary care-effectiveness of strategies for improving implementation of complex interventions: Systematic review of reviews. *BMJ Open, 5*(12), e009993.

Lessard, S., Bareil, C., Lalonde, L., Duhamel, F., Hudon, E.,….Levesque, L. (2016). External facilitators and interprofessional facilitation teams: A qualitative study of their roles in supporting practice change. Implementation Science, 11, 97. Retrieved online: https://implementation-science.biomedcentral.com/articles/10.1186/s13012-016-0458-7.

Li, S. A., Jeffs, L., Barwick, M., & Stevens, B. (2018). Organizational contextual features that influence the implementation of evidence-based practices across healthcare settings: A systematic integrative review. *Systematic Reviews, 7*(1), 72.

Lorinkova, N. M., Pearsall, M. J., & Sims, H. P. (2013). Examining the differential longitudinal performance of directive versus empowering leadership in teams. *Academy of Management Journal, 56*(2), 573–596.

Medves, J., Godfrey, C., Turner, C., Paterson, M., Harrison, M., MacKenzie, L., & Durando, P. (2010). Systematic review of practice guideline dissemination and implementation strategies for healthcare teams and team-based practice. *International Journal of Evidence-Based Healthcare, 8*, 79–89.

Metz, A. (2016). *Practice profiles: A process for capturing evidence and operationalizing innovations*. Chapel Hill, NC: National Implementation Research Network, University of North Carolina at Chapel Hill.

Metz, A., & Bartley, L. (2012). Active implementation frameworks for program success: How to use implementation science to improve outcomes for children. *Zero to Three Journal, 34*(4), 11–18.

Metz, A., & Bartley, L. (2015). Co-creating the conditions to sustain the use of research evidence in public child welfare. *Child Welfare, 94*(2), 115.

Metz, A., & Bartley, L. (2016). Co-creating the conditions to sustain the use of research evidence in public child welfare. *Child Welfare, 94*, 115–139.

Metz, A., Bartley, L., Ball, H., Wilson, D., Naoom, S., & Redmond, P. (2015). Active implementation frameworks for successful service delivery: Catawba County child wellbeing project. *Research on Social Work Practice, 25*, 415–422.

Metz, A., Naoom, S. F., Halle, T., & Bartley, L. (2015). *An integrated stage-based framework for implementation of early childhood programs and systems (OPRE Research Brief 2015–48)*. Washington, DC: Office of Planning, Research and Evaluation, Administration for Children and Families, U.S. Department of Health and Human Services.

Metz, A., Louison, L., Ward, C., & Burke, K. (2017). *Active implementation practitioner profile. The National Implementation Research Network*. Chapel Hill, NC: University of North Carolina.

Meyers, D. C., Durlak, J. A., & Wandersman, A. (2012). The quality implementation framework: A synthesis of critical steps in the implementation process. *American Journal of Community Psychology, 50*(3–4), 462–480.

Moullin, J. C., Ehrhart, M. G., & Aarons, G. A. (2017). The role of leadership in organizational implementation and sustainment in service agencies. *Research on Social Work Practice*. 1049731517718361.

Neilsen, K., Randall, R., & Christensen. (2017). Do different training conditions facilitate team implementation? A quasi-experimental mixed methods study. *Journal of Mixed Methods Research, 11*, 223–245.

Permanency Innovations Initiative Training and Technical Assistance Project. (2016). *Guide to developing, implementing, and assessing an innovation.* Washington, DC: U.S. Department of Health and Human Services, Administration for Children and Families, Children's Bureau.

Powell, B. J., Waltz, T. J., Chinman, M. J., Damschroder, L. J., Smith, J. L., Matthieu, M. M., … Kirchner, J. E. (2015). A refined compilation of implementation strategies: Results from the expert recommendations for implementation (ERIC) project. *Implementation Science, 10*, 21.

Rycroft-Malone, J., Seers, K., Chandler, J., Hawkes, C. A., Crichton, N., Allen, C., … Strunin, L. (2013). The role of evidence, context, and facilitation in an implementation trial: Implications for the development of the PARIHS framework. *Implementation Science, 8*, 28.

Singer, S. J., Benzer, J. K., & Hamdan, S. U. (2015). Improving health care quality and safety: The role of collective learning. *Journal of Healthcare Leadership, 7*, 91.

Saldana, L., & Chamberlain, P. (2012). Supporting implementation: The role of community development teams to build infrastructure. *American Journal of Community Psychology, 50*, 334–346.

Sorgenfrei, M., & Wrigley, R. (2005). *Building analytical and adaptive capacities for organizational effectiveness.* Oxford, UK: INTRAC.

Sprigg, C., Jackson, P., & Parker, S. (2000). Production teamworking: The importance of interdependence and autonomy for employee strain and satisfaction. *Human Relations, 53*, 1519–1543.

Stirman, S. W., Kimberly, J., Cook, N., Calloway, A., Castro, F., & Charns, M. (2012). The sustainability of new programs and innovations: a review of the empirical literature and recommendations for future research. *Implementation science, 7*(1), 17.

Supplee, L., & Metz, A. (2015). Opportunities and challenges in evidence-based social policy. *Social Policy Report, 28*(4), 1–16.

Vargo, S. L., & Lusch, R. F. (2004). Evolving to a new dominant logic for marketing. *Journal of Marketing, 68*(1), 1–17. https://doi.org/10.1509/jmkg.68.1.1.24036

Wageman, R., Hackman, J. R., & Lehman, E. V. (2005). Team diagnostic survey: Development of an instrument. *The Journal of Applied Behavioral Science, 41*(4), 1–27.

Chapter 9
Advancing Implementation Science Measurement

Cara C. Lewis and Caitlin Dorsey

Advancing Implementation Science Measurement[1]

Regardless of the field of study, measurement is perhaps one of the most challenging components of research design and simultaneously the most important, given that "science is measurement" (Siegel, 1964). With implementation science in its infancy, the field is beset with measurement issues that stunt the growth of its advancing knowledge base. In order to confidently test hypotheses, implementation scientists must hone in on key constructs for evaluation and then identify existing measures that exhibit strong psychometric properties and are feasible and appropriate to the context. Consider the following *Vignette 1*:

Dr. I. Care About Psychometrics was writing a grant proposal in which she intended to compare the effectiveness of standardized versus tailored approaches to implementing measurement-based care (MBC) for depression in community mental health settings. Loosely guided by the Exploration, Preparation, Implementation and Sustainment (EPIS) Framework (Aarons et al., 2012), Dr. Psychometrics hypothesized that contextual factors (e.g., organizational readiness, culture, and climate), as

---

[1] Refer Glossary on Page 247

C. C. Lewis (✉)
Kaiser Permanente Washington Health Research Institute,
MacColl Center for Healthcare Innovation, Seattle, WA, USA

Department of Psychiatry and Behavioral Sciences, School of Medicine,
University of Washington, Seattle, WA, USA
e-mail: Cara.C.Lewis@kp.org

C. Dorsey
Kaiser Permanente Washington Health Research Institute,
MacColl Center for Healthcare Innovation, Seattle, WA, USA
e-mail: Caitlin.N.Dorsey@kp.org

© Springer Nature Switzerland AG 2020
B. Albers et al. (eds.), *Implementation Science 3.0*,
https://doi.org/10.1007/978-3-030-03874-8_9

well as practitioner attitudes, would mediate the success of the tailored condition on MBC fidelity and penetration. She had discovered many organization-level assessments and practitioner attitudinal measures in her literature search; however, she was under a tight deadline and not able to investigate their psychometric properties as carefully as she would have liked. Fortunately, her colleague, a seasoned implementation scientist, narrowed her search and recommended using the Texas Christian University Organizational Readiness for Change (TCU-ORC; Lehman, Greener, & Simpson, 2002) and the Evidence-Based Practice Attitudes Scale (EBPAS; Aarons, 2004). Her quick scan of the literature demonstrated that both had been used significantly in previous studies (e.g., TCU-ORC = 570 citations; EBPAS = 569 citations), which she believed suggested that these measures must have at least reasonable psychometric strength, and both offered national (United States of America) norms to which she could compare her sample. Dr. Psychometrics was somewhat concerned about the number of items in the two measures (TCU-ORC = 129 items; EBPAS = 18 items), but she felt that she could justify this combined survey length to reviewers.

As the *Vignette 1* highlights, the challenges faced by Dr. Psychometrics and implementation scientists more broadly include (a) selecting a theory to guide one's work; (b) honing in on key constructs for evaluation; (c) deciding upon key measurement approaches (e.g., quantitative, qualitative or mixed methods); (d) locating existing measures from the expansive literature landscape; (e) assessing the quality of existing measures to select the optimal instrument or determining an alternative approach when no measures exist; and (f) (potentially) refining measurement to limit investigator and respondent burden and maximizing relevance. These measurement challenges are often amplified in the case of new fields (Martinez, Lewis, & Weiner, 2014). However, significant progress has been made in the past decade to assuage many of these measurement issues in implementation science. For instance, a comprehensive review of models, frameworks, and theories was conducted by Tabak, Khoong, Chambers, & Brownson in 2012 and an associated interactive website was created to help researchers select from the 60+ that exist (http://www.dissemination-implementation.org/content/aboutUs.aspx). Additionally, careful guidance is available regarding when, why, and how mixed methods may be appropriate for an implementation study (Palinkas et al., 2010). Furthermore, a recent review of measurement resources directs researchers to the numerous systematic reviews and living web-based repositories for ease of access to existing measures (Rabin et al., 2016); these same resources typically provide some kind of assessment of the measure's psychometric properties. Moreover, new, high-quality measures are published each month (e.g., Aarons, Ehrhart, & Farahnak, 2014; Ehrhart, Aarons, & Farahnak, 2014), filling the gaps that are revealed by systematic reviews. Most recently, the pragmatic measures construct is gaining traction as a critical feature of measures that highlights the importance of limiting burden and producing actionable results, for example (Glasgow & Riley, 2013; Boyd et al., 2017). We raised these issues in *Vignette 1* and begin this chapter by highlighting key resources for the reader, given that these are often the most salient measurement issues to implementation scientists. However, consistent with the mission of this book, this chapter will prioritize a new set of issues inherent to Dr. Psychometrics' situation that have received little attention in the extant literature. That is, despite this exceptional progress made in a relatively short period of time, the potential to advance the field of implementation science remains limited by several critical unaddressed questions. The field needs to come together on solutions in order to advance cumulative knowledge and ensure that our science efficiently informs the practice of implementation.

The ultimate goal of our field's science is to identify effective and efficient strategies to support community/provider agencies to integrate evidence-based practices (PAR-13-055: Dissemination and Implementation Research in Health (R01) n.d.) and/or improve service delivery through data-based decision-making (e.g., Johnson, Collins, & Wandersman, 2013). To maximize the impact of our work and achieve this lofty goal, implementation stakeholders (i.e., those engaged in and affected by the practice of implementation) such as policy-makers, agency administrators, or intermediaries (e.g., trainers, internal and external facilitators, implementation practitioners, and purveyors) need to be able to take our empirical findings and apply them independently. Consider the following *Vignette 2:*

Dr. Make It Pragmatic is the director of a community mental health center seeking to implement measurement-based care (MBC) for depressed patients. Through his attendance at a community mental health network conference, he recently learned that MBC is an evidence-based practice and that by integrating it into his clinics, he will be able to engage in data-based decision-making to inform subsequent clinical program changes (Lewis, Scott, et al., 2015). At the same conference, he learned about the field of implementation science and how it might be able to inform his process. Dr. Pragmatic had attended a series of talks about the importance of ensuring organizational readiness prior to beginning an implementation and decided to start by conducting a needs assessment to see if his clinics would be in a position to benefit from MBC training. Unfortunately, the organizational assessment measure that was discussed at the conference cost thousands of dollars, but he was able to find a free measure online that came equipped with a scoring guide and national norms for comparison, the Texas Christian University Organizational Readiness to Change scale (Lehman et al., 2002). He selected only four (i.e., communication, stress, change, and leadership) of the 18 scales that looked most relevant to his purpose, given that the entire scale was simply too long for his staff to complete.

Some may have read *Vignette 2* and thought that Dr. Pragmatic is ahead of the curve in thinking about how to approach clinical program change. Indeed, it may be premature to think that the science is in such a place to guide stakeholders in independent implementation practice. However, we believe that this is an appropriate goal and that measures can be an avenue to this end (Lewis, Stanick, et al., 2015). In order to move the field in this direction, as *Vignette 2* highlights, the challenges faced by Dr. Pragmatic and implementation stakeholders more broadly include parallel issues to those raised for implementation scientists. One of the major differences is that stakeholders have a hard(er) time accessing the science; even if the articles are published in open access journals, they are written for academics (complete with entirely new set of jargon) and often require significant time to read and synthesize the literature (a luxury stakeholders do not have). In addition, there is currently little guidance pointing toward key factors that predict implementation success and almost no literature regarding the pragmatic nature of implementation measures (Lewis, Fischer, et al., 2015).

Taken together, both researchers and stakeholders continue to face significant implementation measurement challenges. Ironically, these very challenges are only widening the science–practice gap the field aims to close. Glasgow et al. (2012) proposed five D&I values that should be prioritized to move the field of implementation science forward, working to close the aforementioned gap: (1) rigor and relevance (i.e., the use of rigorous research methods that address critical questions in relevant contexts), (2) efficiency and speed (i.e., the use of efficient methods to study D&I), (3) collaboration (i.e., the use of interdisciplinary research teams and research–practice collaborations), (4) improved capacity (i.e., a necessary increase in the capacity to train future D&I researchers and share advances made through implementation science with all stakeholders); and (5) cumulative knowledge (i.e., the need to create resources and funds of accessible knowledge about D&I research and its findings). The ultimate goal of D&I science is for advances to become readily available for practice partners to use with their unique populations and settings. Adherence to these five core values with respect to measurement will move the field closer to achieving this goal.

This chapter will begin to grapple with the following key issues:

- When is it time to put a measure on the shelf? There are numerous measures in frequent use that do not have established psychometric properties or have evidenced poor psychometrics. Confidence in one's findings from these measures is thus undermined.
- Can we adopt a core set of common measures? The majority of measures are generated for one-time use. Without common use of measures, it is challenging for the field to build a cumulative knowledge base.
- What is the minimal set of reporting standards for psychometric properties? As there are no agreed-upon reporting standards, authors provide little information regarding measures, the construct they assess, their quality, how they were revised, etc. Accordingly, it is difficult to determine the quality of the study.
- How can psychometrically validated measures be used to inform implementation practice? Measures are not routinely used in "real-world" clinical practice despite their potential to be independently employed to guide stakeholder decision-making. Instead, we see implementation scientists generating high-cost strategies and associated measures that are prohibitive in most practical contexts.

This set of issues was raised because resolution is needed to build a cumulative knowledge base and enhance the relevance of our science for our community partners. Each section will begin with a discussion of the implications of the question raised, and then provide an overview of related and recent advances in the field as well as the limitations of published work, followed by recommendations for future directions. However, first, a more thorough overview of the state of implementation science measurement is warranted.

The Current State of Implementation Science Measurement

To our knowledge, seven papers summarize the state of implementation science measurement via systematic reviews and related synthesis approaches. These reviews range from focusing on a single construct (e.g., organizational readiness to change, Weiner, Amick, & Lee, 2008; fidelity, Ibrahim & Sidani, 2015) to those that cover an entire framework and its associated 33 constructs (e.g., Lewis, Fischer, et al., 2015). The focus, approach, and results of each review will be summarized in this section, as the state of implementation science measurement will inform responses to the central questions of this chapter.

First, in 2008, Weiner and colleagues conducted a comprehensive review of 106 peer-reviewed articles and 43 instruments relevant to organizational readiness for change, which they define as "the extent to which organizational members are psychologically and behaviorally prepared to implement organizational change" (Weiner et al., 2008). In their initial review, the authors found discrepancies between conceptual models of organizational readiness for change, as well as limited evidence across the 43 identified measures to support their reliability ($N = 33$; 76.74%) and validity (face/content [$N = 25$; 58.14%], predictive [$N = 15$; 34.88%], concurrent [$N = 9$; 20.93%], convergent [$N = 9$; 20.93%], and discriminant [$N = 7$; 16.28%]). Additionally, the authors found few rigorous empirical studies testing the capacity of organizational readiness for change and how it predicted overall implementation success. Weiner updated his review of organizational readiness for change measures for this book (see Chap. 6, this book); yet, his conclusions about existing measures did not change; 8 years did not render stronger evidence of reliability (i.e., internal consistency) or validity (i.e., structural validity) for the identified measures. However, he did find four additional measures that have promising psychometric properties; yet, none had been tested for predictive validity. Finally, 76% of measures had only been used in a single study.

In 2009, Hrisos et al. (2009) conducted a systematic review investigating proxy measures of clinical behavior (e.g., review of medical records or interviewing the clinician) in an attempt to locate a link between these types of measures and how clinicians are actually performing in practice. Fifteen papers met criteria for inclusion, as they contained checklists of discrete clinical activity (i.e., behaviors that could be coded as yes or no), ranging from 1 to 168 behaviors observed in each study. While it is essential for these proxy measures to be both reliable and valid, only four studies were found to use suitable statistical methods for points of comparison. Additionally, these authors found that only eight out of the 15 (53.33%) checklists reported on the interrater reliability of their generated scores. Five additional reports stated that they evaluated interrater reliability, claiming these scores to be "good"; however, no statistics were provided.

Jumping to 2012, Emmons, Weiner, Fernandez, & Tu (2012) identified and evaluated 36 measures spanning across the constructs of leadership ($N = 16$) (i.e., "the ability of an individual to influence, motivate, and enable others to contribute toward the effectiveness and success of organizations of which they are members"; House et al., 1999), vision ($N = 2$) (i.e., "an idea of a valued outcome which represents a higher order goal and a motivating force at work"; Farr & West, 1990), managerial relations ($N = 1$) (i.e., "alliances between groups within an organization to promote change"; Zuckerman, Shortell, Morrison, & Friedman, 1990), organizational climate ($N = 14$) (i.e., "organizational members' perceptions of their work environment"; Emmons et al., 2012) and absorptive capacity ($N = 3$) (i.e., "an organization's ability to access and effectively use information"; Emmons et al., 2012). Only the constructs of leadership ($N = 4$) and organizational climate ($N = 12$) demonstrated both reliability and some form of validity (construct, translation, face, content, criterion-related, predictive, concurrent, convergent, and/or discriminant) (total $N = 16$; 44.44%). Across all five constructs, the authors found that (1) no measure was used in more than one study, (2) most studies did not include reports of the measure's psychometric properties, (3) some were based on a single response per unit, and (4) the levels of the instrument and analysis were not always compatible. Given these four issues, the authors noted that they were unable to offer any recommendations for using the identified measures to evaluate any of the five constructs.

In 2013, Chaudoir, Dugan, & Barr (2013) employed a systematic review, ultimately identifying 62 measures assessing constructs within the organization (e.g., leadership effectiveness, culture or climate), provider (e.g., physicians, psychologists or allied health professionals), innovation (e.g., relative advantage or quality of evidence), structural (e.g., physical environment, social climate or public policies), and patient (e.g., health-relevant beliefs, motivation, or personality traits) level domains outlined by Durlak and Dupre (2008). Their item-level analysis of psychometrics centered only on predictive validity (without establishing reliability or construct validity) and revealed that almost half of the identified measures ($N = 30$; 48.39%) did not include an assessment of criterion validity in their original validation studies or in any other studies that cited using the measure. Of the measures that did assess predictive validity ($N = 32$; 51.61%), only adoption ($N = 29$ out of 32; 90.1%) and fidelity ($N = 5$ out of 32; 15.6%) were represented as implementation outcomes of interest. Their review also uncovered that the constructs at the level of the organization, provider, and innovation had the greatest number of measures, while the structural and patient-level constructs were less saturated. Additionally, of the 62 measures identified in their review, 21 (33.87%) only had one associated citation.

In 2014, the Society for Implementation Research Collaboration (SIRC; formerly the Seattle Implementation Research Conference series; see Lewis et al., (2016) for history and mission of SIRC) developed the Instrument Review Project. This work aimed to close critical measurement gaps through a systematic review of quantitative instruments relevant to the field's most highly cited frameworks, the Consolidated Framework for Implementation Research (CFIR; Damschroder et al., 2009) and the Implementation Outcomes Framework (IOF; Proctor et al., 2009). The SIRC Instrument Review Project has identified over 420 instruments to date, with great variability in the number of measures distributed across constructs. For example, within the knowledge and beliefs construct, belonging to the CFIR domain characteristics of individuals, there were 56 identified instruments, whereas the CFIR's outer setting domain contained a mere four measures across its four constructs, with the constructs external policy and incentives and peer pressure containing no measures. With respect to the IOF, 104 measures have been identified (Lewis, Fischer, et al., 2015), with only one instrument with corresponding data available for internal consistency, structural validity, predictive validity, norms, responsiveness, and usability (all psychometric properties assessed in the study's rating criteria). Across all the measures, the proportion of instruments that rated "good" or "excellent" for reliability was 47%, for structural validity 17%, for predictive validity 9%, for norms 53%, for responsiveness 2%, and for usability 89%.

Moving to 2015, Ibrahim and Sidani conducted a descriptive review of instruments assessing the implementation outcome of fidelity, which is the competent and reliable delivery of an intervention as intended in the original design (Bellg et al., 2004; Carroll et al., 2007; Stein, Sargent, & Rafaels, 2007). These authors identified 21 studies assessing the construct, with most measures developed to assess the fidelity of a specific intervention. Across the 21 measures, acceptable levels of reliability and validity were identified through utilizing Streiner & Norman (2008)'s methodological framework. Almost all ($N = 19$; 91%) of the identified measures reported on reliability, broadly speaking. Thirteen (68.4%) evaluated internal consistency, 13 (68.4%) reported on interrater reliability, whereas none of the studies included reported on test–retest reliability. The measures that assessed internal consistency had a concerning spread of Cronbach's alpha values, ranging from unacceptable (0.47) to excellent (0.98). Most ($N = 18$; 86%) of the measures contained an evaluation of validity, broadly speaking. Of those that evaluated validity, 11 (61.1%) reported on construct validity, whereas ten (56%) reported on content validity.

Also in 2015, Chor, Wisdom, Olin, Hoagwood, & Horwitz (2015) identified 118 measures that assessed 27 predictors (e.g., government policy and regulations, social climate, risk, individual characteristics) of adoption, which is "the complete or partial decision to proceed with the implementation of an innovation as a distinct process preceding but separate from actual implementation", outlined by Wisdom, Chor, Hoagwood, & Horwitz (2014) in their review of theories and constructs implicated in innovation adoption. In building upon Wisdom et al., (2014)'s narrative synthesis by replicating their search strategy, Chor et al., (2015) found that the measures were unevenly distributed across the predictors, with external environment (i.e., extra-organizational environment's influences on adoption; Wisdom et al., 2014) housing the most measures ($N = 10$) and the predictors of affiliation with organizational culture (i.e., fit between individual staff and organizational culture; Wisdom et al., 2014), feedback on execution and fidelity (i.e., individualized feedback on the execution and fidelity of adopting an innovation; Wisdom et al., 2014), and social network (i.e., social linkages fostered among individual staff; Wisdom et al., 2014) containing the fewest measures ($N = 1$). The authors observed multiple definitions of a single predictor in addition to multiple forms of measurement. With respect to psychometric properties of the 118 measures, only 62

(52.54%) had available evidence of validity and reliability; no distinctions or nuances were provided regarding the psychometric ratings and so it is unclear which set of properties were represented in each measure's associated literature.

A recent environmental scan and literature review by Rabin et al. (2016) revealed 11 (total $N = 17$) additional implementation science measures resources, of which six of the 17 (35.29%) provided information pertaining to the psychometric properties of measures and were summarized above. One additional, but unique, measures resource entitled "the Grid Enabled Measures (GEM) project" is a living repository that focuses on accumulating behavioral, social science, and other scientific measures, with a special section on Dissemination and Implementation. As of 2012 (Rabin et al., 2012), GEM housed 1202 measures, organized by construct with definitions ($N = 383$) and their theoretical foundation ($N = 174$) provided in some, but not all cases (i.e., for the minority of cases, given that the resource relies upon crowd sourcing). GEM offers the option of users to provide information about psychometric properties, but this is not systematically reported or monitored for accuracy. Although GEM and the other resources do not provide a formal synthesis of the state of implementation science measurement as a systematic review offers, the resources are immensely valuable to the research and practice communities.

Taken together, these reviews and resources provide ample insight into the numerous instrumentation issues with which the field of implementation science grapples. For instance, even though a measure cannot be valid without first establishing its reliability, reliability reporting in the above reviews ranged from 53.33% (Hrisos et al., 2009) to 76.74% (Weiner et al., 2008). In Emmons et al. (2012)'s review of measures assessing key organizational-level constructs, only 44.44% of measures demonstrated both reliability and validity compared to 52.54% in Chor's review of measures of constructs predicting adoption. Finally, when considering more nuanced yet still critical elements of reliability and validity (e.g., structural validity, sensitivity to change), results from the SIRC Instrument Review Project (Lewis, Fischer, et al., 2015) revealed that only one measure out of 104 (0.01%) provided information relevant to all six evidence-based assessment (EBA) criteria applied in their study.

These systematic reviews and measurement resources are critical to advancing the cumulative knowledge of the field. Simultaneously, these syntheses reveal significant gaps in the literature and pervasive measurement issues including discrepancies in how constructs are conceptualized, a paucity of evidence for measure reliability and validity, and extreme variation in the amount of attention/measure development associated with different implementation constructs. The result of these ongoing measurement issues is that our science rests on shaky ground threatening the confidence we may have in our findings. However, perhaps the wrong question has plagued the field, the question of whether and which measures have psychometric strength. Perhaps the more pressing questions now are "When is it time to put a measure on the shelf?" and "Can we adopt a core set of common measures?"

When Is It Time to Put a Measure on the Shelf? Can We Adopt a Common Set of Measures?

Despite these major advances in implementation science measurement evaluation and synthesis, there is little guidance to answer the question, "When is it time to put a measure on the shelf?" Said differently, when should resources be allocated to creating a new measure of a construct versus attempting to (re)establish psychometric strength in an existing measure? The only accessible data to help answer this question pertain to the recent reporting of measures used for single use. Specifically, this one-time use of measures phenomenon was reported on in four of the seven systematic reviews (Chaudoir et al., 2013; Emmons et al., 2012; Lewis, Fischer, et al., 2015; Weiner et al., 2008) discussed above. For example, in Emmons et al.'s (2012) review of 36 measures focusing on organizational-level constructs, the authors found that none of the measures had been used in more than one study. Also, results from the SIRC Instrument Review Project revealed that across 104 measures of implementation outcomes, 53 (50.96%) had only one article citing its use. Similarly, in Weiner's updated review of organizational readiness to change measures (see Chap. 6 of this book), 76% of the included measures were used in a single study. In Chaudoir et al.'s (2013) review, 33.87% of the measures included had a single associated citation. The simplest explanation is that these one-time use measures have simply gone overlooked, given that only recently have implementation science measurement reviews of multiple constructs been published.

However, drawing on the example in *Vignette #1* provides some evidence that implementation scientists are not making informed decisions about measure use based on existing evidence of psychometric strength, but that awareness of a measure and other pragmatic qualities such as cost, may lead to overuse of measures that actually should be shelved. Specifically, the Texas Christian University Organizational Readiness for Change measure (Lehman et al., 2002) referenced in the vignette is one of the most widely used (cited in 570 publications), least validated, and unreliable measures of organizational readiness to change. It remains in high circulation likely due to its growing popularity (greater citations breed greater use), free status (no charge), associated national norms, and the capacity to select from 23 subscales. However, it is clear from Weiner's recent analysis (see Chap. 6 of this book) that years of repeated use have not led to stronger evidence of reliability and validity (i.e., it is "adequate" at best, but "minimal" evidence for the majority of the psychometric properties). To be clear, the poorly performing psychometrics of this measure across studies warrants great concern that the findings in these articles are tenuous and may not be reflective of the interpretations put forth.

Careful attention to this specific issue in the context of the aforementioned systematic reviews allows the evaluation of an alternative hypothesis that single use measures are appropriately "shelved" or abandoned because of failure to demonstrate psychometric strength. For instance, we reanalyzed data from the SIRC Instrument Review Project and found that of the 53 measures with a single citation, the average evidence-based assessment (EBA) rating score (*more information on the specifics of this rating criteria can be found in subsequent sections*) was 7.10 ($SD = 3.59$) out of a possible 24. Those with two to nine citations ($N = 39$) had an average EBA score of 10.08, measure packets containing 10–19 citations ($N = 5$) demonstrated an average EBA rating of 11.90, while finally, those with 20 or more citations ($N = 2$) revealed an average EBA score of 13.50. An independent samples *t*-test was conducted to compare the EBA ratings for measures with a single citation ($N = 53$) and measures with more than one citation ($N = 46$). A significant difference was observed wherein the EBA ratings for measures with a single citation were lower ($M = 7.10$, $SD = 3.59$) than measures with more than one citation ($M = 10.42$, $SD = 3.86$); $t(97) = 4.43$, $p < 0.0001$. Moreover, when our team was contacting measure developers to gain permission to include measures or measure items for posting on our website, the most common reason for declining our request was "poor psychometrics."

Unfortunately, we were unable to conduct this same reanalysis with the three other reviews that provided information regarding the one-time measure use phenomenon due to their limited reporting of psychometric properties in the published manuscripts. In the 2013 review by Chaudoir et al., predictive validity was the only psychometric property included in their review. Predictive validity was evaluated in a dichotomous fashion, absent of any data that could be incorporated into a reanalysis; the authors only indicated (yes/no) if the measure evaluated this property. If the measure did evaluate predictive validity, the associated implementation outcome was listed, as well as if it was statistically significant (yes/no). Of the measures that had only one associated citation ($N = 21$), there were only six (28.57%) that demonstrated statistically significant evidence of predictive validity. Conversely, for measures with more than one citation ($N = 41$), only 16 (39.02%) of these did *not* evaluate predictive validity. In Weiner's update of his 2008 review (see Chap. 6 of this book), 76 measures assessing organizational readiness were rated using the same Evidence-Based Assessment (EBA) criteria as the SIRC Instrument Review Project (Lewis, Fischer, et al., 2015). His analysis provided additional evidence of the connection between predictive validity and the number of times a measure has been used. Weiner found that measures assessing organizational readiness for change used across more than one study demonstrated stronger psychometric properties; in fact those with repeated use were more likely to receive excellent ratings for predictive validity (i.e., "two or more medium-strong correlations or associations between the measure, or the scales that comprise it, and adoption or implementation outcomes", see Chap. 6 of this book). Further analysis and cross-comparisons are warranted in order to determine if this same conclusion is present across all EBA criteria. Finally, we were unable to conduct any sort of comparison analysis in the Emmons et al., (2012) review of organizational measures because all measures were limited to a single use. However, fewer than one-half of the included measures contained any report of psychometrics ($N = 16$, 44.44%), with these reports questionable at best. For example, concerns have been raised over the factor structures and reliability of the organizational climate measures, with statistics for each falling below required thresholds of acceptability. In some, there is some evidence to suggest that single use measures are those that are appropriately shelved due to a poor showing of psychometrics. To explore this issue further, we urge those conducting systematic reviews of measures to consider including this analysis in future studies or at least provide numerical data on psychometric ratings to allow others to test this hypothesis.

However, it is also possible that measures are used only once because of specific item language that limits their generalizability. Indeed, some theories (e.g., Theory of Planned Behavior, TPB; Ajzen, 1991) of behavior change posit that context-, population-, or intervention-specific language is necessary to accurately evaluate the relation between a construct and criterion. According to Francis et al. (2004)'s manual for constructing questionnaires based on TPB, researchers should follow a nine-step approach: (1) define the population of interest; (2) concretely define the behavior under investigation; (3) design how to best measure intention to engage in the new behavior; (4) determine the most commonly perceived advantages and disadvantages of performing the new behavior; (5) identify the people who have the most influence over the approval or disproval of the behavior; (6) determine the perceived barriers and facilitators of the behavior; (7) create items assessing all TPB constructs using information gleaned in steps 1 through 6; (8) pilot the measure and refine the items; and (9) assess test–retest reliability. However, it is unclear if this level of specificity is necessary across implementation science constructs, theories, models, and frameworks, given that the broad-reaching Evidence Based Practice Attitudes measure (Aarons, 2004) has demonstrated predictive validity in numerous studies (e.g., Beidas et al., 2015), for example.

This approach of developing context/population/intervention-specific measures may be important and yet it presents formidable challenges with respect to synthesizing findings across studies. Indeed, the ultimate goal of SIRC's Instrument Review Project is to create a consensus battery or core set of common measures for use to promote ease of cross-study comparison capabilities. If the field came together in this way, there would be new potential for great progress. For instance, SIRC's measure repository will eventually seek to collect study data (across research teams) to identify robust predictors of implementation outcomes. Moreover, a database of this nature would provide the power and thus the opportunity to apply more advanced analytic approaches, such as item response theory, which would allow for truly pragmatic measurement approaches in which one could adaptively administer implementation measures by using only discriminative items. However, we are far from realizing this goal, in part because achieving consensus on a standard set of measures is difficult for any field. For instance, the National Quality Forum has endorsed over 700 healthcare performance measures in the last decade (NQF: Prioritizing Measures n.d.). Moreover, although the benefits of a consensus battery for advancing implementation science are obvious, it is possible that the practice of implementation will require measure specificity to inform tailoring of strategies to contextual factors. Nonetheless, this set of questions warrants greater attention by the field.

Despite the limited empirical guidance available to address the two questions guiding this section, we recommend the following. First, acknowledge that reliability is a feature of the measure *as it functions in your particular study*. Therefore, it is inappropriate to assume that since it demonstrated reliability previously, the measure is sound; rather, it is your responsibility to establish evidence of reliability in your sample and report on this in the service of being transparent with the reader. Second, recall this lesson from your introduction to psychology course: measures cannot be deemed valid if not proven first to be reliable (Kimberlin & Winterstein, 2008). If you are underpowered or underresourced to examine a measure for its structural validity (i.e., a measure of unidimensionality), for instance, you can be certain that it is not structurally valid if the scale (or set of subscales) does not demonstrate internal consistency. Third, do not trust your peers! Just because peer-reviewed articles have resulted in citing a previously mentioned measure 570 times does not mean that the measure is psychometrically sound. Fourth, look to one of the seven aforementioned resources for synthesized, cross-study information regarding reliability and validity to make an informed decision based on the psychometric status of a measure over time. A critical note: only a few of these systematic reviews provide a nuanced representation of the psychometric properties (e.g., none, minimal, adequate, good, excellent; Lewis, Fischer, et al., 2015), whereas others offer a binary "yes" or "no" statement about having reliability or validity, for instance, which is much less useful and should be considered with caution (e.g., Chor et al., 2015).

Given the limited discussion in the literature of the one-time use phenomenon, we propose two final recommendations in relation to shelving a measure based on its evidence of reliability and validity. First, we contend that a measure with less than adequate reliability evidence across five unique studies should be considered for the shelf. Second, if validity assessments across five unique studies do not suggest that the measure, and its associated subscales, evaluate empirically distinct concepts, we suggest it be shelved. We suggest this approach of accumulating evidence about poor psychometrics prior to shelving a measure because the absence of psychometric reporting does not equate with poor psychometrics. In fact, our field is failing when it comes to psychometric reporting of measures, a critical issue that we will grapple with next. Ideally, if readers embrace these recommendations, we will emerge with a focused set of measures with strong evidence of psychometric properties across studies. One final recommendation is that researchers employ generalizable measures to encourage use across studies or administer both specific and general measures of a construct in the same study to empirically test which approach is optimal.

What Is the Minimal Set of Reporting Standards for Measurement?

There are currently no established reporting standards specific to measurement as it is used in implementation science. Because of this, we find that authors tend to provide little information about the constructs they seek to assess, the measures used in their studies, their quality, how they were revised, and how they performed with respect to reliability and validity. This lack of information should raise red flags for readers, as one could interpret this as indicative of the (poor) quality of the study.

Reporting standards are commonly used as a mechanism for enhancing the transparency, replicability, and quality of research. In addition, by promoting "complete" reporting of a minimum standard across a single type of study, readers are better able to critically appraise and interpret the findings. Indeed, reporting standards (often referred to as "guidelines") are so popular, the EQUATOR (The EQUATOR Network | Enhancing the QUAlity and Transparency Of Health Research n.d.) has been formed and provides a searchable database of standards that address the following study types: randomized trials, observational studies, systematic reviews, case reports, qualitative research, diagnostic/prognostic studies, quality improvement studies, economic evaluations, and animal preclinical studies and study protocols. Reporting standards can be useful in the development phases of a study as well as for tracking purposes during study implementation, but they are traditionally most critical during the reporting phase of one's work. Reporting standards typically are endorsed by journals. If endorsed, authors are expected to conform to the standards for reporting set in place, making it relatively easy for reviewers and editors to ensure that reporting is complete, transparent, and replicable, oftentimes using a checklist approach during the review process.

To improve accessibility and enhance endorsement rates, these standards of reporting are often published in numerous journals. For instance, the revised CONSORT statement for randomized clinical trials has a total of 75 endorsement citations with uptake by 15 journals.[2] A recent Cochrane review summarized the impact of the 1996 or 2001 CONSORT statement and concluded that CONSORT has significantly influenced the completeness of reporting; however, the authors of the Cochrane review noted that journals are not communicating clearly enough about their endorsement of CONSORT rendering suboptimal completeness of reporting (Turner, Shamseer, Altman, Schulz, & Moher, 2012). A parallel standard of reporting is currently being established for implementation science: Standards for reporting phase IV implementation studies (STaRI; Pinnock et al., 2015), which will hopefully raise the quality of the science produced by our field.

Perhaps unsurprisingly, almost all ($N = 8$, 80%) of the standards listed above include mention of measurement reporting guidelines, but the standard is so minimal that only one guideline included mention of both of the foundational psychometric properties – reliability and validity. Specifically, the SPIRIT guidelines for study protocols (Chan et al., 2013) included an explicit mention of these foundational psychometric properties by stating "…a description of study instruments

[2]Ann Int Med. 2010;152(11):726–32. PMID: 20335313; BMC Medicine. 2010;8:18. PMID: 20334633; BMJ. 2010;340:c332. PMID: 20332509; J Clin Epidemiol. 2010;63(8): 834–40. PMID: 20346629; Lancet. 2010;375(9721):1136 supplementary webappendix; Obstet Gynecol. 2010;115(5):1063–70. PMID: 20410783; Open Med. 2010;4(1):60–68.; PLoS Med. 2010;7(3): e1000251. PMID: 20352064; Trials. 2010;11:32. PMID: 20334632

(e.g., questionnaires, laboratory tests) along with their reliability and validity, if known" should be included in the final report. Most all other guidelines simply stated the need to report "results of any other analyses performed," which clearly leaves room for the author to omit any discussion of measurement psychometrics (Schulz, Altman, & Moher, 2010). For details regarding the measurement-related standards available across the ten sets, please see Table 9.1.

Recall, reliability is the extent to which a measure (or its set of items) produces the same results (on repeated administrations). As noted in the previous section, in order for measures to be valid, they must first be deemed reliable. Validity is the quality of the inferences, claims, or decisions drawn from the scores of an instrument. Psychometric properties, such as reliability and validity, allow us to have confidence in the findings produced in research studies. Therefore, one could argue that measures should be determined to be both reliable and valid in the target population or practice setting. However, in new fields, it is especially unlikely that reliable and valid measures are available for the many constructs under investigation. Unfortunately, given the complete lack of measurement reporting standards, we cannot tell if the summaries of systematic reviews explored in the first section of this chapter reflect the actual state of the evidence or the lack of reporting on psychometric properties in implementation science-related journals. Therefore, we argue that measurement reporting standards need to be established, disseminated, and endorsed for the field of implementation science.

Although there are no current measurement reporting standards, particularly for implementation science, Zumbo & Chan's (2014) review of related fields revealed seven tools that support the systematic *rating* of measure and methodological quality of measurement studies. The majority of these tools were designed to guide the evaluation and synthesis of measures to inform measure selection for research or clinical administration, with the exception of the COSMIN (i.e., COnsensus-based Standards for the selection of health Measurement INstruments). The COSMIN is a checklist for evaluating a study's methodological quality of measurement properties in health measurement instruments; the authors indicate that it can serve the dual purpose of reporting standards that journals may adopt to determine whether critical design aspects and statistical methods related to measurement are clearly reported (Mokkink et al., 2010). Unfortunately, the COSMIN is specific to measure development and/or evaluation studies and there is no guidance as to which psychometric and design properties are essential for reporting outside of the measure development context, such as in a typical implementation evaluation. Thus, there remains a critical unmet need to put forth minimal standards of reporting for measures used in the evaluation of implementation efforts.

In order to inform a minimal set of reporting standards for the field, we first reviewed several of the existing and related tools for evaluating measurement quality (from a recently published review, not an exhaustive list) to identify the common psychometric qualities of interest. This step was taken because (a) foundational measurement properties do not differ between fields and (b) in setting minimal standards for reporting, it is paramount to ensure that key psychometrics used in evaluating measures are included. Ten criteria emerged as "most common" when using

Table 9.1 Comparison of reporting standards inclusion of measurement issues

Reporting standard	Study type	Measurement standards
CONSORT (Schulz, Altman, & Moher, 2010)	Randomized Trials	1. "Results of any other analyses performed, including subgroup analyses and adjusted analyses, distinguishing pre-specified from exploratory"
		2. "Generalisability (external validity, applicability) of the trial findings"
STROBE (Von Elm et al., 2007)	Observational Studies	1. "Report other analyses done—e.g., analyses of subgroups and interactions, and sensitivity analyses"
		2. "Discuss the generalisability (external validity) of the study results"
PRISMA (Moher, Liberati, Tetzlaff, & Altman, 2009)	Systematic Reviews	"Give results of additional analyses, if done (e.g., sensitivity or subgroup analyses, meta-regression)"
CARE (Gagnier et al., 2013)	Case Reports	No mention
SRSQ(O'Brien, Harris, Beckman, Reed, & Cook, 2014)	Qualitative Research	"Techniques to enhance trustworthiness and credibility of data analysis (e.g., member checking, audit trail, triangulation); rationale"
STARD (Bossuyt et al., 2015)	Diagnostic/ Prognostic Studies	No mention
SQUIRE 2.0 (2015) (Ogrinc et al., 2015)	Quality Improvement Studies	"Factors that might have limited internal validity such as confounding, bias, or imprecision in the design, methods, measurement, or analysis"
CHEERS (Husereau et al., 2013)	Economic Evaluations	"Describe all analytical methods supporting the evaluation. This could include methods for dealing with skewed, missing, or censored data; extrapolation methods; methods for pooling data; approaches to validate or make adjustments (such as half cycle corrections) to a model; and methods for handling population heterogeneity and uncertainty"
ARRIVE (Kilkenny, Browne, Cuthill, Emerson, & Altman, 2010)	Animal Pre-Clinical Studies	"Report the results for each analysis carried out, with a measure of precision (e.g., standard error or confidence interval)"
SPIRIT (Chan et al., 2013)	Study Protocols	"Plans for assessment and collection of outcome, baseline, and other trial data, including any related processes to promote data quality (e.g., duplicate measurements, training of assessors) and a description of study instruments (e.g., questionnaires, laboratory tests) along with their reliability and validity, if known. Reference to where data collection forms can be found, if not in the protocol"

the criterion that the property is included in at least 50% of the identified tools, whereas only three emerged when requiring that the majority (more than half; i.e., 62.5%) included the psychometric property. This latter, more parsimonious approach yielded the following psychometric properties as central to the reporting process (see the Glossary for definitions): internal consistency, construct validity, and criterion validity. It is unsurprising that these three psychometric properties emerged given the following. Internal consistency is the only form of reliability that is relevant across measure types (unlike interrater reliability) and study designs (unlike test–retest reliability). Construct validity is the most basic form of validity that provides evidence that the instrument assesses what it claims to measure. Criterion validity reveals the extent to which a measure is related to an outcome, either concurrently or in a predictive fashion. It would be rare for a measure to be included in a study without exploring its relation to other variables of interest. Thus, for any minimal measurement reporting standard, we argue that these three psychometric properties should be included. Importantly, in setting this reporting standard, we urge researchers to carefully specify construct and criterion validity with respect to the relevant theoretical underpinnings and conceptual relations. This practice will help ensure advancing existing theories and cumulative knowledge. For full definitions of the various types of validity and reliability commonly found in measurement reporting standards, please see the Glossary found at the end of this chapter.

Second, we reviewed the issues and limitations that emerged from our overview of the current state of implementation science measurement, a previous publication on instrumentation issues in implementation science (Martinez et al., 2014) and the findings from the recent publication referencing measurement resources (Rabin et al., 2016) to determine if any of the issues raised could be addressed by encouraging completeness of reporting moving forward. For instance, we believe that the issue of homonymy, synonymy, and instability (Gerring, 2001) can be addressed through measure reporting standards (i.e., through provision of construct labels and definitions), as can the limited use of theories, frameworks, and models (i.e., through citing those that provide definitions or nomological networks in the service of establishing construct validity). By requiring minimal reporting standards, we also hope to, at least partially, address the problem raised regarding one-time use measures because we will be able to determine whether this problem is manifest solely due to poor psychometrics.

Specifically, to address issues of homonymy, synonymy, and instability (Gerring, 2001) as well as content validity, we recommend that a minimal reporting standard be that the constructs purportedly measured are carefully named and defined, and theories, models, or frameworks from which the definitions were pulled are referenced. Additionally, authors should provide a full list of survey items, as it is difficult to judge content validity based solely on the sample items provided in text. Importantly, authors need to justify why the construct of interest aligns with the data source tapped. That is, not all constructs are best evaluated by self-report, which is most appropriate when seeking attitudes, beliefs, and perspectives of participants. Some constructs such as the implementation outcome of fidelity is best assessed via direct observation to avoid gaining a biased self-perception. To address the one-time use phenomenon, authors are encouraged to indicate clearly the stage of measure development (e.g., needs additional evidence, unable to evaluate structural validity).

Authors also need to report on the characteristics of the measures they are using in their studies. First, authors must answer the question, "Who is going to respond to the measure?" This can be answered through specifying the target or level of measurement (e.g., individual, team, and organizational), as well as the compilation or aggregation method of the resulting data if appropriate. Next, authors need to specify the timing of the measure administration. When will it be administered to participants? For instance, is the measure specific to only one phase of the study or is it time-sensitive so that other study phases depend upon the results of the measure? Finally, the scoring procedure (e.g., summing versus averaging, equal versus unequal weighting) for the measure and the rationale for the specified approach must be included in the final write-up. Once a description of the measure characteristics has been defined, authors should include statistical analyses relevant to checking the performance of their measure. At the very minimum, authors need to include reports of internal consistency (to reflect one assessment of reliability) and structural validity (to reflect one assessment of construct validity) in their reports.

While formal reporting standards relevant for implementation science are under construction (Pinnock et al., 2015), we anticipate that like the extant reporting standards, little attention will be paid to measurement. We hope readers will incorporate the recommendations summarized in Table 9.2 as our team works to refine and disseminate these into formal measurement reporting standards for implementation science.

Our aim is to promote standardization of findings presented in measure validation and other empirical studies as well as to improve transparency of measurement approaches employed. Both Drs. Psychometric and Pragmatic introduced in the vignettes at the beginning of this chapter would greatly benefit from this work. Ultimately, we hope that this process will refine the peer-review process (Zumbo & Chan, 2014), enhance ease of replication, expedite the speed with which poor-quality measures are shelved, and enable the field to adopt and advance a consensus battery of measures. In sum, we will all benefit from higher quality research once there is uptake and adherence to measurement reporting standards in implementation science (Cobo et al., 2011).

Table 9.2 Summary of reporting standards recommendations

Reporting standard recommendations
Carefully name and define constructs, as well as reference the theories, models, or frameworks from which the definitions were pulled
Provide a full list of survey items
Justify why the construct(s) of interest aligns with the data source tapped
Clearly indicate the stage of measure development
Report on the characteristics of the measures: target population (who), timing of the measure administration (when) and scoring procedure and rationale
Statistical analyses relevant to checking the performance of the measure: internal consistency, structural validity, construct validity, and criterion validity

Conclusions and Future Directions: Can Psychometrically Strong Measures Be Pragmatic?

In conclusion, although Dr. I. Care About Psychometrics seeks to prioritize use of measures with sound fundamental properties, she is faced with a field in which few high-quality measures appear to exist. The majority of the extant measures have only been used in a single study and have poor psychometrics, but even some measures used in hundreds of studies are of poor quality. Fortunately, there are seven systematic reviews of implementation science measures (Chaudoir et al., 2013; Chor et al., 2015; Emmons et al., 2012; Hrisos et al., 2009; Ibrahim & Sidani, 2015; Lewis, Fischer, et al., 2015; Weiner et al., 2008) and a recent study that provides an overview of measurement resources (Rabin et al., 2016). However, without minimal reporting standards for measurement, it is unclear how challenged the field really is, as it could be that existing measures are simply underdeveloped and/or underperforming, or it could be that measures are on track for development but authors are simply not reporting on quality-related details. Regardless, Dr. Psychometrics is convinced that the next critical step for the field is to develop, disseminate, and have journals endorse minimal measurement reporting standards.

Unfortunately, Dr. Make It Pragmatic faces not only the concerns of Dr. Psychometric, but also concerns about the utility of measures in the implementation practice space. He knows that he needs measures with strong psychometric properties, but he also requires that they be low cost, actionable, brief, believed in by his staff, and easy to use (i.e., administer, score, and interpret) (Glasgow & Riley, 2013). He has such a limited budget for improving clinical care that he cannot afford technical assistance for the full implementation process (from exploration to preparation to implementation to sustainment; Aarons et al., 2012) and so he is hopeful that measures could be useful tools to guide him through each stage. However, the field is not quite there, and in fact, he worries that the work of many implementation scientists is increasingly far removed from the underresourced realities of his practice world.

Indeed, the field of implementation, both science and practice, has a long way to go with respect to advancing psychometrically strong and pragmatic measurement approaches. Our team is currently working to address three critical gaps via the following aims. First, to establish a stakeholder-driven operationalization of pragmatic measures and develop reliable, valid rating criteria for assessing the construct (Lewis, Weiner, Stanick, & Fischer, 2015). Our intention is to develop, disseminate, and seek endorsement of minimal reporting standards from the rating criteria that emerge in hopes that scientists will consider pragmatic measure dimensions in measure development, application, analysis, and reporting. Second, to develop reliable, valid, and pragmatic measure of three critical implementation outcomes: acceptability, appropriateness, and feasibility. The three constructs are critical implementation outcomes that predict adoption and require psychometrically strong measures. Finally, to identify measures that assess constructs in the Consolidated Framework for Implementation Research (Damschroder et al., 2009) and the Implementation

Outcomes Framework (Proctor et al., 2009) that are both psychometrically and pragmatically strong. Our goal is that through these aims, measures will begin to be developed with both science and practice in mind.

Acknowledgments Research reported in this publication was supported by the National Institute of Mental Health under Award Number R01MH106510-01 granted to PI: CC Lewis.

Glossary

Absorptive Capacity (*pg. 232*) An organization's ability to access and effectively use information (Emmons et al., 2012)

Adoption (*pg. 233*) The complete or partial decision to proceed with the implementation of an innovation as a distinct process preceding but separate from actual implementation (Wisdom et al., 2014)

Barrier (*pg. 237*) Factor that obstructs changes in targeted professional behaviors or healthcare delivery processes, such as the cost and complexity of the intervention (Krause et al., 2014)

Collaboration (*pg. 230*) One of five core tenets of dissemination and implementation (D&I) research proposed by Glasgow et al. (2012), defined as the use of interdisciplinary research teams and research-practice collaborations (Glasgow et al., 2012)

Concurrent Validity (*pg. 231*) The degree to which an instrument distinguishes groups it should theoretically distinguish. Concurrent validity is not demonstrated if there is no reasonable hypothesized difference among groups on the instrument (Weiner et al., 2008)

Construct Validity (*pg. 232*) The degree to which inferences can legitimately be made from an instrument to the theoretical construct that it purportedly measures (Weiner et al., 2008)

Content Validity (*pg. 231*) The ability of the selected items to reflect the variables of the construct in the measure (Zamanzadeh et al., 2015)

Convergent Validity (*pg. 231*) The degree to which an instrument performs in a similar manner to other instruments that purportedly measure the same construct (e.g., two measures show a strong positive correlation). Convergent validity is most often assessed through confirmatory factor analysis (Weiner et al., 2008)

Criterion Validity (*pg. 232*) An empirical check on the performance of an instrument against some criteria (Weiner et al., 2008)

Cumulative Knowledge (*pg. 230*) One of five core tenets of dissemination & implementation (D&I) research proposed by Glasgow et al. (2012), defined as the need to create resources and funds of accessible knowledge about dissemination & implementation (D&I) research and its findings (Glasgow et al., 2012)

Discriminant Validity (*pg. 231*) The degree to which an instrument performs in a different manner to other instruments that purportedly measure different constructs. Discriminant validity is most often assessed through confirmatory factor analysis (Weiner et al., 2008)

Efficiency (*pg. 230*) One of five core tenets of dissemination & implementation (D&I) research proposed by Glasgow et al. (2012), defined as the use of efficient methods to study dissemination & implementation (D&I) (Glasgow et al., 2012)

Facilitator (*pg. 237*) Factor that enables changes in targeted professional behaviors or healthcare delivery processes, such as the cost and complexity of the intervention (Krause et al., 2014)

Fidelity (*pg. 228*) The competent and reliable delivery of an intervention as intended in the original design (Ibrahim & Sidani, 2015)

Homonymy (*pg. 242*) Models that define the same construct in different ways (i.e., two discrepant definitions for the same term) (Martinez et al., 2014)

Implementation Outcomes (*pg. 232*) Effects of deliberate and purposive actions to implement new treatments, practices, and services (Proctor et al., 2009)

Improved Capacity (*pg. 230*) One of five core tenets of dissemination & implementation (D&I) research proposed by Glasgow et al. (2012), defined as a necessary increase in the capacity to train future dissemination & implementation (D&I) researchers and share advances made through implementation science with all stakeholders (Glasgow et al., 2012)

Intermediary (*pg. 229*) Known as trainers, internal and external facilitators, implementation practitioners and purveyors. Intermediaries provide training and consultation and otherwise assist community settings to implement evidence-based practices (Lewis et al., 2016)

Internal Consistency (*pg. 233*) Refers to whether several items that propose to measure the same general construct produce similar scores

Inter-rater Reliability (*pg. 231*) A measure of reliability used to assess the degree to which different judges or raters agree in their assessment decisions (Reliability and Validity n.d.)

Leadership (*pg. 229*) The ability of an individual to influence, motivate, and enable others to contribute toward the effectiveness and success of organizations of which they are members (House et al., 1999)

Managerial Relations (*pg. 232*) Alliances between groups within an organization to promote change (Zuckerman et al., 1990)

Mixed Methods (*pg. 228*) Focus on collecting, analyzing and merging both quantitative and qualitative data into one or more studies. The central premise of these designs is that the use of quantitative and qualitative approaches in combination provides a better understanding of research issues than either approach alone (Robins et al., 2008)

Norms (*pg. 228*) The sample size, and the mean (M) and standard deviation (SD) for the instrument results (C. C. Lewis, Fischer, et al., 2015)

Organizational Climate (*pg. 232*) Organizational members' perceptions of their work environment (Emmons et al., 2012)

Organizational Readiness for Change (*pg. 231*) The extent to which organizational members are psychologically and behaviorally prepared to implement organizational change (Weiner et al., 2008)

Penetration (*pg. 228*) The integration of a practice within a service setting and its subsystems (Proctor et al., 2009)

Pragmatic Measure (*pg. 228*) One that has relevance to stakeholders and is feasible to use in most real-world settings to assess progress (Glasgow & Riley, 2013)

Predictive Validity (*pg. 232*) The degree to which the instrument can predict or correlate with an outcome of interest measured at some time in the future (Lewis, Fischer, et al., 2015)

Predictor (*pg. 233*) Variable that may anticipate implementation effectiveness (Jacobs et al., 2015)

Proxy Measure (*pg. 231*) Indirect measures of clinical practice, such as a review of medical records or interviewing the clinician (Hrisos et al., 2009)

Qualitative Methods (*pg. 228*) Used to explore and obtain depth of understanding as to the reasons for success or failure to implement evidence-based practice or to identify strategies for facilitating implementation (Teddlie & Tashakkori, 2003)

Quantitative Methods (*pg. 228*) Uused to test and confirm hypotheses based on an existing conceptual model and obtain breadth of understanding of predictors of successful implementation (Teddlie & Tashakkori, 2003)

Reliability (*pg. 231*) The extent to which a measure (or its set of items) produces the same results (on repeated measures)

Responsiveness (*pg. 233*) The ability of an instrument to detect clinically important changes in the construct it measures over time (Lewis, Fischer, et al., 2015)

Rigor and Relevance (*pg. 230*) One of five core tenets of dissemination & implementation (D&I) research proposed by Glasgow et al. (2012), defined as the use of rigorous research methods that address critical questions in relevant contexts (Glasgow et al., 2012)

Social Network (*pg. 233*) The pattern of relations and interactions that exist among people, organizations, communities, or other social systems (Valente, 1996)

Stakeholder (*pg. 229*) An individual, group, or organization who may affect, be affected by, or perceive itself to be affected by a decision, activity, or outcome of a project, program, or portfolio

Structural Validity (*pg. 233*) The degree to which all the test items rise and fall together; or to which, by contrast, perhaps, one set of test items rise and fall together in one pattern, and another group of test items rises and falls in a different pattern (Lewis, Fischer, et al., 2015)

Synonymy (*pg. 242*) Models that define different constructs the same way (i.e., two unique terms assigned the same definition) (Martinez et al., 2014)

Test-retest Reliability (*pg. 233*) A measure of reliability obtained by administering the same test twice over a period of time to a group of individuals. The scores from Time 1 and Time 2 can then be correlated in order to evaluate the test for stability over time ("Reliability and Validity," n.d.)

Theory of Planned Behavior (*pg. 237*) States that people's behavior is determined by their intention to perform a given behavior (Casper, 2007)

Translation Validity (*pg. 232*) The degree to which an instrument accurately translates (or carries) the meaning of the construct (Weiner et al., 2008)

Usability (*pg. 233*) The ease of administration, which is calculated by the total number of items on the measure being rated (Lewis, Fischer, et al., 2015)

Validity (*pg. 231*) The quality of the inferences, claims or decisions drawn from the scores of an instrument

Vision (*pg. 232*) An idea of a valued outcome which represents a higher order goal and a motivating force at work (Farr & West, 1990)

References

Aarons, G. A. (2004). Mental health provider attitudes toward adoption of evidence-based practice: The Evidence-Based Practice Attitude Scale (EBPAS). *Mental Health Services Research, 6*(2), 61–74.

Aarons, G. A., Ehrhart, M. G., & Farahnak, L. R. (2014). The implementation leadership scale (ILS): Development of a brief measure of unit level implementation leadership. *Implementation Science, 9*(1), 1–10.

Aarons, G. A., Green, A. E., Palinkas, L. A., Self-Brown, S., Whitaker, D. J., Lutzker, J. R., ... Chaffin, M. J. (2012). Dynamic adaptation process to implement an evidence-based child maltreatment intervention. *Implementation Science, 7*(1), 1–9.

Ajzen, I. (1991). The theory of planned behavior. *Organizational Behavior and Human Decision Processes, 50*(2), 179–211.

Beidas, R. S., Marcus, S., Aarons, G. A., Hoagwood, K. E., Schoenwald, S., Evans, A. C., ... Mandell, D. S. (2015). Individual and organizational factors related to community clinicians' use of therapy techniques in a large public mental health system. *JAMA Pediatrics, 169*(4), 374–382.

Bellg, A. J., Borrelli, B., Resnick, B., Hecht, J., Minicucci, D. S., Ory, M., ... Czajkowski, S. (2004). Enhancing treatment fidelity in health behavior change studies: Best practices and recommendations from the NIH Behavior Change Consortium. *Health Psychology, 23*(5), 443–451.

Bossuyt, P. M., Reitsma, J. B., Bruns, D. E., Gatsonis, C. A., Glasziou, P. P., Irwig, L., et al. (2015). STARD 2015: An updated list of essential items for reporting diagnostic accuracy studies. *Radiology, 277*(3), 826–832.

Boyd, M. R., Powell, B. J., Endicott, D., & Lewis, C. C. (2017). A method for tracking implementation strategies: an exemplar implementing measurementbased care in community behavioral health clinics. Behavior Therapy, Advance online publication. https://doi.org/10.1016/j.beth.2017.11.012.

Carroll, C., Patterson, M., Wood, S., Booth, A., Rick, J., & Balain, S. (2007). A conceptual framework for implementation fidelity. *Implementation Science, 2*(1), 1–9.

Casper, E. S. (2007). The theory of planned behavior applied to continuing education for mental health professionals. *Psychiatric Services, 58*(10), 1324–1329.

Chan, A.-W., Tetzlaff, J. M., Altman, D. G., Laupacis, A., Gøtzsche, P. C., Krleža-Jerić, K., et al. (2013). SPIRIT 2013 statement: Defining standard protocol items for clinical trials. *Annals of Internal Medicine, 158*(3), 200–207.

Chaudoir, S. R., Dugan, A. G., & Barr, C. H. (2013). Measuring factors affecting implementation of health innovations: A systematic review of structural, organizational, provider, patient, and innovation level measures. *Implementation Science, 8*(1), 1–20.

Chor, K. H. B., Wisdom, J. P., Olin, S.-C. S., Hoagwood, K. E., & Horwitz, S. M. (2015). Measures for predictors of innovation adoption. *Administration and Policy in Mental Health and Mental Health Services Research, 42*(5), 545–573.

Cobo, E., Cortés, J., Ribera, J. M., Cardellach, F., Selva-O'Callaghan, A., Kostov, B., et al. (2011). Effect of using reporting guidelines during peer review on quality of final manuscripts submitted to a biomedical journal: Masked randomised trial. *BMJ, d6783,* 343.

Damschroder, L. J., Aron, D. C., Keith, R. E., Kirsh, S. R., Alexander, J. A., & Lowery, J. C. (2009). Fostering implementation of health services research findings into practice: A consolidated framework for advancing implementation science. *Implementation Science, 4*(1), 1–15.

Durlak, J. A., & DuPre, E. P. (2008). Implementation matters: A review of research on the influence of implementation on program outcomes and the factors affecting implementation. *American Journal of Community Psychology, 41*(3–4), 327–350.

Ehrhart, M. G., Aarons, G. A., & Farahnak, L. R. (2014). Assessing the organizational context for EBP implementation: The development and validity testing of the Implementation Climate Scale (ICS). *Implementation Science, 9*(1), 1–11.

Emmons, K. M., Weiner, B., Fernandez, M. E., & Tu, S.-P. (2012). Systems antecedents for dissemination and implementation: A review and analysis of measures. *Health Education & Behavior: The Official Publication of the Society for Public Health Education, 39*(1), 87–105.

Farr, J. L., & West, M. A. (1990). *Innovation and creativity at work: Psychological and organizational strategies*. Chichester, Wiley.

Francis, J. J., Eccles, M. P., Johnston, M., Walker, A., Grimshaw, J., Foy, R., … Bonetti, D. (2004). Constructing questionnaires based on the theory of planned behaviour. *A Manual for Health Services Researchers, 2010*, 2–12.

Gagnier, J. J., Kienle, G., Altman, D. G., Moher, D., Sox, H., & Riley, D. (2013). The CARE guidelines: Consensus-based clinical case reporting guideline development. *Journal of Medical Case Reports, 7*(1), 1–6.

Gerring, J. (2001). *Social science methodology: A criterial framework*. Cambridge, Cambridge University Press.

Glasgow, R. E., & Riley, W. T. (2013). Pragmatic measures: What they are and why we need them. *American Journal of Preventive Medicine, 45*(2), 237–243.

Glasgow, R. E., Vinson, C., Chambers, D., Khoury, M. J., Kaplan, R. M., & Hunter, C. (2012). National Institutes of Health approaches to dissemination and implementation science: Current and future directions. *American Journal of Public Health, 102*(7), 1274–1281.

House, R. J., Hanges, P. J., Ruiz-Quintanilla, S. A., Dorfman, P. W., Javidan, M., Dickson, M., et al. (1999). Cultural influences on leadership and organizations: Project GLOBE. *Advances in Global Leadership, 1*(2), 171–233.

Hrisos, S., Eccles, M. P., Francis, J. J., Dickinson, H. O., Kaner, E. F. S., Beyer, F., & Johnston, M. (2009). Are there valid proxy measures of clinical behaviour? A systematic review. *Implementation Science, 4*(1), 1–20.

Husereau, D., Drummond, M., Petrou, S., Carswell, C., Moher, D., Greenberg, D., … Loder, E. (2013). Consolidated health economic evaluation reporting standards (CHEERS) statement. *Cost Effectiveness and Resource Allocation, 11*(1), 1–6.

Ibrahim, S., & Sidani, S. (2015). Fidelity of intervention implementation: A review of instruments. *Health, 7*(12), 1687–1695.

Jacobs, S. R., Weiner, B. J., Reeve, B. B., Hofmann, D. A., Christian, M., & Weinberger, M. (2015). Determining the predictors of innovation implementation in healthcare: A quantitative analysis of implementation effectiveness. *BMC Health Services Research, 15*(1), 1–13.

Johnson, K., Collins, D., & Wandersman, A. (2013). Sustaining innovations in community prevention systems: A data-informed sustainability strategy. *Journal of Community Psychology, 41*(3), 322–340.

Kilkenny, C., Browne, W. J., Cuthill, I. C., Emerson, M., & Altman, D. G. (2010). Improving bioscience research reporting: The ARRIVE guidelines for reporting animal research. *PLoS Biology, 8*(6), e1000412.

Kimberlin, C. L., & Winterstein, A. G. (2008). Validity and reliability of measurement instruments used in research. *American Journal of Health-System Pharmacy, 65*(23), 2276–2284.

Krause, J., Van Lieshout, J., Klomp, R., Huntink, E., Aakhus, E., Flottorp, S., et al. (2014). Identifying determinants of care for tailoring implementation in chronic diseases: An evaluation of different methods. *Implementation Science, 9*(1), 1–12.

Lehman, W. E. K., Greener, J. M., & Simpson, D. D. (2002). Assessing organizational readiness for change. *Journal of Substance Abuse Treatment, 22*(4), 197–209.

Lewis, C., Darnell, D., Kerns, S., Monroe-DeVita, M., Landes, S. J., Lyon, A. R., et al. (2016). Proceedings of the 3rd Biennial Conference of the Society for Implementation Research Collaboration (SIRC) 2015: Advancing efficient methodologies through community partnerships and team science. *Implementation Science, 11*(1), 1–38.

Lewis, C. C., Fischer, S., Weiner, B. J., Stanick, C., Kim, M., & Martinez, R. G. (2015). Outcomes for implementation science: An enhanced systematic review of instruments using evidence-based rating criteria. *Implementation Science, 10*, 1–17.

Lewis, C. C., Scott, K., Marti, C. N., Marriott, B. R., Kroenke, K., Putz, J. W., … Rutkowski, D. (2015). Implementing measurement-based care (iMBC) for depression in community mental health: A dynamic cluster randomized trial study protocol. *Implementation Science, 10*(1), 1–14.

Lewis, C. C., Stanick, C. F., Martinez, R. G., Weiner, B. J., Kim, M., Barwick, M., & Comtois, K. A. (2015). The society for implementation research collaboration instrument review project: A methodology to promote rigorous evaluation. *Implementation Science, 10*(1), 1–10.

Lewis, C. C., Weiner, B. J., Stanick, C., & Fischer, S. M. (2015). Advancing implementation science through measure development and evaluation: A study protocol. *Implementation Science, 10*(1), 1–18.

Martinez, R. G., Lewis, C. C., & Weiner, B. J. (2014). Instrumentation issues in implementation science. *Implementation Science, 9*(1), 1–9.

Moher, D., Liberati, A., Tetzlaff, J., & Altman, D. G. (2009). Preferred reporting items for systematic reviews and meta-analyses: The PRISMA statement. *Annals of Internal Medicine, 151*(4), 264–269.

Mokkink, L. B., Terwee, C. B., Patrick, D. L., Alonso, J., Stratford, P. W., Knol, D. L., … De Vet, H. C. (2010). The COSMIN checklist for assessing the methodological quality of studies on measurement properties of health status measurement instruments: An international Delphi study. *Quality of Life Research, 19*(4), 539–549.

NQF: Prioritizing Measures. (n.d.). Retrieved 30 June 2016, from http://www.qualityforum.org/prioritizing_measures/

O'Brien, B. C., Harris, I. B., Beckman, T. J., Reed, D. A., & Cook, D. A. (2014). Standards for reporting qualitative research: A synthesis of recommendations. *Academic Medicine, 89*(9), 1245–1251.

Ogrinc, G., Davies, L., Goodman, D., Batalden, P., Davidoff, F., & Stevens, D. (2015). SQUIRE 2.0 (Standards for QUality Improvement Reporting Excellence): Revised publication guidelines from a detailed consensus process. *The Journal of Continuing Education in Nursing, 46*(11), 501–507.

Palinkas, L. A., Aarons, G. A., Horwitz, S., Chamberlain, P., Hurlburt, M., & Landsverk, J. (2010). Mixed method designs in implementation research. *Administration and Policy in Mental Health and Mental Health Services Research, 38*(1), 44–53.

PAR-13-055: Dissemination and Implementation Research in Health (R01). (n.d.). Retrieved 30 June 2016, from http://grants.nih.gov/grants/guide/pa-files/PAR-13-055.html

Pinnock, H., Epiphaniou, E., Sheikh, A., Griffiths, C., Eldridge, S., Craig, P., & Taylor, S. J. C. (2015). Developing standards for reporting implementation studies of complex interventions (StaRI): A systematic review and e-Delphi. *Implementation Science: IS, 10*(1), 1–10.

Proctor, E. K., Landsverk, J., Aarons, G., Chambers, D., Glisson, C., & Mittman, B. (2009). Implementation research in mental health services: An emerging science with conceptual, methodological, and training challenges. *Administration and Policy in Mental Health and Mental Health Services Research, 36*(1), 24–34.

Rabin, B. A., Lewis, C. C., Norton, W. E., Neta, G., Chambers, D., Tobin, J. N., … Glasgow, R. E. (2016). Measurement resources for dissemination and implementation research in health. *Implementation Science, 11*(1), 1–9.

Rabin, B. A., Purcell, P., Naveed, S., Moser, R. P., Henton, M. D., Proctor, E. K., … Glasgow, R. E. (2012). Advancing the application, quality and harmonization of implementation science measures. *Implementation Science, 7*(1), 1–11.

Reliability and Validity. (n.d.). Retrieved June 30, 2016, from https://www.uni.edu/chfasoa/reliabilityandvalidity.htm

Robins, C. S., Ware, N. C., Willging, C. E., Chung, J. Y., Roberto Lewis-Fernández, M. D., et al. (2008). Dialogues on mixed-methods and mental health services research: Anticipating challenges, building solutions. *Psychiatric Services, 59*(7), 727–731.

Schulz, K. F., Altman, D. G., & Moher, D. (2010). CONSORT 2010 statement: Updated guidelines for reporting parallel group randomised trials. *BMC Medicine, 8*(1), 1–9.

Siegel, S. (1964). *Decision and choice: Contributions of Sidney Siegel.* New York, NY: McGraw-Hill.

Stein, K. F., Sargent, J. T., & Rafaels, N. (2007). Intervention research: Establishing fidelity of the independent variable in nursing clinical trials. *Nursing Research, 56*(1), 54–62.

Streiner, D. L., & Norman, G. R. (2008). *Health measurement scales: A practical guide to their development and use* (4th ed.). New York, NY: Oxford University Press.

Tabak, R. G., Khoong, E. C., Chambers, D. A., & Brownson, R. C. (2012). Bridging research and practice: Models for dissemination and implementation research. *American Journal of Preventive Medicine, 43*(3), 337–350.

Teddlie, C., & Tashakkori, A. (2003). Major issues and controversies in the use of mixed methods in the social and behavioral sciences. *Handbook of Mixed Methods in Social & Behavioral Research*, (1st ed.). Thousand Oaks, Sage, 3–50.

The EQUATOR Network | Enhancing the QUAlity and Transparency Of Health Research. (n.d.). Retrieved from http://www.equator-network.org/

Turner, L., Shamseer, L., Altman, D. G., Schulz, K. F., & Moher, D. (2012). Does use of the CONSORT statement impact the completeness of reporting of randomised controlled trials published in medical journals? A Cochrane review. *Systematic Reviews, 1*(1), 1–7.

Valente, T. W. (1996). Social network thresholds in the diffusion of innovations. *Social Networks, 18*(1), 69–89.

Von Elm, E., Altman, D. G., Egger, M., Pocock, S. J., Gøtzsche, P. C., Vandenbroucke, J. P., et al. (2007). The Strengthening the Reporting of Observational Studies in Epidemiology (STROBE) statement: Guidelines for reporting observational studies. *Preventive Medicine, 45*(4), 247–251.

Weiner, B., Amick, H., & Lee, S.-Y. (2008). Conceptualization and measurement of organizational readiness for change: A review of the literature in health services research and other fields. *Medical Care Research and Review., 65*(4), 379–439.

Wisdom, J. P., Chor, K. H. B., Hoagwood, K. E., & Horwitz, S. M. (2014). Innovation adoption: A review of theories and constructs. *Administration and Policy in Mental Health and Mental Health Services Research, 41*(4), 480–502.

Zamanzadeh, V., Ghahramanian, A., Rassouli, M., Abbaszadeh, A., Alavi-Majd, H., & Nikanfar, A.-R. (2015). Design and Implementation Content Validity Study: Development of an instrument for measuring Patient-Centered Communication. *Journal of Caring Sciences, 4*(2), 165–178.

Zuckerman, H. S., Shortell, S. M., Morrison, E. M., & Friedman, B. (1990). Strategic choices for America's Hospitals. JSTOR.

Zumbo, B. D., & Chan, E. K. (2014). *Validity and validation in social, behavioral, and health sciences.* Cham, Springer.

Chapter 10
Implementing Implementation: Integrating the Measurement of Implementation and Effectiveness in Complex Service Systems

Wei Wu Tan, Colleen Jeffreys, and Arno Parolini

Implementation science is concerned with sustaining evidence-based practices in real-world contexts. At its core sits the drive to understand the determinants of successful implementation and identify ways to continuously improve practice, with the ultimate goal of providing services to bring about optimal outcomes for clients. As such, the added value of implementation science lies in its direct relevance to practice, making it impossible to separate implementation research from operational contexts such as case management or business process management.

With this perspective in mind, this chapter describes a framework that will enable implementation stakeholders to measure implementation success over time and to learn about causal mechanisms of implementation in complex service systems, focusing on the issue of creating an integrated multi-purpose data system. We begin by viewing implementation as part of a system component and describe a causal approach of implementation research within a service delivery system. Such an approach depends on putting in place a high-quality data system that integrates research with operational components to form a holistic view of stakeholder incentives in what we denote as the Implementation Space. To ensure that implementation success and causal mechanisms can be measured, it is critical that the total implementation space is considered from the beginning so that data can be purposefully collected, stored and used. We also discuss the process of learning from the perspective of the Plan-Do-Study-Act (PDSA) cycle of continuous quality improvement

---

W. W. Tan (✉) · A. Parolini
Department of Social Work, The University of Melbourne, Melbourne, VIC, Australia

California Child Welfare Indicators Project, School of Social Welfare,
University of California at Berkeley, California, USA
e-mail: ww.tan@unimelb.edu.au; arno.parolini@unimelb.edu.au

C. Jeffreys
Department of Social Work, The University of Melbourne, Melbourne, VIC, Australia
e-mail: colleen.jeffreys@unimelb.edu.au

© Springer Nature Switzerland AG 2020
B. Albers et al. (eds.), *Implementation Science 3.0*,
https://doi.org/10.1007/978-3-030-03874-8_10

(CQI), showing how this can be mapped onto the implementation system. Finally, we briefly discuss the role of funding bodies and government during this transformation.

Viewing Implementation as Systems Component

Since the advent of implementation science as a distinct field of study more than two decades ago (Chambers, 2012), a great deal of research has focused on describing the implementation processes and identifying key implementation factors at various levels and contexts. This has led to a number of implementation models and frameworks which aim to guide practitioners in the implementation of evidence-based practices (Tabak, Khoong, Chambers, & Brownson, 2012).

A common trait of all these models and frameworks is the recognition that implementation is a process involving a large array of contextual factors operating at multiple levels. For example, the Consolidated Framework for Implementation Research (CFIR) synthesises existing theories and consolidates them into five major domains with a total of 37 constructs (Damschroder et al., 2009). The Exploration, Preparation, Implementation, Sustainment (EPIS) framework prescribes four implementation phases, each influenced by groups of inner and outer contextual factors (Aarons, Hurlburt, & Horwitz, 2011). Both these frameworks describe an interconnected system consisting of intervention characteristics, inner context, outer context, individuals involved and implementation strategies, among others.

The need to view implementation as a system component in accordance with the frameworks is increasingly recognised. Systems-based approaches have received attention in recent implementation related literature (Maglio & Mabry, 2011; Chambers et al., 2012; Holmes et al., 2014; Roberts, 2015). As Chambers (2012) points out, after a decade of maturation, implementation science is currently undergoing a transition where the focus has shifted from testing the effectiveness of individual interventions towards sustainment of implementation strategies within complex dynamic systems of care.

In a similar vein, Proctor (2014) suggested that implementation research be directed towards three areas in the future: (1) scaling up of EBPs to broaden their reach and impact, (2) addressing multiple levels of changes in service systems, and (3) adopting and sustaining of multiple EBPs by large systems of care in order to serve clients routinely facing complex problems.

Dynamic systems, however, are characterised by complex structures and multifaceted interactions of system parts. Researchers and practitioners are, therefore, confronted with the challenge of how to measure implementation success. It has been recognised that implementation success can only be measured by taking into account client outcomes, system outcomes and implementation outcomes (Proctor et al., 2011). Thus, implementation success is also contingent on intervention effectiveness, and measurement requires a systems approach that acknowledges interventions and their implementation as integral parts of dynamic service systems with multiple stakeholders, including service providers, practitioners and clients. Furthermore, researchers face methodological challenges, as traditional approaches to establishing causality, such as randomised controlled trials (RCTs) and Hybrid Designs (Curran, Bauer, Mittman, Pyne, & Stetler, 2012), are often unable to capture multilevel dynamic measures of implementation success within complex systems.

In an attempt to fill this gap, Parolini, Tan, and Shlonsky (2019) developed a formal method to describe the causal linkages between implementation success and intervention effectiveness as parts of a system, framing implementation from a decision-making perspective. This approach views implementation as a collection of strategies to introduce and sustain an intervention in a system. These strategies are both the results and drivers of decisions made by agents at different levels across the phases of implementation. This concept is illustrated in Fig. 10.1 using the EPIS framework (Aarons et al., 2011) as an organising structure. The arrow at the bottom represents the decision junctures across the first three implementation phases (Exploration, Adoption Decision/Preparation and Active Implementation). The three circles at the top represent contextual and client variables, feeding into each decision juncture. In the spirit of the conceptual model, the approach integrates the last phase, Sustainment, with the concept of Continuous Quality Improvement (CQI), as shown by the arrow feeding back to the client variables, inner context variables and outer context variables.

This multilevel decision juncture approach enables researchers to identify causal links between the effects of individual implementation components and strategies, measures of effectiveness and potential barriers such as low fidelity by using methods such as choice modelling, structural models and causal inference. Such a systems perspective operates under the principle that change can only be effected by understanding the causal mechanisms acting within a system. That is, simply

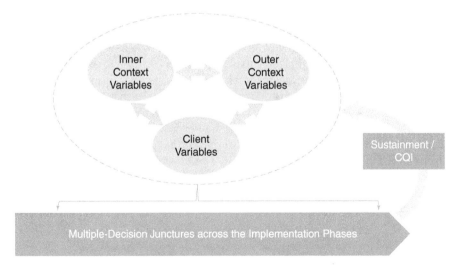

Fig. 10.1 The multilevel decision juncture approach. (Source: Adapted from Parolini et al. (2019))

finding associations between factors is insufficient for truly understanding the underlying processes and their direct and indirect effect on implementation and effectiveness outcomes. Rather, specific testing of these relationships must be driven by theories about the causal relationships between the factors.

To this end, Parolini et al. (2019) illustrated the process of causal analysis[1] in implementation systems based on the three tasks proposed by Heckman and Vytlacil (2007). They demonstrated the approach using a hypothetical case study of a youth mental health intervention with simulation data generated based on empirical studies in the health service research and implementation literature. They successfully illustrated the use of non-experimental data and quantitative methods to identify the effect of implementation strategies on implementation, system and effectiveness outcomes, and they also established a comparison of their approach with traditional experimental approaches. The demonstrated approach is particularly useful when implementing EBPs in complex delivery systems or when conducting RCTs is not an option.

In the following sections, we describe how researchers should purposefully collect, store and use data based on the study of Parolini et al. (2019) to ensure that implementation success can be measured and causal mechanisms can be studied in a complex dynamic service system. Specifically, we focus on practical issues in implementation research, including (i) how implementation success and intervention effectiveness can be integrated in a single research study from a practical perspective (section "Integration of Implementation in Research Designs") and (ii) what a data system that supports implementation research would look like (section "Integrating Implementation with Data Systems"). We also deliberate on viewing implementation sustainment through the lens of CQI (section "Viewing Implementation Sustainment through the Lens of CQI").

Throughout our discussion, we will pay particular attention to the interplay of research foci of implementations scientists and operational priorities of organisations and practitioners delivering services to clients. Implementation is ultimately a matter of practice environments and is concerned with processes to improve the uptake of evidence-based practices to improve clients' outcomes within a service delivery system. However, implementation science is based on research, and therefore, also has a focus on developing theories of change and investigating components of the implementation space that may not be of direct relevance to practitioners in their everyday working environment. A lack of overlap between research foci and operational priorities at different levels of the system is likely to cause friction and can be a significant driver of low fidelity and Type 3 error (Cook & Dobson, 1982; Dobson & Cook, 1980; Rezmovic, 1982). This concept is illustrated in Fig. 10.2, where we show operational priorities and research foci as two separate spaces in a diagram. Together, they define the Implementation Space which represents the full set of stakeholder interests in the implementation system.

---

[1] Elaboration of the difference between causal effects and structural parameters is beyond the scope of this chapter. Readers are referred to more technical papers highlighting that both can be identified within structural systems (Heckman & Vytlacil, 2005; Pearl, 2009; White & Chalak, 2013).

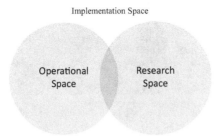

Implementation Space

Fig. 10.2   Implementation space

As illustrated in Fig. 10.2, the two spaces overlap to a degree that depends on the particular research question and study design. The shift of focus in implementation research recommended by practitioners such as Chambers (2012) and Proctor (2014) and the causal approach suggested by Parolini et al. (2019) necessitates the integration of implementation research into real-life practice settings, with an emphasis on sustainment or CQI. This implies a large overlap between the research space and the operational space. In fact, as we draw our attention to the investigation of systems behaviours over time, seamless integration of research and operational spaces into a single system that accounts for stakeholder preferences across all levels becomes all the more important. To this end, the following sections describe a framework of implementation research in a practice environment for ongoing learning about systems behaviour and implementation success.

Integration of Implementation in Research Designs

As outlined in the previous section, every systems level change initiative must consider the whole implementation space to avoid unexpected systems resilience. For implementation, this entails framing implementation efforts within a system of diverse actors whose potentially conflicting interests drive dynamics within the environment. Such complexity highlights the dangers of a narrowly focused research question that ignores stakeholders' diverse interests at different levels, which may lead to unexpected effects.

Unanticipated effects of interventions are well studied and represented as model components in systems disciplines such as Economics and System Dynamics where they are often referred to as *externalities* (e.g. Mas-Colell, Whinston, & Green, 1995) or *policy resistance* (e.g. Sterman, 1994, 2006). Including them in models requires consideration of operational priorities and strategic interests of a wide range of stakeholders. In implementation models, this entails treating implementation itself as an intervention in a system, thus linking implementation success and programme effectiveness within a single research framework. In this section, we provide an overview of an approach to achieve this integration from a practical perspective.

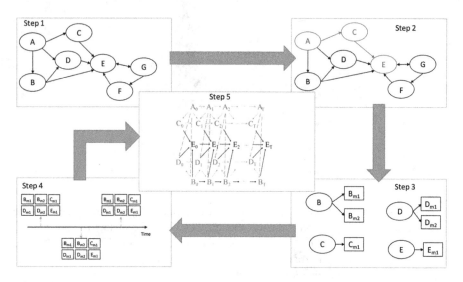

Fig. 10.3 Five-step process of integrated analysis for implementation research

Focusing on the drivers of implementation and outcomes, we propose a general framework for integrated implementation research that consists of five steps. These steps overlap with the approach described in Parolini et al. (2019) and Heckman and Vytlacil (2007), but we focus particularly on practical aspects of data collection during latter stages. Figure 10.3 illustrates our staged process in a schematic form. In the diagrams, ovals represent constructs not directly observable, while rectangles represent measurements, that is, variables included in the analysis. Throughout the whole process, the research question, or hypotheses, should be the centre of attention. In other words, the research question should inform all steps of the process.

Step 1. Developing a Theoretical Model of the Implementation System

This step is in line with Task 1 of the staged process described in Heckman and Vytlacil (2007). The researchers start out with a theoretical model of the system which specifies causal links (arrows in Fig. 10.3, Step 1) between elements of the system and highlights what constructs enter the model at which points (ovals in Fig. 10.3, Step 1). Framed in terms of the multilevel structural decision approach of Parolini et al. (2019), the theoretical model provides a clear understanding of the drivers of each decision made in the process of implementation. Obviously, it would be impossible to capture the complete system in a single model as the number of elements to include is likely to be very large. Hence, it is absolutely crucial that researchers are very clear about the specific questions they want to investigate. It is unlikely that a useful and practically relevant model can be developed without a clear understanding of what one is looking for. So, the first step of every research plan is to develop precise research questions or hypotheses that can be tested.

Once the focus of the study has been established, the next step is to describe the system of mechanisms that generates the outcomes of interest. Using the decision theoretic context of Fig. 10.1, we would build a model of a system in which actors make choices that are influenced by personal and contextual characteristics.

It is important to emphasise that this theory is not merely a product of algorithmic selection of covariates based on correlations, as in a widely applied erroneous approach observed in structural equation models (Bollen & Pearl, 2013). Pearl (2009) and Heckman and Vytlacil (2007), among others, emphasise that the model described in this step represents a precise theory of the mechanisms acting within the system and should be based on existing evidence and expert knowledge rather than simply observing data and making assumptions based on associations. A particularly valuable source of information for model development is the various frameworks for implementation that provide detailed insights into the different components which may hinder or promote implementation endeavours (e.g.Aarons et al., 2011 ; Damschroder et al., 2009). Most importantly, the model should not be driven by the data that happen to be available to the researcher. This critical point clearly separates the structural systems approach described here from data-driven models focusing on prediction.

Step 2. Identifying What Data Are Needed to Answer the Questions of Interest

Once a credible theoretical model has been developed, the next step is to identify the effects of interest within the model. In other words, we examine whether the effect of an intervention or implementation strategy can actually be identified, given what we know about the system. At this step, we operate under the assumption of a hypothetical population that is large enough to justify asymptotic assumptions and we are not concerned with sample size. Since the techniques involved in Steps 1 and 2 are well beyond the focus of this article, we will not treat them here in more detail, other than symbolically highlighting the process of identification by colouring a segment of the diagram in Step 2 of Fig. 10.3. Readers interested in the technical details may refer to the related literature (Heckman & Pinto, 2015; Heckman & Vytlacil, 2007; Pearl, 2009; White & Chalak, 2013). An important outcome of Step 2 for practical research planning is that this process highlights variables (including confounders) that will need to be included in, or excluded from, the analysis (Pearl, 2009; White & Lu, 2011).

Step 3. Choosing the Right Measures at the Right Level

The choice of measurements is indicated in Fig. 10.3 with the matching of the ovals to the rectangles. While Step 2 is concerned with the identification of parameters and consequently provides a direct way to select variables based on a rigorous theoretical model, we have so far only specified structural constructs that may or may not be directly observable. Without reliable measurement of factors in the theoretical model, inferences about the effects of implementation and conclusions regarding implementation success are no more than subjective statements.

Yet, choosing suitable measures is far more than a trivial task, as is evidenced by a large and growing literature devoted to measuring implementation constructs (Chaudoir, Dugan, & Barr, 2013; Lewis et al., 2015), including measures of implementation success at different levels of the system (Proctor et al., 2011).

As a first principle, measures used in quantitative analyses should have known properties and well-established reliability and validity. For implementation research, this is especially important, with many ongoing efforts seeking to establish standardised measurements of factors not directly observable in different settings of the implementation space (e.g. Fernandez et al., 2018).

In addition to considering reliability and validity, it is crucial to choose measures that capture information at the right level. While this may seem to be a trivial statement, we have observed that it is often a substantial barrier in practice. As a general rule, researchers should aim to apply measures that capture the variation at the level at which the effect of interest is anticipated. For example, to investigate intervention adoption within an organisation, the optimal level of measurement would not be at the organisational level or provider level but actually at the client level. Through aggregation of client-level measurements, one can then derive an organisational-level measure that is more accurate than assessment at higher levels of the system. In a similar vein, Implementation Climate (Ehrhart, Aarons, & Farahnak, 2014) should be measured at the employee level and subsequently aggregated to derive an organisational-level representation of the supportive environment for evidence-based practice. This highlights the fact that the level of measurement may not be identical to the level at which outcomes are defined. Furthermore, to capture implementation success within systems, measures of implementation will need to be collected in addition to other relevant personal and contextual information as described in the section "Integrating Implementation with Data Systems".

This also accentuates the importance of appropriate sampling frames for implementation measures. As an example, let us assume that we want to investigate the effects of an intervention and, in particular, how differences in the implementation fidelity of this intervention affect outcomes. Depending on the study design and system model, implementation measures may be confounders, moderators, mediators, or instrumental variables for the treatment effect of the intervention. In any case, the sampling frame for implementation measures will have considerable impact on the inference drawn from analyses. For example, if implementation fidelity is only assessed for a subset of the analysis sample, then inference is dependent on assumptions of extrapolation equivalent to those in the case of missing values. Hence, it is preferable that, where possible, measures that are important to assess implementation are administered to the total analysis sample.

Step 4. Choosing the Right Frequency of Measurement

To maintain a focus on system behaviour and continuous quality improvement, collection of data across time, represented by the repeated sets of rectangles in Step 3 of Fig. 10.3, is indispensable. Again, the theoretical model developed in Step 1 should be used as a guide to decide the frequency of measurement. This is a crucial step as the frequency of data collection directly impacts the identification of effects in the system. For example, consider the situation shown in Fig. 10.4 where the aim is to identify the effect of variable A on variable B. The subscripts on these variables in the top panel represent the time points of measurement.

If measurement is done, for example, only yearly instead of half-yearly, the originally recursive system in the top panel of Fig. 10.4 will be transformed into a non-recursive system at the data level. In other words, the directionality of the causal effect can no longer be identified from the data because this information is not preserved at the annual aggregate level. This example illustrates how choices regarding the timing of measurements can directly influence the conclusions drawn from research findings, as often highlighted in relation to cross-sectional study designs.

Step 5. Using Data to Answer the Questions

Once a theoretical model has been developed (Step 1), causal effects have been identified (Step 2), appropriate measures have been selected (Step 3) and administered at suitable intervals (Step 4), we can learn about the causal mechanisms and

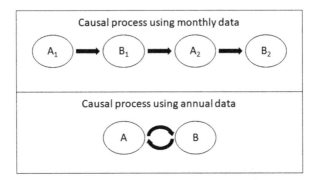

Fig. 10.4 The effects of measurement frequency on parameter identification

overall system behaviour over time. It is only during this final step that sample size and variation will have to be considered. At this stage, researchers should conduct ex ante power analyses, based on previous evidence, to determine the necessary sample sizes in cases where it is not feasible to collect data from the total population.

However, the actual estimation of systems parameters is beyond the focus of this article, and readers interested in the technical details may refer to the related literature (e.g. Skrondal & Rabe-Hesketh, 2004).

Integrating Implementation with Data Systems

The section "Integration of Implementation in Research Designs" delineates a 5-step implementation research framework that facilitates the investigation of causal mechanisms of implementation in service systems setting. This section deals with the practical issue of implementing an actual data system that enables the application of the 5-step framework.

As outlined in the previous section, there must be, by definition, a large overlap between the research space and the operational space in implementation science. Consequently, the realisation of a data system to capture implementation success and intervention effectiveness is in itself an undertaking that requires careful implementation. This calls for a well-considered, flexible, and high-quality data system that caters fully to the complete implementation space, including research foci and operational priorities. In fact, a truly integrated implementation space requires the integration of implementation with data systems.

Traditionally, data collection systems are often classified into two categories: (1) administrative databases which are built with a focus on operational domains such as case management, reporting and strategic planning; and (2) research data collection systems with a focus on measures of relevance to a particular research question, such as attitudes, standardised scales, etc. However, in reality, database designs can be very flexible and can easily accommodate the needs of both categories of data systems mentioned above.[2]

In this section, we describe the design principles for high-quality hybrid data systems that combine the elements of a research data collection system with an operational administrative database system. We also provide an example of a simplified service delivery data model that integrates research foci and operational priorities. We approach this complex topic from the perspective of an optimal scenario, where a data system is designed by service agencies to fulfil their operational responsibilities as well as to learn about ways to optimise practice and business

---

[2] For example, most customer relationship management systems today are built on a modular basis that support the flexibility to expand the functionalities of data systems based on the needs of businesses. While standard solutions are most likely not able to fully cater to the multifaceted needs of a service delivery systems described here, module-based designs are easily implementable in data systems specially designed for the purposes described here.

processes. While our framework may be seen as ambitious, it represents the optimal benchmark for integration of research and operational components within a single data system that supports a culture of continuous quality improvement and organisational learning over time. However, the realisation of an integrated data system may be subject to system restrictions in many settings (e.g. funding or existing data collection systems). In such cases, the overall structure of the data system outlined in this section would remain unchanged, but individual data components may be collected from different systems and linked using a variety of approaches. Hence, we will focus on the optimal scenario where we are able to design a comprehensive data system from scratch and acknowledge that alternative ways of generating data sets for different purposes can be interpreted as approximations to our benchmark model.

Data Systems as Key Factor to Measuring Implementation Success

The quality of any analytics or research is predicated on the quality of the data available for the analysis, as the old adage 'garbage in garbage out' indicates. When research data needs are an afterthought, and researchers must rely on whatever is available in the operational administrative data set, there are immediate limitations placed on what can be evaluated and our confidence in the findings. In such cases, the overlap between research space and operational space is effectively small, regardless of the intention to integrate the two. One can say without exaggeration that data systems are key to measuring implementation success and, therefore, should be designed taking into account the 5-step framework described above.

Our perspective shares some commonalities with the areas of information management (e.g. Krcmar, 2005) and knowledge management (e.g. Maier, 2007), where data systems are an integral part of the translation of implicit knowledge and attitudes held by practitioners into explicit knowledge available to the organisation and researchers to effect change and improve processes.

While there are different perspectives on data quality dimensions, in general, the major considerations for any data system to promote the collection of quality data include the following four dimensions (Pipino, Lee, & Wang, 2002; Wand & Wang, 1996):

- Completeness – the extent to which data are of appropriate breadth, depth and scope (Wang & Strong, 1996, p.32).
- Correctness – the extent to which data are accurate, reliable and free of errors (Wang & Strong, 1996, p.31).
- Consistency – the extent to which data are always represented in the same manner and remain compatible with legacy data (Wang & Strong, 1996, p.32).
- Timeliness – the extent to which the currency of the data is appropriate and the data are still useful (Wang & Strong, 1996, p.32).

Completeness

To address the completeness dimension of data quality, we should consider the requirements of all stakeholders involved at various levels in the implementation project. These stakeholders can generally be divided into three main groups – researchers, operational/management, and providers and their clients.[3] By considering their data needs from the outset, a more complete data model can be designed and implemented. It is important that all necessary data fields required for both operational and research purposes are designed into the data system and populated from the start of the data collection process. At a detailed level, this also requires that all necessary data fields are set to mandatory in the data system and cannot be skipped, preventing missing values. In situations where not all relevant data can be collected and input within a single data repository, planning should include concepts and solutions for complementing data collection with data linkage to other data systems to fill information gaps where necessary (e.g. Wulczyn et al., 2017).

Correctness

To address the correctness dimension of quality, we need to ensure that 'free text' data entry fields are limited to notes and that data variables have a discrete list of valid values for selection (including not applicable, declined to answer and not known) or a defined range of values with both upper and lower limits, thus preventing invalid values.

Where linkage of data repositories is necessary to achieve completeness, these considerations would be part of the data system design stage to ensure acceptable reliability of linkage results, for example, by using consistent identifier structures. An important issue to consider is that in cases where data linkage is required, completeness and correctness of data are no longer within the control of the database administrator or researcher but depend on business rules and external data quality assurance measures installed in the external systems to be linked.

Consistency

To address the consistency dimension of quality, logic built into the data system should reflect business rules that describe important relationships between data variables both within and across data systems. Thus, data system logic should be employed to ensure uniformity of equivalent data variables throughout the data systems and also enforce necessary dependencies between data variables. For example,

---

[3] A fourth group of stakeholders are funding bodies and government. However, we defer the discussion on this group to the end of this section as in most cases, it may not be directly involved in the implementation project itself. Generally, the role of this group is more likely to be that of a policy maker or a data user with an interest in impact assessment or policy.

a business rule could be implemented in all data systems that dates are always recorded in the DD/MM/YYYY format as opposed to the alternative MM/DD/YYYY format, thus avoiding ambiguity around dates such as 1/12/2001 which are valid in both formats but represent quite different dates. Similarly, data integrity can be maintained over time by preventing deprecated variables and values from being deleted or overwritten.

Timeliness

To address the timeliness dimension of quality, data systems need to be designed to encourage the timely collection of data through good user interface (UI) design which promotes ease of use. This can be encouraged through facilities such as calendaring of appointments, automatic scheduling and reminders of key data collection events such as client assessments.

In addition to the four dimensions described above, an often-overlooked aspect of data quality is the impact of the provider's workload at the point of data collection. Time pressure and caseload of providers are an important consideration with regard to data quality since the priority of providers is to meet the needs of the client, not necessarily the administrative needs of the organisation. Under time pressure, the minimal amount of data required to satisfy the data system will typically be collected unless the providers can see that there are benefits to themselves in collecting the full data needed and are assisted in doing so in a timely and efficient manner. If the workload of the providers can be addressed through the design of intuitive and responsive user interfaces that follow typical case workflows, thus supporting and assisting them in their day-to-day work, we would expect the quality of the data collected to improve. Simple mechanisms such as reminders for client appointments and assessments, drop-down list of pre-loaded values, and lookup lists can provide value for the provider staff.

Figure 10.5 defines how the different data requirements of the three project streams – Research, Operation/Administration and Service Delivery – should inform the design of the data system that supports implementation

- The *Research* stream covers the evaluation requirements and involves measures and outcomes that need to be collected at set intervals throughout the evaluation (e.g. base-line, follow-up, case close), following the 5-step implementation research framework described in the section "Integration of Implementation in Research Designs".
- The *Administrative* stream centers primarily on operational and management reporting and performance targets across clients, programmes, outlets and workgroups.
- The *Service Delivery* stream focuses on front-line delivery of service to clients by providers, covering areas such as client lists, case notes, appointments and reviews.

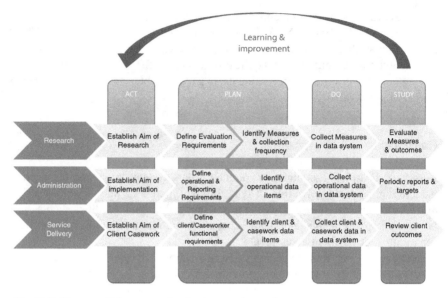

Fig. 10.5 Three parallel streams of an implementation project

By overlaying the Plan-Do-Study-Act (PDSA) cycle developed by Deming (1986) onto the three streams in Fig. 10.5, we can construct a learning and improvement cycle that is informed by and serves all three streams of the implementation space.

A Simplified Service Delivery Data Model

We provide an example of a simplified service delivery data model from which we can see how following an integrated and complementary planning and developmental process, the needs of all stakeholders can be met. Figure 10.6 shows the Entity Relationship Diagram (ERD) of the data model, where research data and operational data are presented in different colours. Although the data entities can be identified as either supporting the research or the operational requirements, they are still inter-related and together form an integrated foundation for the data system. It is the totality of this system that informs the implementation space and will be used in the 5-step implementation research framework.

In some cases, there is overlap between the data requirements of all stakeholders such as with the Client, Service Activity and Program Schedule entities. The Client entity is central to any data system centred on service delivery, while the Service Activity entity records contact time between the provider and the client as well as scheduled dates for both providing services and assessments. The scheduling of programme events that supports the providers in service delivery and assessment of intervention outcomes are both facilitated by the Program Schedule entity. This entity has a central role in the collection of data by the providers for both service provision and research purposes in a timely manner.

An important difference to traditional administrative database systems is that measures of implementation, client outcomes and other variables of importance to the research space are embedded in the data system (AssesMeasure) and are directly related to other entities within the model (AssessForm). These elements can be designed as individual components, or modules, and can be collected at different times. For example, a measure of programme fidelity could be administered at the end of a service episode for each client or a scale to measure implementation climate within the organisation could be administered annually as part of staff satisfaction surveys.[4]

The generic design presented in Fig. 10.6 highlights the advantages of a modular multipurpose data system, namely their flexibility. Given appropriate planning during the design phase, these data systems can be adapted over time to accommodate changing demands of stakeholders across the system. This is a crucial advantage compared to standard solutions since stakeholder priorities, such as research questions or focus areas for quality improvement, are likely to change as the implementation system evolves. For example, it is straightforward to introduce additional measurement scales to the system in Fig. 10.6 by expanding the AssessMeasure and AssessForm entities as required. While standard products, such as readily available customer relationship management solutions, may often be attractive to provider agencies due to shorter development times and lower costs at the onset, purpose-built flexible hybrid data systems may offer considerable efficiencies over the product lifecycle, especially if flexibility of content or reporting structures is anticipated.

The extent of such comparative advantages will depend on the expected changes to the data system required in the future, and the costs of alternative options (e.g. standard software) including costs related to managing data system compatibility and data quality issues, etc.[5] Hence, decisions regarding flexibility of data systems should be driven by the expected costs and benefits over the lifecycle (e.g. Total-Cost-of-Ownership; see Krcmar, 2005) of alternative products.

We now consider the role of funding bodies and government agencies who are also stakeholders either as funders, data users, programme designers or policy makers. While funding bodies and government agencies may not be directly involved in the implementation project itself, they do have the ability to influence the dissemination of flexible data systems either directly or indirectly. Direct influences include financing agencies to implement evidence-based practices and develop hybrid data systems, or providing a centrally developed data system maintained by government

---

[4] Concerns about anonymity for such measurements could be easily accommodated by restricting the content of reporting functions to aggregate measures or to report individual-level measures with de-identified data only. Alternatively, measures could be administered without linking the information to a particular identification key, that is, the data are truly anonymous but are still stored within the same data system and therefore available for CQI endeavours.

[5] In this context, costs are not restricted to monetary costs but also include opportunity costs as defined in the economic literature.

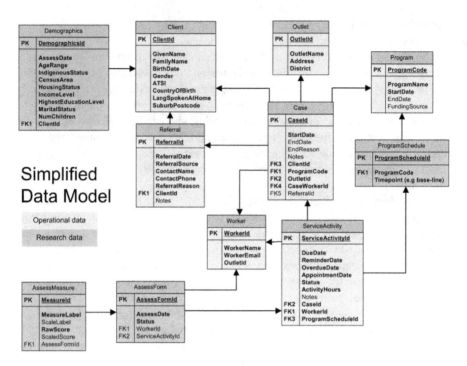

Fig. 10.6 A simplified data model of service delivery

that is accessible to agency staff. Indirectly, government and funding bodies could enhance the dissemination of flexible systems through integrating data on implementation success into minimum data set collections.

In most cases, this group of stakeholders play the role of a regulator or data user with an interest in impact assessment or policy. As such, routine progress reports would have to be generated for them. However, data needed for such purposes are not likely to differ from what we have considered above.

Viewing Implementation Sustainment Through the Lens of CQI

By collecting data at all levels and across all three streams over time, the data system described above allows iterative learning about implementation as part of the service delivery system. When carried out iteratively, the 5-step model of causal inquiries, based on this data system, facilitates information for implementation sustainment and CQI. From the outset, we have presented the Sustainment phase of implementation as a CQI process, as shown in Fig. 10.1. This emphasis on sustainment and improvement through iterative learning is in accordance with the principles of Deming's Plan-Do-Study-Act (PDSA) cycle of CQI (Deming, 1986).

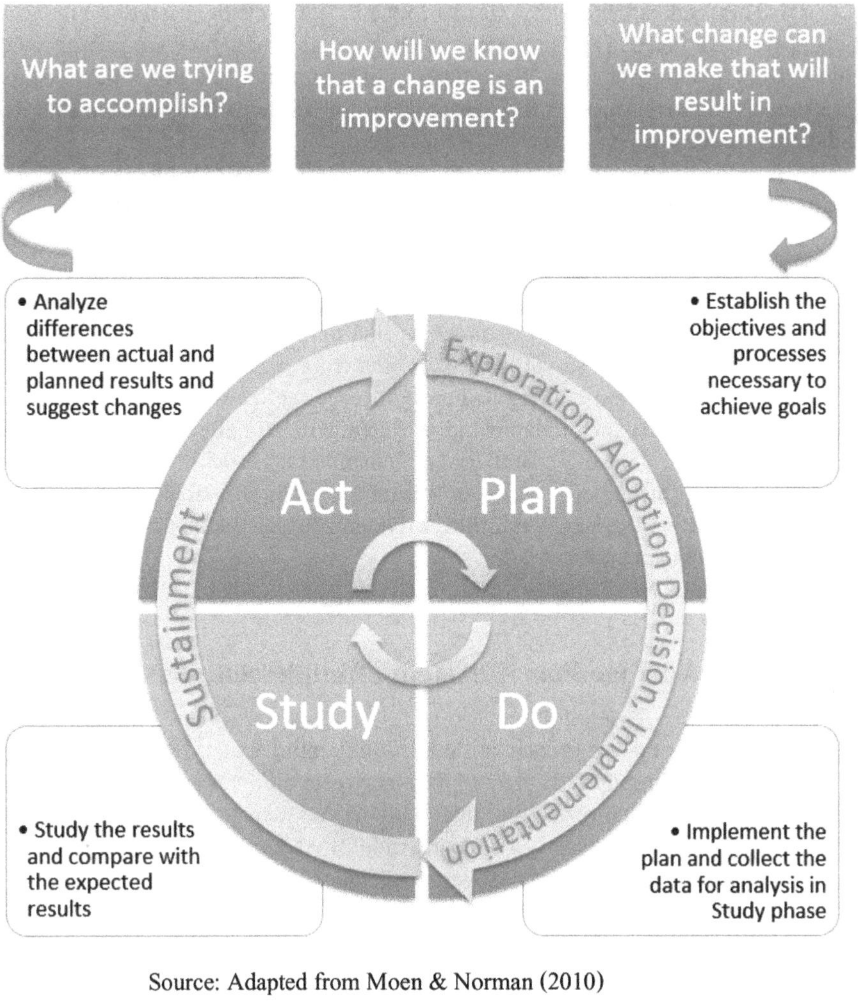

What are we trying to accomplish?

How will we know that a change is an improvement?

What change can we make that will result in improvement?

• Analyze differences between actual and planned results and suggest changes

Exploration

Adoption Decision

Implementation

Sustainment

Act

Plan

Study

Do

• Establish the objectives and processes necessary to achieve goals

• Study the results and compare with the expected results

• Implement the plan and collect the data for analysis in Study phase

Source: Adapted from Moen & Norman (2010)

Fig. 10.7. Model for improvement. (Source: Adapted from Moen & Norman (2010))

Originally formulated as a Plan-Do-Check-Act (PDCA) cycle (Deming, 1950), the PDSA cycle was a revised formulation which emphasises studying rather than checking and, therefore, places the emphasis on learning as well as improvement (Moen & Norman, 2010). The PDSA cycle, shown in Fig. 10.7, further evolved into a Model for Improvement, which incorporates three fundamental questions (Langley, Nolan, & Nolan, 1994) central to the model for improvement, providing the focus for the continuous improvement and learning process driven by the PDSA cycle, as shown at the top of Fig. 10.7.

In our 5-step approach, learning occurs through an iterative process of evaluation, with sustainment portrayed as a quality improvement process where previous experiences provide feedback to the system between cycles of evaluation as a form of CQI. This feedback process is similar to the PDSA cycle delineated in Fig. 10.7, where we have inserted the implementation phases to show how the two perspectives can be mapped together. When high-quality data collected in a timely fashion are used in conjunction with the causal structural model, it provides insights for adjusting the strategy or operation.

An important aspect of continuous improvement is the establishment of ongoing value for stakeholders across the implementation space. From this perspective, the research focus is directly linked to the organisational focus through data quality and research translation. Another characteristic of our model is that each stream by itself is subject to implementation and consequently CQI. For example, research projects need to be implemented into the practice environment, data systems are implemented to facilitate client service provision, and reporting systems are implemented into managerial decision-making to improve process effectiveness and efficiency. These interventions to the implementation system will have effects on the data quality which forms a core ingredient for implementation research that, in turn, will provide valuable insights for the other streams. Overall, a systems perspective on implementation emphasises a multilevel dynamic CQI structure that has effects within and across streams.

Bringing It All Together: A System of Implementation

The central tenet of our approach, as detailed in Parolini et al. (2019) and expanded here to include high-quality data systems, is the recognition of implementation as a system component, acknowledging interventions and their implementation as integral parts of dynamic service systems with multiple stakeholders. As such, we need to recognise that any project involving implementation should not be just about research, service delivery or administrative needs, but a synthesis of all three. Therefore, data systems which form an integral part of the implementation system must be designed with considerable stakeholders input at all three levels at the design phase and as the project progresses, to ensure that the project delivers outcomes for everyone involved and continues to deliver.

Stakeholder engagement is one of the major requirements for a successful data project (Kimball, Ross, Thornthwaite, Mundy, & Becker, 2008). In order to succeed, any system of implementation must deliver value to stakeholders across all three streams shown in Fig. 10.5. Each of these groups should be catered for and encouraged to participate in the requirement gathering and design process. Using this approach, a data system that adds value to each stakeholder and encourages ongoing participation in the implementation cycle can be built, thus paving the way for the 5-step implementation research framework introduced in this article.

As the field of implementation science matures and research moves towards sustainment of implementation strategies within complex dynamic systems of care, the integration of implementation research into real-life practice settings will become increasingly important. In this chapter, we have addressed critical issues such as how implementation success and intervention effectiveness can be integrated into a single research study from a practical perspective, and what a data system that supports implementation research in a real-world practice context would look like. Such issues are best pursued by prospectively planning implementation research in an integrated fashion and embedding these concepts within data systems that support continuous quality improvement and practice optimisation across all domains of the implementation space.

References

Aarons, G. A., Hurlburt, M., & Horwitz, S. M. (2011). Advancing a conceptual model of evidence-based practice implementation in public service sectors. *Administration and Policy in Mental Health and Mental Health Services Research, 38*(1), 4–23. https://doi.org/10.1007/s10488-010-0327-7

Bollen, K. A., & Pearl, J. (2013). Eight myths about causality and structural equation models. In S. L. Morgan (Ed.), *Handbook of causal analysis for social research* (pp. 301–328). Dordrecht: Springer Netherlands. https://doi.org/10.1007/978-94-007-6094-3_15

Chambers, D. (2012). Foreword. In R. C. Brownson, G. A. Colditz, & E. K. Proctor (Eds.), *Dissemination and implementation research in health: Translating science to practice* (pp. vii–xix). Oxford: Oxford University Press.

Chambers, D., Wilson, P., Thompson, C., Harden, M., Coiera, E. (2012) Social Network Analysis in Healthcare Settings: A Systematic Scoping Review. PLoS ONE 7(8):e41911

Chaudoir, S. R., Dugan, A. G., & Barr, C. H. (2013). Measuring factors affecting implementation of health innovations: A systematic review of structural, organizational, provider, patient, and innovation level measures. *Implementation Science, 8*(1), 22. https://doi.org/10.1186/1748-5908-8-22

Cook, T. J., & Dobson, L. D. (1982). Reaction to reexamination: More on type III error in program evaluation. *Evaluation and Program Planning, 5*(2), 119–121. https://doi.org/10.1016/0149-7189(82)90018-0

Curran, G. M., Bauer, M., Mittman, B., Pyne, J. M., & Stetler, C. (2012). Effectiveness-implementation hybrid designs: Combining elements of clinical effectiveness and implementation research to enhance public health impact. *Medical Care, 50*(3), 217–226. https://doi.org/10.1097/MLR.0b013e3182408812

Damschroder, L. J., Aron, D. C., Keith, R. E., Kirsh, S. R., Alexander, J. A., & Lowery, J. C. (2009). Fostering implementation of health services research findings into practice: A consolidated framework for advancing implementation science. *Implementation Science, 4*, 50. https://doi.org/10.1186/1748-5908-4-50

Deming, W. E. (1950). *Elementary principles of the statistical control of quality: A series of lectures.* Nippon Kagaku Gijutsu Remmei. Retrieved from https://books.google.com.au/books?id=8k5DGQAACAAJ

Deming, W. E. (1986). *Out of the crisis.* Cambridge, MA: Cambridge University Press. Retrieved from https://books.google.com.au/books?id=4qw8AAAAIAAJ

Dobson, D., & Cook, T. J. (1980). Avoiding type III error in program evaluation: Results from a field experiment. *Evaluation and Program Planning, 3*(4), 269–276. https://doi.org/10.1016/0149-7189(80)90042-7

Ehrhart, M. G., Aarons, G. A., & Farahnak, L. R. (2014). Assessing the organizational context for EBP implementation: The development and validity testing of the Implementation Climate Scale (ICS). *Implementation Science, 9*(1), 157. https://doi.org/10.1186/s13012-014-0157-1

Fernandez, M. E., Walker, T. J., Weiner, B. J., Calo, W. A., Liang, S., Risendal, B., ... Kegler, M. C. (2018). Developing measures to assess constructs from the inner setting domain of the consolidated framework for implementation research. *Implementation Science, 13*(1), 52. https://doi.org/10.1186/s13012-018-0736-7

Heckman, J. J., & Pinto, R. (2015). Causal analysis after Haavelmo. *Econometric Theory, 31*(1), 115–151. https://doi.org/10.1017/S026646661400022X

Heckman, J. J., & Vytlacil, E. (2005). Structural equations, treatment effects, and econometric policy evaluation. *Econometrica, 73*(3), 669–738. https://doi.org/10.1111/j.1468-0262.2005.00594.x

Heckman, J. J., & Vytlacil, E. J. (2007). Chapter 70 Econometric evaluation of social programs, part I: Causal models, structural models and econometric policy evaluation. In J. J. Heckman & E. E. Leamer (Eds.), *Handbook of econometrics, Vol. 6* (pp. 4779–4874). North Holland: Elsevier. https://doi.org/10.1016/S1573-4412(07)06070-9

Holmes, B.J., Finegood, D.T., Riley, B.L., Best, A. (2014). Systems thinking in dissemination and implementation research. In R. C. Brownson, G. A. Colditz, & E. K. Proctor (Eds.), *Dissemination and Implementation Research in Health: Translating Science to Practice* (pp. 175–91). New York; Oxford: Oxford University Press.

Kimball, R., Ross, M., Thornthwaite, W., Mundy, J., & Becker, B. (2008). In Tom (Ed.), *The data warehouse lifecycle toolkit: Practical techniques for building data warehouse and business intelligence systems* (2nd ed.). Indianapolis: Wiley.

Krcmar, H. (2005). *Informations management* (4th ed.). Berlin, Germany: Springer.

Langley, G. J., Nolan, K. M., & Nolan, T. W. (1994). The Foundation of Improvement. *Quality Progress, 27*(6), 81–86.

Lewis, C. C., Stanick, C. F., Martinez, R. G., Weiner, B. J., Kim, M., Barwick, M., & Comtois, K. A. (2015). The society for implementation research collaboration instrument review project: A methodology to promote rigorous evaluation. *Implementation Science, 10*(1), 2. https://doi.org/10.1186/s13012-014-0193-x

Maglio, P.P., & Mabry, P.L. (2011). Agent-based models and systems science approaches to public health. Am J Prev Med, 40(3):392–394.

Maier, R. (2007). *Knowledge management systems: Information and communication technologies for knowledge management* (3rd ed.). Berlin, Germany: Springer.

Moen, R. D., & Norman, C. L. (2010). Circling back. *Quality Progress, 11*, 20.

Mas-Colell, A., Whinston, M. D., & Green, J. R. (1995). *Microeconomic theory*. New York: Oxford University Press.

Parolini A., Tan W.W., Shlonsky A. (2019). Decision-based models of the implementation of interventions in systems of healthcare: Implementation outcomes and intervention effectiveness in complex service environments. *PLOS ONE 14*(10): e0223129. https://doi.org/10.1371/journal.pone.0223129

Pearl, J. (2009). *Causality: Models, reasoning, and inference* (2nd ed.). New York: Cambridge University Press.

Pipino, L. L., Lee, Y. W., & Wang, R. Y. (2002). Data quality assessment. *Communications of the ACM, 45*(4). https://doi.org/10.1145/505248.506010

Proctor, E. (2014). Dissemination and Implementation Research. In *Encyclopedia of social work*. Oxford University Press. Retrieved from http://socialwork.oxfordre.com/view/10.1093/acrefore/9780199975839.001.0001/acrefore-9780199975839-e-900

Proctor, E., Silmere, H., Raghavan, R., Hovmand, P., Aarons, G., Bunger, A., ... Hensley, M. (2011). Outcomes for implementation research: Conceptual distinctions, measurement challenges, and research agenda. *Administration and Policy in Mental Health and Mental Health Services Research, 38*(2), 65–76. https://doi.org/10.1007/s10488-010-0319-7

Rezmovic, E. L. (1982). Program implementation and evaluation results: A reexamination of type III error in a field experiment. *Evaluation and Program Planning, 5*(2), 111–118. https://doi.org/10.1016/0149-7189(82)90017-9

Roberts, M. S. (2015) Dynamic Simulation in Health Care Comes of Age. Value in Health 18 (2):143–144

Skrondal, A., & Rabe-Hesketh, S. (2004). *Generalized latent variable modeling: Multilevel, longitudinal, and structural equation models*. Boca Raton, FL: Chapman & Hall/CRC.

Sterman, J. D. (1994). Learning in and about complex systems. *System Dynamics Review, 10*(2–3), 291–330. https://doi.org/10.1002/sdr.4260100214

Sterman, J. D. (2006). Learning from evidence in a complex world. *American Journal of Public Health, 96*(3), 505–514. https://doi.org/10.2105/AJPH.2005.066043

Tabak, R. G., Khoong, E. C., Chambers, D. A., & Brownson, R. C. (2012). Bridging research and practice. Models for dissemination and implementation research. *American Journal of Preventive Medicine, 43*, 337–350.

Wand, Y., & Wang, R. Y. (1996). Anchoring data quality dimensions in ontological foundations. *Communications of the ACM, 39*(11), 86–95. https://doi.org/10.1145/240455.240479

Wang, R. Y., & Strong, D. M. (1996). Beyond accuracy: What data quality means to data consumers. *Journal of Management Information Systems, 12*(4), 5–33. https://doi.org/10.1080/07421222.1996.11518099

White, H., & Chalak, K. (2013). Identification and identification failure for treatment effects using structural systems. *Econometric Reviews, 32*(3), 273–317. https://doi.org/10.1080/07474938.2012.690664

White, H., & Lu, X. (2011). Causal diagrams for treatment effect estimation with application to efficient covariate selection. *The Review of Economics and Statistics, 93*(4), 1453–1459. https://doi.org/10.1162/REST_a_00153

Wulczyn, F., Clinch, R., Coulton, C., Keller, S., Moore, J., Muschkin, C., … Barghaus, K. (2017). *Establishing a standard data model for large-scale IDS use* (actionable intelligence for social policy, expert panel report). Actionable intelligence for social policy, University of Pennsylvania. Retrieved from https://www.aisp.upenn.edu/wp-content/uploads/2016/07/Data-Standards.pdf

Chapter 11
The Scale-Up of Linked Multilevel Interventions: A Case Study

Fred Wulczyn and Sara Feldman

Introduction

In this chapter, we describe the scale-up and impact of a *linked multilevel intervention* in a public child welfare system (the Project).[1] Linked multilevel interventions are interventions with multiple components that target one or more levels within the systems that affect health and other service outcomes (Trickett & Beehler, 2013). In health care, multilevel interventions are gaining traction (Huang, Drewnoski, Kumanyika, & Glass, 2009; Scott et al., 2013; Trickett & Beehler, 2013), but there are very few references to multilevel interventions in the child welfare literature despite the obvious parallels. Families with children in the child welfare system face challenges across multiple life domains, and the systems designed to serve those families are administratively and financially interdependent. Single prong interventions that address one level of the service system while ignoring the interdependencies may simply be less effective in the long run. In this chapter, we describe one attempt to align the interdependencies in ways that improve the chances an intervention will have its intended effect.

The setting for this study is a large urban child welfare system where leadership, working with the private sector, sought to increase permanency rates (i.e., reunification, adoption, and guardianship) and placement stability. Both outcomes are central to the ways in which the effectiveness of child welfare systems is judged. The main clinical interventions selected by the public child welfare agency were *Keeping*

---

[1] This chapter is based on an evaluation report prepared for the public child welfare agency that developed the linked interventions. Additional information about those reports is available from the authors. In addition, see Chamberlain, Feldman, Wulczyn, Saldana, and Forgatch (2016).

F. Wulczyn (✉) · S. Feldman
Center for State Child Welfare Data, Chapin Hall Center for Children,
University of Chicago, Chicago, IL, USA
e-mail: fwulczyn@chapinhall.org

© Springer Nature Switzerland AG 2020
B. Albers et al. (eds.), *Implementation Science 3.0*,
https://doi.org/10.1007/978-3-030-03874-8_11

Foster Parents Supported and Trained (KEEP) and *Parenting Through Change* (PTC).[2] Each intervention targets caregiver skills, and both have been named as evidence-based interventions (EBIs).[3]

In addition, agency leadership linked the EBIs to *administrative and fiscal changes* intended to reinforce the EBI*s*. On the administrative side, the public agency required their private sector partners to lower caseloads, to alter the role of supervisors, and to reduce the number of children placed in a single foster home at any one time. Caseloads were reduced in order to make time for the new work case-workers were asked to do as part of the intervention. Similarly, supervisory routines were altered so that supervisors could spend more time building the capacity of their staff to engage families in high-quality, goal-focused casework. As for fiscal changes, the public agency funded the EBI scale-up and other investments with savings from the expected reductions in foster care utilization. Fiscal strategies that rely on reinvestment are increasingly common in child welfare (Wulczyn, 2000; Wulczyn & Orlebeke, 2000). For example, the federal Title IV-E Waiver Programs (the Waivers) rely on reinvestment as a way to funnel resources out of the foster care program and into nonplacement services.[4] In this project, funds were recycled as part of an effort to upgrade the process, quality, and capacity to deliver better foster care services (Wulczyn, Alpert, Orlebeke, & Haight, 2014). The EBIs linked to the administrative changes and the reinvestment strategy represent the multilevel intervention.

The chapter is divided into four parts. Part one focuses on the EBI and its implementation. In its fiscal model, the public agency projected an impact large enough to generate the resources needed to finance the EBI scale-up and reduced caseloads. For that reason, EBI training involved virtually all of the caseworkers and supervisors working in the five private agencies selected for the project. It was a significant logistical undertaking. The Oregon Social Learning Center (OSLC), which is where both KEEP and PTC were developed, was brought in by the public agency to conduct the training.

The second and third parts of the chapter focus on findings from the evaluation. We first describe the implementation study and then turn our attention to the outcomes study. The chapter closes with a summary of lessons learned.

---

[2] Although the public agency implemented both KEEP and PTC as a paired intervention – KEEP targets foster parents and PTC was focused on bio-parents – we limit our discussion of the interventions to KEEP in order to better focus on the multilevel, linked nature of the intervention. We speculate that the expected, at-scale effect of the EB intervention depends on its alignment with the other forces in the so-called system that affect performance and outcomes. This is similar to the EPIS model of EB implementation (Aarons, Hurlburt, & Horwitz, 2011), but it differs in important ways. In the EPIS model, the issue is how various multilevel factors affect the implementation of an EBP. In our case, the multiple levels are conceptualized as part of the intervention itself.

[3] For more information about KEEP, see http://www.cebc4cw.org/program/keeping-foster-and-kin-parents-supported-and-trained/. For more information about PTC, see http://www.cebc4cw.org/program/parenting-through-change/

[4] For information on the Title IV-E Waiver program, please see http://www.acf.hhs.gov/programs/cb/programs/child-welfare-waivers (accessed on July 7, 2016).

Linked Multilevel Interventions

As already noted, the Project called for EBIs linked to both administrative and fiscal changes. Taken together, each part of the intervention was designed to work in unison with the others in an effort to generate a self-reinforcing process of change that would have a positive effect on permanency rates and placement stability. Details of the interventions and their interdependencies are described below.

KEEP

KEEP is a training and support intervention developed with direct input from caregivers (e.g., foster parents and relative foster parents). KEEP targets the following outcomes: (a) decreasing the number of foster care placement disruptions (lateral moves and step-ups to group care placements), (b) improving child behavioral and emotional problems, and (c) increasing the number of positive placement changes (e.g., reunification, adoption) by (d) increasing caregiver skills and confidence. KEEP has been found to be effective at achieving these outcomes in randomized controlled trials (Chamberlain et al., 2008; Price, Chamberlain, Landsverk, & Reid, 2009) and quasi-experimental studies (Greeno et al., 2016). More specifically, KEEP has been shown to improve outcomes such as placement stability and behavioral and emotional improvements for children in foster and kinship care (Chamberlain et al., 2008; Price et al., 2008).

A major principle of KEEP is that foster and kinship parents can serve as key agents of change for children. This is accomplished by strengthening caregivers' confidence and skills, so they can change their child's behaviors, teaching effective parent management strategies, and providing the caregivers with support. As such, KEEP targets foster/kinship parents specifically, and the intervention is delivered in the context of a foster/kinship parent group, where foster parents interact with one another guided by two group facilitators. KEEP groups were in addition to the regular preservice training that all foster parents receive from the CWS system. Parents are encouraged to conduct a home practice each week relative to the session content. Each session begins by debriefing the home practice with parents and tailoring the KEEP strategies to the situation at their home with their child(ren).

To learn the model, facilitators participate in a 5-day experiential training that includes information about the program's theory and practice in the delivery of group sessions. During training, each trainee role plays facilitating several key sessions while other trainees act as foster/kinship parents. KEEP is delivered in 16 weekly group meetings (90 min each) and includes detailed manuals for group facilitators (lead and co-lead) and for foster/kin parents. Facilitators tailor the session content based on issues and ideas raised by the group participants.

Fidelity to the KEEP curriculum is monitored closely. Fidelity is measured across three dimensions including (1) content, (2) process, and (3) structure using a standardized rating protocol (Facilitator Adherence Rating; FAR). During groups, the facilitators record each session using a laptop with software that enables the recording to be uploaded to a secure website. KEEP expert consultants view the recordings, rate them using the FAR, and identify areas for reinforcement and feedback. The recordings then are used in weekly consultation meetings (1.5 h each). Prior to the consultation, facilitators complete a session review form with questions about what went well and challenges experienced. They also complete weekly forms on parent attendance and engagement ratings. Each of these measures informs the consultation process.

Administrative Interventions

As part of the Project, the public agency introduced four administrative changes. First, the public agency asked each of the private agencies to *reduce worker caseloads* to no more than 12 active cases. This change was designed to give workers more time to spend with children, parents, and foster parents. During that time, caseworkers were expected to align their interactions with the EBIs. Because workers already spend considerable time fulfilling regulatory and other requirements, the lower caseloads created the space in the workweek to absorb the new expectations without undermining the usual casework demands.

Second, supervisors were asked to *spend more time building the capacity of their staff*, particularly in the areas of high-quality, goal-focused work. To do this, caseworkers and supervisors alike were trained in *R3*, a training program built on the social learning principles used with both KEEP and PTC. Social learning theory posits that people modify their behavior by observing reinforcement received by others, and that all individuals exist within and respond to their environments in an adaptive way (i.e., the behaviors that are reinforced for will increase in frequency).

Third, the public agencies imposed a limit of *3 children in a foster home*, except in cases involving large sibling groups. This requirement was based on the notion that a foster parent's capacity to provide care is affected by the number of foster children living in the home. By limiting the number of children, the public agency was hoping to leverage caregiver skills by reducing workload in the foster home.

Last, the public agency, in its oversight of the private agencies, reinvigorated the *attention paid to Adoption and Safe Families Act timelines* that specify when agencies should shift their attention from reunification to adoption. In essence, when children have been in placement for 15 out of the 22 most recent months, the reasonable efforts threshold that directs agencies to focus their efforts on reunification is lowered, allowing for greater attention on adoption. This component of the multi-level intervention was meant to address the protracted adoption process described for the public agency by federal reviewers during the Child and Family Service Reviews.

Fiscal Intervention

The fiscal intervention was relatively straightforward. In most places around the country, private agencies are reimbursed by the public agency using a fee-for-service method (Wulczyn & Orlebeke, 2000; Wulczyn & Orlebeke, 2006). A fee-for-service method provides reimbursement for the service provided. Fee-for-service systems work well when the demand for services is rising and providers need assurances that their expansion will be funded. At other times, when demand for services is shrinking or when government partners want better outcomes for the dollar spent, fee-for-service systems pose significant disincentives relative to the business as usual model (Wulczyn, 2000). The dynamic tension is best expressed this way. Nongovernmental organizations (NGOs) work under contract with government agencies. Over the course of a fiscal year, their budgets are developed in relationship to the expected demand for the services they provide. Annual budget projections are based on historical assumptions that balance revenue, expenditures, and demand (Wulczyn & Halloran, 2017). When government partners move to improve outcomes, as in the case of EBP implementation, the desired goal represents a reduction in demand for services (e.g., shorter length of stay or fewer admissions), all else being equal. Reductions in demand for services run counter to revenue/expenditure equilibria used by the agency to develop their budget. As such, the objectives behind the implementation of an EBP are often misaligned with an agency's fiscal dynamics.

For the Project, the EBP/fiscal dynamic was addressed in this way. Lower caseloads and EBP training – the core investments in the project – were financed with the savings the EPBs and other innovations were intended to stimulate. Normally, because the expected increase in permanency rates weakens an agency's ability to invest in the capacity needed to accomplish the goal, the fiscal consequences are hard to overcome. By funneling the savings back into the agencies through the rate structure, the private agencies acquired the capacity to respond to the expectations set by the public agency.

Synergies Within the Multilevel Interventions

When scaling up EBIs, it is often the case that too little thought is given to the ways in which action on one part of the system connects to the broader system and the potential for contradictory dynamics. In this Project, leaders saw and acted on the interdependencies. Perhaps, the most important link across levels tied the EBI to the fiscal strategy. EBIs almost always involve teaching the workforce new skills. However, those skills are set against the demands of a job that is already taxing in terms of requirements that cannot be set aside in favor of something new: the new and the old have to coexist. To make room for the EBIs, leadership lowered caseloads and then paid for the lowered caseload with savings the EBIs and other changes were expected to generate. The deliberate attempt to link the intervention across clinical, administrative, and fiscal domains was a distinguishing feature of the Project and its theory of change.

Evaluation

The evaluation, which was carried out under separate contract, was designed to examine whether the Project was implemented as designed and whether the project achieved its intended impact. The public agency asked the evaluator (Chapin Hall) to address the following research questions:

- What were the organizational contexts into which Project was implemented? What changes were needed to accommodate the new practice requirements?
- To what extent was the model implemented as intended? How did staff experience the demands of implementation?
- What was the impact of the Project on the stability of children's placements?
- What was the impact of the Project on children's time in care prior to permanency?

Four sources of data inform the way in which we answered these questions. First, Chapin Hall research staff conducted one-on-one interviews with system stakeholders over the course of the pilot year, including provider agency staff ($n = 16$), public agency staff ($n = 12$), and the developers of the clinical models ($n = 7$). The interviews were designed to get an in-depth description of the implementation experience from various perspectives, particularly as it relates to changes in the process of care, the quality of care, and the extent to which the necessary capacity adjustments were made to support implementation efforts. An inductive (grounded) approach was used to analyze the interview data.

The second source of data comes from an online survey administered to case planning and supervisory staff from the five participating provider agencies. Staff completed the survey at two points in time: toward the middle of the first year and then again toward the end of the first year. The survey was designed to gauge implementation levels from the perspective of case planners and supervisors – those closest to the work on the ground. The survey also included questions about employee job satisfaction and the extent to which job satisfaction changed under the Project. The total response rate for the Time 1 survey was 53% ($n = 108$; 85 case planners and 23 supervisors, representing four of the five pilot agencies). The total response rate for the Time 2 survey was 52% ($n = 68$; 56 case planners and 12 supervisors, representing all five pilot agencies).

The third source of data comes from a web-based fidelity management system known as FIDO, which holds implementation and fidelity data related to KEEP. Data from FIDO were used in conjunction with administrative records, the fourth source of data. The administrative data include information related to children's placements in out-of-home care. Together, FIDO and the administrative data were used to create an analytic data file that allowed for a comprehensive understanding of overall system performance while also identifying any Project-specific effects.

Implementation

The evaluation was organized around three basic questions: was the process of care followed; was the quality of care up to the expected standard; and was the capacity needed to meet process and quality standards available (Wulczyn et al., 2014). The *process of care* refers to the steps followed during the time family members/children are engaged with services. In the case of the Project, the process changes were dictated by the intervention design and changes in how supervisors used their time, among others. The *quality of care* generally refers to how well something is done. In the Project context, observable changes in caseworkers' interactions with caregivers are a prime example of the way in which quality of care was expected to change under the Project model. In practice, process and quality are closely aligned in that adherence to the process of care is in and of itself an indicator of quality, especially if the underlying process protocols are supported by an evidence base that links the process and programmatic content to outcomes. *Capacity* refers to whether there are sufficient resources in the system to implement a new initiative in a manner that is consistent with new requirements. In general, capacity has human, structural, and operational meaning. Ensuring staff can manage new workload demands associated with an initiative, securing the availability of required tools and resources, and the ability of organizations to bring their operations into alignment given the new demands represent the kind of capacity changes agencies were asked to make. With complex multilevel initiatives, implementation effort will depend on the extent to which stakeholders attend to, coordinate, and mutually reinforce the various process, quality, and capacity investments that have been made.

Process of Care

The extent to which the Project changed the process of care for agencies, particularly as it relates to casework with parents, foster parents, children, and adolescents, depended, in part, on the nature of what had been in place at each agency before the onset of the Project. To varying degrees, the provider agencies that participated in the Project pilot had in place a process of care that included a variety of programs designed to provide parents, foster parents, and adolescents with training and support across a range of well-being domains. In large part, these business-as-usual programs were not evidence based in the traditional sense, but were implemented with an eye toward the perceived needs of each agency's population. Generally speaking, program attendance was sporadic; the agency representatives who participated in interviews described a situation where core groups (of foster parents, parents, or youth) would cycle through the range of programs being offered at the agency, without much variation.[5]

The process of care changes required by KEEP was generally well received by the agencies. The potential value added to the agency and, more specifically, to the children, families, and caseworkers that would be most directly affected by the changes was understood from the very beginning of the Project period. Prior to the Project, case planners were more likely to collect reports about parents' progress in meeting their treatment goals rather than playing an integral part in that process. Under the Project, case planners were better equipped to conduct comprehensive and actionable assessments and to see themselves as active agents in helping families through the process of change.

An important piece of context for considering the changes introduced under the Project is that prior to the Project, under the business as usual model, agency staff did not expect to facilitate the various caregiver training and support programs offered by their agency. In some cases, caseworkers or supervisors would help facilitate a parent training session or support group. In other cases, agencies hired dedicated staff to take responsibility for organizing and running a particular training program, as was commonly the practice for group work with adolescents. But, generally, this aspect of service delivery was not a part of the day-to-day casework routine.

In this respect, the process by which agencies – and caseworkers in particular – engaged and worked with families changed a great deal. Under the Project, *all* case planners and supervisors received comprehensive training designed to help them work differently with families from the outset. The training (and associated expectations) offered under the Project represented a major shift for case planners, whose training was typically limited to on-the-job training specific to the functional aspects of their role (the "how-to" of casework in a foster care agency).

Staff at all five agencies completed their KEEP training largely within expected timeframes, noteworthy given the time intensiveness of the trainings (five full days for each model) and the challenges associated with providing case coverage for staff during training periods. According to the survey data collected after case planning and supervisory staff had been trained in these two models, case planners' reactions to KEEP training were mostly favorable and they generally left the trainings feeling prepared to facilitate a group.

By and large, the agencies began enrolling parents in KEEP groups immediately following the completion of the training. Although the agencies attempted to enroll foster parents in KEEP strategically (i.e., focusing first on parents of children who

---

[5] Foster parent training is required for all foster parents on an ongoing basis. In this respect, each of the participating provider agencies had a process in place for training foster parents. The content of the training offered by KEEP, though, was different than what was being offered by the agencies prior to the Project.

had recently been placed in care), ultimately logistics ruled the day, with groups being filled with foster parents who were able to attend on a given day or at a given time.

The potential for KEEP to help caregivers connect to and support their children was identified by all of the senior staff that participated in interviews. KEEP provided staff with a concrete set of tools to use in their work with parents and foster parents. Although the work associated with running KEEP groups was not insignificant, the general message from senior staff was that case planners were excited by the new skills they had acquired. Further, foster parents were observed to be forming connections with agency staff in ways that stood out from what had been observed prior to the Project.

Quality of Care

The five agencies chosen to participate in the Project varied in terms of their prior experience using evidence-based models in their day-to-day practice with families. However, all five agencies espoused a commitment to using evidence-based models as a way to improve their work with children and families. In the case of the Project, the agencies saw the invitation to participate in the Project pilot as an opportunity to be at the forefront of progressive change, to help shape a new approach to providing foster care services. It was viewed as an opportunity to develop the body of empirically validated interventions specific to improving the safety, permanency, and overall well-being outcomes of children in foster care and their families.

Senior agency staff were also excited about the idea of *providing more core services in-house*, particularly a caregiver skills program. Having agency staff directly provide these services led workers to be more accountable for engaging clients (parents, foster parents, and youth) in services and for the quality of the services being provided.

When designing the Project, Children's Services and the model developers emphasized the importance not only of implementing evidence-based interventions for children in out-of-home care, but also of doing so in a way that would allow the provider agencies to track the extent to which the new models were being implemented with fidelity, a core indicator of service quality. Fidelity ensures the core elements that drive the desired change in client outcomes have the opportunity to exert their influence.[6]

One of the key features of the Project, and KEEP, in particular, was the rigorous fidelity protocols that directed regular, detailed feedback on the extent to which facilitators are adhering to model standards. The FIDO database, a newly designed data management system, enabled agency staff to track the KEEP experiences of caregivers. For KEEP, FIDO tracked not only the number of sessions

---

[6] McHugo et al. (2007).

each individual attended but also the fidelity ratings assigned to each facilitator by trained consultants who observed facilitators in action via video upload. For KEEP participants, FIDO tracked attendance and fidelity data as well as information from the Parent Daily Report (PDR), which monitors foster parents' stress levels related to specific behavior problems displayed by the foster child in their home.

In this way, the data contained in FIDO allowed the model developers and agency staff to observe the association between participation in KEEP and changes in care-giver behavior, foster parent stress, and the frequency of identified child behavior problems. Once FIDO data were linked to an administrative database that contains information about children's placements in out-of-home care, it was easier to under-stand how participation in the interventions was affecting caregivers and child outcomes.

Adhering to the fidelity protocols associated with KEEP (completing the Parent Daily Report and data entry into FIDO) required considerable time and effort on the part of the providers. As detailed in the following section on capacity, the agencies also needed to invest resources to build up internal IT infrastructures to allow for adherence to the fidelity protocols associated with KEEP.

Keeping up with the volume of data entry associated was a significant challenge for the agencies that, over time, they have become increasingly able to manage. The same holds for the utilization of the FIDO-originated reports. At the outset, compli-ance was low but improved steadily and significantly over time, as the new activities associated with KEEP became more routine.

Capacity

In many respects, the capacity changes brought about by the Project were the most significant. In this context, capacity can be thought of in three ways. The first has to do with staffing, with the questions being: What effect did the Project have on staff caseloads and staff workloads? Did the change in caseload requirements offset the increase in skills training and workload requirements? The second way to think about capacity has to do with the structures of the organization. The question is, did the agencies have or create the internal structures required to implement the Project? For the Project, the main consideration has to do with structures related to informa-tion technology. The third way to think about capacity has to do with the operations of the agency, in which case we ask, how did the operations of the agency change as the agency worked to adhere to the requirements set forth by the Project? Each of these questions is considered below.

Staffing

Developing and refining both group facilitation and clinical skills – in training, in groups, and in day-to-day practice – takes a lot of time and dedication. Quite simply, the magnitude of the implementation effort (i.e., the added workload) posed real challenges for staff who also needed to monitor the day-to-day compliance-related activities that remained a part of foster care service provision. This was certainly the case for new case planners, who also required training in the core responsibilities of the job.

Much of the stress associated with managing the new workload was to be mitigated by reductions in caseload to no more than 12 active cases per case planner. However, interview and survey data suggest that caseload reductions were not automatic once the Project went live at the agencies; rather, it was a process that developed over the course of the first year. Just about all of the senior staff we interviewed noted that prior to the Project, average caseloads were somewhere between 15 and 20 cases per case planner. Similarly, about 63% of the case planners who participated in the survey indicated that prior to the Project they had caseloads in excess of 12 active cases. Several months into the first year, just about 45% of case planners indicated a caseload in excess of 12 active cases. By the end of the first year, this figure was lower, with 7% of case planners reporting a caseload over 14 active cases and a substantial portion of case planners reporting a caseload of between 12 and 14 cases.[7]

Supervisors' workload also increased in important ways under the Project. First, supervisors generally took on more case planners as supervisees than had been the case prior to the Project. As discussed above, the reductions in caseloads happened over time, so that at the beginning of the pilot period, many supervisors were left feeling overwhelmed by the volume of cases for which they were now being held accountable.

Second, staff supervision changed under the Project. Whereas supervision between supervisors and case planners may have focused on the administrative tasks associated with casework within a highly regulated child welfare services environment, under the Project supervisors were also expected to incorporate core concepts from the clinical models (tracking engagement of foster parents in KEEP; monitoring case progress, in part, through the use of the Parent Daily Report, etc.) as well as modeling for case planners the concepts taught through the casework practice model.

It is also important to note that several agencies reported higher-than-usual turnover during the early parts of the Project pilot period. On the one hand, managing a foster care program with less than optimal staffing is difficult. It is even more difficult when simultaneously working with staff to implement numerous labor-intensive clinical models. On the other hand, senior staff from the agencies who reported notable

---

[7]At the time of the second survey, 34% of responding case planners reported a caseload between 12 and 14 active cases.

turnover ultimately saw it as an opportunity to make use of enhanced interviewing approaches and ensure vacancies were filled with individuals who fit the *new* case planner and supervisor roles, given the changes made under the Project.

Structural Capacity

The Project required the agencies to reevaluate the structure of their organizations with respect to information technology and data support. The fidelity protocols required the agencies to have various pieces of technology that would enable video recordings of groups and other clinical sessions to be uploaded to model consultants. Many of the agencies struggled, at least initially, to get the necessary IT structures in place so that they could adhere to the fidelity protocols. New pieces of equipment needed to be purchased by some agencies; across agencies, staff needed to identify who would be responsible for providing tech support to groups on a regular basis. Managing data entry into FIDO, while initially thought to be a task that case planners would manage, turned out to be more labor intensive than originally understood, requiring agencies to rethink how data entry and data cleaning were managed.

There were also physical resource challenges that needed to be solved. For example, agencies had to quickly figure out how to allocate meeting space given the range of key activities now required. For larger agencies, this posed less of a problem, but for smaller agencies, this challenge was particularly acute.

Operational Capacity

The Project required the agencies to make significant shifts in the way staff were organized into what were termed "pods," with one supervisor and the six case planners they would be supervising constituting a single pod. Pod formations were conceptualized as a way to structure KEEP groups, so that parents and foster parents would be enrolled in a KEEP group facilitated by someone associated with the same pod as their case planner (if not the case planner themselves). Structuring staff into pods meant, for most agencies, a major overhaul to their preproject staffing arrangement. Moreover, the shifting of case planners, case aides, and supervisors – and in some cases the cases they carried – had to be done within a very tight timeframe.

The use of pod formations as a way to structure KEEP caseloads made intuitive sense to those we interviewed, but some questioned the practicality of the approach. As noted above, scheduling and logistics seemed to be the primary factor in terms of how KEEP groups were actually filled, although keeping groups within a given pod was the ultimate goal. Keeping groups "within the pod" became even more difficult when filling groups with new parents or foster parents (i.e., new cases), given the rate of new admissions at each agency. By the end of the pilot period, although staff was still organized into pods, KEEP groups were reportedly being filled without as much consideration to pod assignment as was originally intended.

The Project also required agencies to examine basic features of their operations such as the hours the agency is open and how staff work-time would be structured. To accommodate caregivers, group activities had to be scheduled on evenings or weekends, meaning that worktimes/workdays for staff had to be changed.

Outcomes

To recap, the Project was a set of linked, multilevel interventions that targeted casework practice, caregiver skills, caseloads size, and supervisory practice, among other changes. In this section of the report, we focus on whether the Project affected outcomes for children. For this analysis, we are concerned with answering the following questions:

- Did the Project affect permanency rates?
- Did the Project increase placement stability?

With regard to the analysis, there are two important points to note from the start. The first point worth making upfront is that the Project is a bundle of changes implemented *together* with the expectation that outcomes for children would improve.[8] For this reason, we rely on an Intent-to-Treat (ITT) analysis as the focal point of our outcome analysis. The Intent-to-Treat analysis considers all children who received placement services during the time the Project was active in the agency. We call this exposure. For purposes of the evaluation, exposure commenced when the agency was declared active within the Project. The agency was active when the multilevel components were in place.

Second, because the Project involved linked multilevel interventions implemented simultaneously, it is not possible to tease apart the impact of any one component. In time, it may be important to isolate component-specific effects, but for now, the intention was to bundle all the components into a single intervention. For that reason, we evaluated the Project as a single intervention, using the KEEP implementation date as the date when *all* the intervention components were active.

Methods

To understand the extent to which the linked multilevel interventions had their intended effects on children's outcomes, we constructed an agency-specific person-period data file. The file records the time each child spends with a specific private

---

[8] On a number of occasions, during meetings with the public agency leadership, we were reminded by the public agency that the Project was "so much more" than KEEP or any single EBI. To the public agency, the Project was the bundle of interventions, structural and practice changes in their entirety.

agency. The agency-specific spells (or episodes) are then divided into time intervals (person periods) of a given length; for this analysis, we looked at 3-month periods. Each person period has associated with it a flag indicating (1) whether, for that period the child was exposed to the intervention (i.e., in a home supervised by one of the participating agencies after the agreed upon start date), (2) whether the child was eligible for the clinical models based on whether they were in a regular family foster home, and (3) whether the child's foster parents had participated in the training during that period. The public agency provided the data for the eligibility flag (2, above); data related to the timing of foster parents/parents training (3, above) were pulled from the FIDO database. The person period also included a variable indicating whether a placement move or an exit occurred during that interval. The underlying statistical model evaluates the log odds of movement or exit; the treatment effect is captured by whether person-periods that include treatment are (1) more or less likely to also include a movement and (2) more or less likely to end with an exit to permanency.

Because children are clustered within agencies, we account for the nested structure with a multilevel model. The multilevel model produces properly weighted estimates of the average exit rate to account for the fact that the larger Project agencies contribute more information to the model. The addition of the treatment effect shows the impact of treatment on the average rate. Adding time as a variable in the model (i.e., indicating the year during which the interval was observed) controls for any trends in the underlying data.

Sample

The intervention targeted all children between the ages of 0 and 21 placed in non-specialty family foster homes supervised by the five agencies. The sample includes both children in care at the start of the pilot period (the legacy caseload) and all admissions involving children entering family foster care from the onset of the program forward. In total, there were 4052 children included in the ITT analysis and 91,087 children included in the comparison group. A summary of both groups, by age, is found in Table 11.1.

The agency-specific, person periods provide a concise way to introduce the treatment (i.e., dose) at the specific time it occurs. For the legacy caseload, this method addresses the fact that children were at different points in their placement history when the treatment starts. Because the log odds of exit or placement change differ with respect to how long children have already been in care, the person periods assess the treatment effects after controlling for the timing of the treatment relative to the child's prior history in care.

Table 11.1 Count of agency spells by treatment status, entry year, and age

	Age at beginning of agency spell						Age at beginning of agency spell					
Entry year	< 1	1–5	6–12	13–17	18+	Total	<1	1–5	6–12	13–17	18+	Total
ITT group												
2003	0	2	4	0	0	6	0%	33%	67%	0%	0%	100%
2004	3	1	3	0	0	7	43%	14%	43%	0%	0%	100%
2005	1	3	3	2	0	9	11%	33%	33%	22%	0%	100%
2006	6	12	8	3	0	29	21%	41%	28%	10%	0%	100%
2007	3	22	20	5	0	50	6%	44%	40%	10%	0%	100%
2008	19	28	31	17	0	95	20%	29%	33%	18%	0%	100%
2009	32	54	47	42	1	176	18%	31%	27%	24%	1%	100%
2010	62	126	93	108	8	397	16%	32%	23%	27%	2%	100%
2011	101	163	156	185	41	646	16%	25%	24%	29%	6%	100%
2012	108	266	277	450	91	1192	9%	22%	23%	38%	8%	100%
2013	125	252	242	627	199	1445	9%	17%	17%	43%	14%	100%
Comparison group												
2003	803	1478	1674	3147	509	7611	11%	19%	22%	41%	7%	100%
2004	727	1326	1442	2933	652	7080	10%	19%	20%	41%	9%	100%
2005	602	1318	1304	2909	694	6827	9%	19%	19%	43%	10%	100%
2006	911	2527	2546	3147	832	9963	9%	25%	26%	32%	8%	100%
2007	890	2071	2295	3203	819	9278	10%	22%	25%	35%	9%	100%
2008	1009	2211	2209	3558	864	9851	10%	22%	22%	36%	9%	100%
2009	943	2296	2330	3508	1026	10,103	9%	23%	23%	35%	10%	100%
2010	880	2135	2247	3080	859	9201	10%	23%	24%	33%	9%	100%
2011	763	1686	1689	2659	932	7729	10%	22%	22%	34%	12%	100%
2012	676	1356	1463	2401	812	6708	10%	20%	22%	36%	12%	100%
2013	648	1335	1409	2506	838	6736	10%	20%	21%	37%	12%	100%

Project Effects on Outcomes – Permanency

In this section, we explore whether the Project influenced permanency and stability. We present the results of a multilevel discrete time model that compares the experiences of Project children with the experiences of children from all other agencies operating under the public agencies jurisdiction from 2003 forward – the comparison group. Among children in that group are children served by the agencies prior to the start of the program. The group also includes children served by non-Project agencies operating at the time the Project was active. In addition to knowing when children entered the ITT group, we also know how long they had been in care, the number of prior spells of care, their race/ethnicity, age, and gender. We used these variables to control for case mix differences.

The results for the person periods are not shown separately because they do not factor into the underlying impact analysis. We included them in the analysis because the likelihood of permanency differs by person period. For example, on average 13% of the children leave care during the first person-period. Generally, the likelihood of

Table 11.2 Intent-to-treat: effect of the project on permanent exits from foster care

	Odds ratio	Significance[a]
Person period – not shown separately		
Placement history		
First child spell	Reference	
Second child spell	0.787	***
Third child spell	0.733	***
More than 3 child spells	0.567	***
First agency spell	Reference	
Second agency spell	0.78	***
More than two agency spells	0.553	***
Gender	Reference	
Male	1.028	*
Female	Reference	
Race/ethnicity		
White	Reference	
African American	1.042	*
Hispanic	1.159	
Other races and ethnicities	1.703	
Age at placement		
Under 1	Reference	
1–5 years	1.478	***
6–12 years	1.656	***
13–17 years	0.922	***
>17 years	0.23	***
Agency effect	1.168	*
Period effect	0.644	***
Treatment agency * Period	**1.111**	***

[a]***Significance at the $p < 0.01$ level
*Significance at the $0.01 < p < 0.05$ level

leaving care shrinks with each person period. Because this is consistent with general exit patterns observed elsewhere and across different models used in this study, we elected not to report these findings.

In addition to person-period differences in the rate of exit, prior placement history affected permanency rates in the expected direction – children who returned to care leave their next spell of care more slowly. Demographic attributes also contribute to the rate of permanency: males and older children move to permanency more quickly; African Americans reach permanency at a rate that is slightly higher than what was observed for whites and Hispanics.[9]

---

[9] The interpretation of odds ratios is as follows: Odds ratios greater than 1 imply faster rates of exit to permanency; odds ratios of less than 1 imply slower permanency rates relative to the relevant reference group. For example, males leave care at a rate that is about 3% faster (1.028) than the rate reported for females.

The treatment-related effects are reported in the last three rows of Table 11.2. Given an evaluation design in which we compare permanency rates among children served by the agencies with permanency rates for children in all the other agencies plus the treatment agencies prior to the program start date, we have to contend with two specific issues: (1) how the Project agencies in general compare with all the other agencies and (2) are there any time trends in the data that would obscure the treatment effect.

To capture these effects, we first control for agency and period effects. As reported in Table 11.2, the Project agencies have historically had higher permanency rates (1.168 odds ratio) than other, non-Project agencies. In addition, during the time when the Project became active, exits to permanency were generally slowing down (0.644 odds ratio).

With agency and period effects removed (i.e., a statistical control is used), the treatment effect on the children in the agencies is captured as the interaction between the period and the treatment agency (Treatment agency * Period). The corresponding coefficient shows that when the children exposed to the treatment (ITT) are compared with children served by nonagencies *together* with children served by the agencies but not during the Project, the rate of permanency for children in the ITT group was greater than the rate for all other children in the comparison group (1.111 odds ratio). This difference was small but statistically significant.

The Project Effects on Outcomes – Stability

The stability outcome, presented in Table 11.3, was studied in the same way. There are person-period differences in the likelihood of movement, with the likelihood of movement higher in the earlier person periods. These results are not shown separately. The likelihood of changing placements also depends on demographic characteristics and placement history. These findings were in the expected direction, given the literature as it pertains to these issues (Wulczyn, Kogan, & Harden, 2003).

As before, treatment-related effects are found in the last three rows of Table 11.3. We control again for agency (odds ratio 0.793) and period effects (0.993), both of which indicate a slower rate of movement. The agency-specific, person periods provide a concise way to introduce the treatment (i.e., dose) at the specific time it occurs. For the legacy caseload, this method addresses the fact that children were at different points in their placement history when the treatment starts. Because the log odds of exit or placement change differ with respect to how long children have already been in care, the person periods assess the treatment effects after controlling for the timing of the treatment relative to the child's prior history in care. When these are factored in, the treatment effect (shown as Treatment agency * Period) indicates that the Project did not have a statistically significant effect on placement stability for the ITT group.

Table 11.3 Intent-to-treat: effect of the project on placement stability

	Odds ratio	Significance[a]
Person periods – not shown separately		
Placement history		
First child spell	Reference	
Second child spell	1.01	
Third child spell	1.156	***
More than 3 child spells	1.3	***
First agency spell	Reference	
Second agency spell	0.76	***
More than two agency spells	1.033	
Gender		
Male	0.979	
Female	Reference	
Race/ethnicity		
White	Reference	
African American	1.45	***
Hispanic	1.201	*
Other race category	1.293	***
Age at placement		
Under 1	Reference	
1–5 years	1.45	***
6–12 years	1.553	***
13–17 years	1.598	***
>17 years	0.81	*
Agency effect	0.793	
Period effect	0.993	*
Treatment agency * Period	**0.901**	

[a]***Significance at the $p < 0.01$ level
*Significance at the $0.01 < p < 0.05$ level

Summary

Given its multilevel nature, the Project attempted to change how foster care works. It combines administrative and fiscal changes (caseloads, foster home capacity, workload, supervisory responsibility together with reinvestment) with evidence-based interventions, all in an effort to improve casework practice, improve caregiver responsiveness to the needs of children, and reduce problem behaviors. In turn, fewer placement moves and shorter time in care were expected to reduce the added trauma so often associated with foster care.

The outcome evaluation looked at children served by the agencies from the point children in those agencies were exposed to the Project – a difficult undertaking given the project could have occurred at any time during a child's involvement with the foster care system. A unique feature of our study is the ability to track when the initial dose of the intervention was administered and whether exposure to the treatment affected the likelihood of changing foster homes or leaving the system altogether.

There are few studies, if any, that promise this level of specificity at this scale. For the counterfactual or comparison group, we compared a similar group of children who would have been eligible for the Project had they been placed with a Project agency; we also used children cared for by the Project agencies but at a time prior to the start of the program. Importantly, we applied an array of statistical controls designed to obtain a more accurate measure of children's outcomes if they received foster care services from a project site. With that said, we found small, positive effects on permanency and inconclusive effects on placement stability. As for the magnitude of the treatment effect, the results from the Project remind us – policy-makers, treatment developers, and researchers – that considerable attention has to be paid to the context into which an EBI is being embedded. In particular, the other sources of outcome variation found in natural settings have to be considered when assessing the merits of a given EBI both before and after implementation.

The challenge with linked multilevel interventions is the difficulty one has teasing apart the effects of one component from another. However, the desire to understand which intervention generated the effect misses the point. Foster care programs operate within what is typically called the child welfare system. The multilevel, interactive nature of systems generally, and the child welfare system in particular, is an inescapable feature of the environment in which an EBI is delivered (Wulczyn et al., 2010; Wulczyn & Halloran, 2017). Systems components interact with each other; the interaction between components requires coordination and other actions that are organized in relation to the goals of the system. Each component adapts to and influences the other components (i.e., bidirectional influences are present). Given the nested, interacting nature of systems, there has to be an integration of effort across parts of the system so that interventions across levels of the system are mutually reinforcing with respect to purpose and goals.

EBIs are often implemented as *niche* interventions that are not always well integrated or embedded into existing systems in a way that delivers the expected impact. At the same time, administrative and fiscal interventions on their own will also likely fall short of their goals because they are not linked directly to practice. Caseworkers with fewer cases and more time still need new skills/interventions to do a better job of achieving case goals. Likewise, fiscal reform on its own takes for granted the assumption that stakeholders will make good decisions as to how to use new resources when selecting interventions and managing implementation.

Linked multilevel interventions that tie together policy and fiscal initiatives with new administrative and clinical procedures provide a solution that allows for scale-ups that have the potential to achieve effects at the population level. Further work is needed to determine how the parts of a multilevel intervention come together, whether the results always reflect the interdependencies found within complex systems, and how these findings alter the way implementation proceeds. A major focus of implementation research has been on the factors that affect sustainment of individual EBIs (Aarons, Hurlburt, & Horwitz, 2011). The findings here suggest, however, that pursuit of multilevel interventions may be an important element of the intervention itself. Indeed, without careful integration of EBIs within the natural ecology of the system, it is easy to see why single EBIs, even ones that have reached sustainment, do not and probably cannot deliver the promised population-level, public health benefits.

References

Aarons, G. A., Hurlburt, M., & Horwitz, S. M. C. (2011). Advancing a conceptual model of evidence-based practice implementation in public service sectors. *Administration and Policy in Mental Health and Mental Health Services Research, 38*(1), 4–23.

Chamberlain, P., Feldman, S. W., Wulczyn, F., Saldana, L., & Forgatch, M. (2016). Implementation and evaluation of linked parenting models in a large urban child welfare system. *Child Abuse & Neglect, 53*, 27–39.

Chamberlain, P., Price, J., Leve, L., Laurent, H., Landsverk, J., & Reid, J. (2008). Prevention of behavior problems for children in foster care: Outcomes and mediation effects. *Prevention Science, 9*(1), 17–27. [PMC: 18185995].

Greeno, E. J., Uretsky, M. C., Lee, B. R., Moore, J. E., Barth, R. P., & Shaw, T. V. (2016). Replication of the KEEP Foster and Kinship parent training program in a population of youth with externalizing behavior problems. *Child Abuse & Neglect, 61*, 75–82.

Huang, T. T., Drewnosksi, A., Kumanyika, S., & Glass, T. A. (2009). A systems-oriented multilevel framework for addressing obesity in the 21st century. *Preventing Chronic Disease, 6*(3), A82.

McHugo, G. J., Drake, R. E., Whitley, R., Bond, G. R., Campbell, K., Rapp, C. A., … Finnerty, M. T. (2007). Fidelity outcomes in the National Implementing Evidence-Based Practices Project. *Psychiatric Services, 58*(10), 1279–1284.

Price, J., Chamberlain, P., Landsverk, J., & Reid, J. B. (2009). KEEP foster parent training intervention: Model description and effectiveness. *Child and Family Social Work, 14*, 233–242.

Price, J. M., Chamberlain, P., Landsverk, J., Reid, J., Leve, L., & Laurent, H. (2008). Effects of a foster parent training intervention on placement changes of children in foster care. *Child Maltreatment, 13*(1), 64–75.

Scott, P. A., Meurer, W. J., Frederiksen, S. M., Kalbfleisch, J. D., Xu, Z., Haan, M. N., et al. (2013). A multilevel intervention to increase community hospital use of alteplase for acute stroke (INSTINCT): A cluster-randomised controlled trial. *Lancet Neurology, 12*(2), 139–148.

Trickett, E. J., & Beehler, S. (2013). The ecology of multilevel interventions to reduce social inequalities in health. *American Behavioral Scientist, 57*(8), 1227–1246.

Wulczyn, F. (2000). Federal fiscal reform in child welfare services. *Children and Youth Services Review, 22*, 131–159.

Wulczyn, F., Alpert, L., Orlebeke, B., & Haight, J. (2014). *Principles, language, and shared meaning: Toward a common understanding of CQI in child welfare* (pp. 1–18). Chicago: Chapin Hall Center for Children.

Wulczyn, F., Daro, D., Fluke, J., Feldman, S., Glodek, C., & Lifanda, K. (2010). *Adapting a systems approach to child protection.* New York: UNICEF.

Wulczyn, F., & Halloran, J. (2017). Foster care dynamics and system science: Implications for research and policy. *International Journal of Environmental Research and Public Health, 14*, 1181–1112.

Wulczyn, F., Kogan, J., & Harden, B. (2003). Placement stability and movement trajectories. *Social Service Review, 77*, 212–236.

Wulczyn, F., & Orlebeke, B. (2000). Fiscal reform and managed care in child welfare services. *Policy and Practice of Public Human Services, 58*, 26–31.

Wulczyn, F., & Orlebeke, B. (2006). *Getting what we pay for: Do expenditures align with outcomes in the child welfare system? No. 106* (pp. 1–8). Chicago: Chapin Hall Center for Children at the University of Chicago.

Chapter 12
Closing the Science–Practice Gap in Implementation Before It Widens

Aaron R. Lyon, Katherine A. Comtois, Suzanne E. U. Kerns, Sara J. Landes, and Cara C. Lewis

Introduction

Across social service sectors (e.g., primary care, behavioral health, education, criminal justice, and child welfare), there is increasing evidence for the effectiveness of specific practices and interventions, relative to usual care services (Fedoroff & Taylor, 2001; Simons et al., 2010; Weisz, Jensen-Doss, & Hawley, 2006). Evidence-based practices (EBPs), broadly defined, are therapeutic interventions or service delivery practices that have demonstrated superiority to other interventions, practices, or services as usual in rigorous research trials. Ideally, these practices are supported by meta-analytic or systematic reviews of such trials. Despite decades of research and billions of dollars devoted to developing EBPs, studies have repeatedly identified a intervention "science–practice gap" in which community-based services spanning many fields are unlikely to routinely incorporate EBPs (Becker,

A. R. Lyon (✉) · K. A. Comtois
University of Washington, School of Medicine, Department of Psychiatry and Behavioral Sciences, Seattle, WA, USA
e-mail: lyona@uw.edu

S. E. U. Kerns
University of Washington, School of Medicine, Department of Psychiatry and Behavioral Sciences, Seattle, WA, USA

University of Denver Graduate School of Social Work, Denver, CO, USA

S. J. Landes
University of Arkansas for Medical Sciences, Department of Psychiatry, Little Rock, AR, USA

Central Arkansas Veterans Healthcare System VISN 16 Mental Illness Research, Education, and Clinical Center (MIRECC), Little Rock, AR, USA

C. C. Lewis
Kaiser Permanente Washington Health Research Institute, Seattle, WA, USA

© Springer Nature Switzerland AG 2020
B. Albers et al. (eds.), *Implementation Science 3.0*,
https://doi.org/10.1007/978-3-030-03874-8_12

Smith, & Jensen-Doss, 2013; Cook & Odom, 2013; Fedoroff & Taylor, 2001; García-Izquierdo, Aguinis, & Ramos-Villagrasa, 2010; Garland et al., 2010; Johnston & Moreno, 2016; Kazdin, 2010; Kuller, Ott, Goisman, Wainwright, & Rabin, 2009; McHugh & Barlow, 2010). As a result, the public health impact of the vast body of EBP research has been severely limited. Furthermore, the lack of EBP availability in community service contexts limits patient choice by dramatically restricting access to "gold standard" interventions. In many countries, the most vulnerable and at-risk populations (e.g., economic, racial, or ethnic minority individuals) are frequently at greatest risk for restricted access to the most effective programming and interventions (i.e., EBPs). This has the potential to exacerbate existing service disparities.

Recently, the internationally recognized field of implementation science has emerged to address the issues described above. Implementation science is defined as the scientific study of the uptake and transfer of EBPs into professional practice and public policy (Eccles & Mittman, 2006). Generally, implementation science examines implementation strategies (e.g., training, organizational changes) (Powell et al., 2015) that can optimize both implementation outcomes (e.g., fidelity, reach, feasibility, sustainment; Proctor et al., 2011) and patient outcomes in specific settings (e.g., clinics, schools) (Aarons, Hurlburt, & Horwitz, 2011; Damschroder et al., 2009; Proctor et al., 2009; Proctor et al., 2011).

Despite a burgeoning research base, this chapter details how the field of implementation science is in danger of following a path reminiscent of the one previously traveled by intervention science – a path that has led to a longstanding divide between science and practice. Because the current volume is devoted to advancing both implementation science and implementation practice (Shlonsky, Chap. 1), we present a training agenda intended to curtail the emerging science–practice gap in implementation.

The (Emerging) Science–Practice Gap in Implementation

As the field of implementation has grown and evolved, opportunities for specialization are occurring, and distinct science and practice components have emerged. Specifically, an increasing number of professionals are functioning as *implementation practitioners*, conducting applied work to improve the quality of service systems, but without the primary goal of producing generalizable knowledge. Furthermore, similar to clinical trials research and the practice it aims to inform, there has been relatively limited incorporation of empirical findings from implementation science into routine implementation practice. Simultaneously, implementation science research questions, designs, and instruments have not been sufficiently informed by practitioners who do the day-to-day work of implementation. As a result, implementation science runs the risk of limited obvious or immediate applicability to real-world implementation practice. This may be because, although implementation science and implementation practice are closely intertwined, each carries its own unique set of needs and priorities (Weisz, Ng, & Bearman, 2014). As a result, siloing based on professional identities – including specialized conferences for implementation researchers and others for practitioners – is beginning to occur.

At least four distinct professional roles or identities have emerged, reflecting a range of implementation science and practice priorities. These roles will need to work together more effectively if the growing implementation science–practice gap is to be stymied and closed. These four professional identities are as follows: (a) researchers who emphasize implementation science and the production of generalizable knowledge; (b) intermediaries, the outside consultants, trainers, training organizations, facilitators, or purveyors, who provide the training, facilitation, and consultation on how to implement an EBP; (c) practice leaders, the community practitioners, or agency or organizational directors who invite and coordinate training and implementation efforts within their organizations or systems of care; and (d) policy leaders who fund or set standards and guidelines at a local, regional, or national level. While the first group (researchers) is clearly focused on implementation science, we conceptualize the latter three as groups representing diverse facets of the implementation practice community. In addition, each of these groups has unique training backgrounds, perspectives, motivations, pressures, and goals regarding implementation. For example, researchers may be focused on isolating independent variables to document and understand the factors affecting different approaches to implementation. Intermediaries (sometimes referred to as purveyors) may have a vested interest in disseminating a particular intervention and, in some cases, have a financial interest in doing so. Practice leaders are generally focused on the specific steps and strategies for integrating an intervention within their unique context with the goal of enhanced outcomes for their consumers at the forefront. Policy leaders who fund EBP implementation are often interested in improving access to evidence-based care or maximizing the value of training and implementation resources.

Below, we discuss each of these four groups in more detail and then propose integrated training solutions to the science–practice gap in implementation that draw upon pragmatic research, interprofessional education, and team science to (a) enhance the implementation workforce and (b) create opportunities for implementation scientists and practitioners to more effectively work together. Shared training opportunities are expected to bring science and practice into closer alignment and highlight gaps where implementation practice is not informed by implementation science or where implementation science is not examining the questions most critical to effective implementation practice.

Implementation Practice (IP)

Intermediaries Intermediaries are those engaged primarily in the active application of implementation strategies (Franks & Bory, 2015). Intermediaries are typically the people and organizations who bring EBPs to new organizations. Some intermediaries provide training and consultation in one specific EBP, while others focus on implementing multiple EBPs or on general principles of training, consultation, or capacity building that can be applied to any EBP (e.g., use of technology, systems change, or leadership development). Intermediaries vary in the extent to which they apply implementation strategies themselves (e.g., building local buy-in, constructing an implementation blueprint), with some explicitly applying strategies to ensure that a context is conducive to a new program and others primarily bringing knowledge content and expertise in a single EBP (e.g., providing a training followed by clinical consultation) and relying on local organizations to manage key implementation issues such as conducting readiness assessments or altering organizational policies, incentives, or record systems. Although they are constantly engaged in "implementation practice," most intermediaries do not simultaneously prioritize evaluation of their work, and many are not aware of relevant research or novel evidence-based implementation strategies (Powell et al., 2015). They may, therefore, benefit from increased knowledge of procedures for carrying out well-supported implementation strategies as well as practical methods of routinely evaluating their success.

Practice Leaders The community clinicians, agency directors, or directors of healthcare systems (e.g., provider networks, hospital healthcare systems, Department of Veterans Affairs, Health Maintenance Organizations [HMOs], nongovernmental organizations [NGOs] focused on health) who invite and coordinate training and implementation efforts for clinicians within their systems of care are all examples of practice leaders. These individuals often select EBPs for adoption in their system and may go "above and beyond" their typical clinical and administrative work duties to ensure that implementation is successful (Ehrhart, Aarons, & Farahnak, 2015). There is currently little research to guide practice leaders in this role, and few have received sufficient training to allow them to evaluate or apply the extant implementation research. Often the resources required to purchase an EBP undertake an implementation process, or both can burden an organization with new costs and increased complexity of their service array, making sustainment difficult. Practice leaders are often ill equipped to manage these burdens or to evaluate whether the implementation strategies applied are meeting organizational goals. Nevertheless, as the ultimate gatekeeper of services for patients, it is imperative that practice leaders have an understanding of, influence on, and strong buy-in surrounding the design and execution of implementation research in order to generate and use the data needed to make cost-effective and efficient implementation decisions.

Policy Leaders Unlike an organizational director or intermediary who is focused primarily on the front-line service providers (e.g., clinicians, teachers, and social workers) who are implementing the EBP and local system issues, policy leaders evaluate whether implementation is successful at a local, regional, or even national level, as well as whether service recipients (e.g., clients, students and parents) benefit from the EBP system wide. These policy leaders (e.g., Departments of Behavioral Health, National Health Service, Medicare, Department of Veteran's Affairs, insurance companies) set standards, guidelines, and regulations for the health care they fund and generally provide the financial resources for EBP delivery as well. As such, policy leaders wield a certain degree of influence over organizational directors and intermediaries, but because they are influencing an agency or healthcare system overall and cannot ensure that specific clinical providers will be doing what the policy directs, they are simultaneously limited in their ability to ensure that an EBP reaches its intended recipients. Thus, it is critical for policy makers to understand what training and implementation strategies are effective and worth funding, which are not, and what data are needed to know when to hold an organization accountable for lack of progress versus acknowledging their limits due to other contextual factors.

Implementation Science (IS)

Researchers The majority of researchers who develop EBPs are not engaged in studying how they are implemented (Weisz et al., 2014). Thus, many EBPs (which have been carefully designed based on research evidence) were initially developed without an accompanying set of implementation strategies. Thus, implementation practitioners are using their own experience rather than data to guide implementation. In contrast, implementation researchers tend to be scientists who use quantitative and/or qualitative methods to develop tools, gather data, and produce generalizable knowledge about implementation processes and outcomes. Researchers engaged in implementation science study a range of topics including models and frameworks of implementation, which organizations and clinicians should implement EBPs, training and consultation models, and systemic strategies for facilitating implementation and for sustaining new practices (Powell et al., 2012, 2015). Unfortunately, most implementation research has been conceptually or theoretically driven, and not adequately linked to the perspectives or needs of the practice leaders, policy leaders, and intermediaries who carry out implementation in the real world. Implementation researchers could benefit from improved knowledge and skills surrounding the identification and development of research questions, designs, and instruments that better reflect implementation practice stakeholder perspectives.

Factors Perpetuating the Science–Practice Gap in Implementation

As Weisz et al. (2014) articulated, "we cannot avoid the fact that dissemination and implementation practice is the subject matter of dissemination and implementation science, and a close connection is needed to ensure that practice will be evaluated and guided by science while science is informed by the questions that arise in practice" (p.71). Nevertheless, as articulated above, a gap has begun to form between implementation's science and practice roles, perpetuated by factors such as the limited applicability of traditional research designs to implementation practice and the structure of traditional funding and training resources, each of which carries its own consequences. Below, we detail specifically how (1) continued reliance on research designs and measures that emphasize traditional, protracted, and expensive methodologies, as well as (2) the restriction of implementation science to academic researchers have both served to maintain the gap between implementation practice and implementation science.

First, implementation science continues to be driven by traditional research paradigms that emphasize experimental control; internal validity; psychometrically valid, expensive measurement; and statistical – rather than local – significance. This has occurred despite calls for the use of a more diverse array of research methods (Gaglio, Phillips, Heurtin-Roberts, Sanchez, & Glasgow, 2014; Glasgow, 2013; Glasgow et al., 2012; Palinkas et al., 2011; Proctor et al., 2009). Typical methods – which are largely focused on explanatory models and efficacy designs – are intended to produce generalizable knowledge and causal inferences, but cannot evaluate the needs of local organizations and individuals, the extent to which an implementation project meets those needs, or the processes through which success or failure occurs. Moreover, the lengthy (upwards of hundreds of items) and expensive ($20,000+ USD for one of the best and most useful measures of organizational readiness; Glisson et al., 2008) assessment instruments typically used by researchers are inaccessible to community partners (Martinez, Lewis, & Weiner, 2014). As a result, implementation science is frequently limited to top-down research approaches designed to answer questions posed by academics, rather than employing locally relevant methods to answer questions identified via a collaborative process among a range of stakeholders. For example, it is common practice that an implementation research team will select an EBP first and then work to identify sites where that EBP can be installed. Similarly, assessments of the implementation "readiness" of sites – a common focus of implementation research (Scaccia et al., 2015; Shea, Jacobs, Esserman, Bruce, & Weiner, 2014; Weiner, 2009) – are typically intended to determine whether the conditions in a destination context are conducive to implementing the selected program and potentially shifting the context to meet the needs of the EBP, rather than working with stakeholders to select an EBP that would be readily implemented within their existing context.

Second, implementation science has been dominated by academic researchers with relatively limited meaningful input from – or collaboration with – service providers, service recipients, advocates, and healthcare organizations. Although stakeholder collaborations (e.g., university community) are invariably held up as essential to effective implementation research (Charns, Egede, Rumsfeld, McGlynn, & Yano, 2014), most scientific approaches do not include a method for service providers, recipients, or other stakeholders to gain sufficient perspective on the research and evaluation process to be fully engaged and equal participants. Current training in implementation science is focused exclusively on academic researchers with little emphasis on engaging the additional stakeholder groups who are vital to the relevance and success of implementation projects. Although impressive and successful academic training programs exist (e.g., Training Institute for Dissemination and Implementation Research in Health [TIDIRH] (Meissner et al., 2013), Implementation Research Institute [IRI]) (Proctor et al., 2013), Knowledge Translation Canada Summer Institute (Straus et al., 2011)), their format may inadvertently perpetuate top-down science and unintentionally widen the emerging divide between those conducting implementation research and those involved in real-world practice improvement efforts (Weisz et al., 2014). With a few notable exceptions (e.g., the Patient-Centered Outcomes Research Institute [PCORI], which explicitly requires stakeholder involvement), this structure is also maintained by existing research funding mechanisms, some of which have funded the training programs listed above. Federal funding is often critical to training in implementation (Proctor & Chambers, 2016), but most research grants are only awarded to scientific investigators and research training grants, like those offered by the United States' National Institute of Mental Health (NIMH) or Australia's National Health and Medical Research Council, explicitly stipulate that only academic researchers may participate. As a result, there are few opportunities for training in implementation practice (Proctor & Chambers, 2016). Implementation science would be advanced by training models that encourage increased engagement of intermediaries, practice leaders, and policy leaders in all aspects of the process in a manner consistent with the basic tenets of stakeholder involvement (Selby, Beal, & Frank, 2012).

Strategies for Addressing the Gap

New approaches are needed to slow this growing gap between implementation practice and implementation science. Weisz et al. (2014) have suggested a number of strategies for facilitating better integration, such as incorporating implementation research questions into any demonstration or service project receiving funding. This is an excellent example of how true integration of implementation science into implementation practice might manifest, and this may also help to address the fact that there is simultaneously considerable room for implementation science to better answer critical questions of high importance to implementation practice. However, the issues presented above prevent this kind of integration from becoming a reality. That is, siloed training and unresolved tensions – particularly regarding the interaction between rigorous methods and contextual relevance – must be addressed. To fully realize and expand upon the vision presented by Weisz and colleagues, we argue that the four types of implementation stakeholders detailed previously must be exposed to (a) pragmatic research, (b) team science, and (c) interprofessional education. Below, we detail these components and then present training recommendations that incorporate them and are intended to enhance collaboration among implementation scientists and practitioners.

Pragmatic Research

The integration of implementation practice and implementation science may be facilitated by more deliberately balancing internal and external validity (Weisz et al., 2014). Direction may be taken from Glasgow (2013) who has highlighted the importance of pragmatic research designs. In contrast to dominant implementation science approaches, pragmatic designs emphasize the real-world context and stakeholder perspectives with the goal of accelerating and broadening the impact of science on policy and practice. Pragmatic studies – often contrasted with explanatory trials (Thorpe et al., 2009) – are designed to focus on questions, perspectives, and outcomes important to stakeholders, be conducted in settings similar to those in practice, include samples that resemble those in typical settings, and include real-world comparison conditions (Glasgow, 2013). As a result, their ultimate goal is to produce findings that are both rigorous and relevant to stakeholders (Glasgow & Chambers, 2012).

For true integration of implementation science and implementation practice, pragmatic measures are needed (Glasgow & Riley, 2013). Pragmatic measures are those that are short, simple, and efficient but also psychometrically sound, so that the labor of administration provides maximum value. It is also important that these measures have a high level of face validity and be easily interpretable. They may be used to evaluate key questions at the patient, clinician, and system levels producing information that is actionable. Despite the potential of pragmatic measures to drive quality improvement, address stakeholder issues, and facilitate implementation, their use in implementation science could be greatly improved (Lewis, Weiner, Stanick, & Fischer, 2015).

Because of the emphasis on stakeholder engagement, locally relevant research questions, and rapid identification of benefits, pragmatic research is extremely well aligned with the goals of implementation science and practice. Implementation is primarily concerned with installing innovative practices in new service contexts, which, for behavioral or psychosocial interventions, almost inevitably requires changes in the perspectives, skills, behaviors, and resource allocations of all of the professional roles described above. Unfortunately, opportunities for implementation stakeholders (including researchers) to receive training in using pragmatic designs and measures are virtually nonexistent, expanding the gap between implementation science and practice.

Team Science

True integration of implementation practice and implementation science perspectives requires training structures that promote collaboration among individuals from different professional backgrounds and with different knowledge, skills, and areas of emphasis. Team science is "a collaborative effort to address a scientific challenge that leverages the strengths and expertise of professionals trained in different [disciplines]" (National Cancer Institute, n.d.). Results from investments in large-scale team science programs suggest that collaboration among scientists in different disciplines is essential to solve complex, vexing problems (Stokols, Hall, Taylor, & Moser, 2008). Indeed, over the past two decades, team science has been leveraged to address challenging social, environmental, and public health issues (e.g., global warming, cancer, AIDS) that have highly complex, multifactorial causes (Stokols, Hall, et al., 2008; Stokols, Misra, Moser, Hall, & Taylor, 2008). Research on team science suggests that more knowledge is produced by teams than individuals and that team-based research is cited more often, and thus is of higher impact (Wuchty, Jones, & Uzzi, 2007).

Ironically, implementation science is a field that was developed to inform the integration of EBPs into real-world settings (Eccles & Mittman, 2006), yet the variety of implementation practitioners described above have rarely been included as equal partners. Success in the broader field of implementation science and practice demands cross-disciplinary informed solutions to maximize relevance and public health impact. Collaborative implementation science, thus, requires the best practices of team science to ensure that each stakeholder's perspective is integrated in the service of optimal research design and implementation practice solutions. Best practices for team science are now emerging (e.g., key leadership characteristics, established conflict resolution strategies, cyberinfrastructure for geographically distant teams). However, without formal training to guide and inform cross-disciplinary work, the differences among team members (e.g., with respect to reward structures, perspectives, pressures, and priorities) may inadvertently undermine effective team processes. Conversely, if properly leveraged, team science may lead to efficient advancements in the extent to which implementation science is able to address pragmatic questions.

Interprofessional Education

Team science is a process for developing research in a cross-disciplinary team format. Interprofessional education (IPE) is a comparable process for cross-disciplinary teaching and learning. While complimentary, IPE differs from team science in that team science is focused on producing collaborative scientific products, whereas IPE is a method of facilitating professional development. Team science reflects practices in which implementation science and practice professionals may engage. IPE is a training model through which to instill these skills and practices.

IPE is rooted in adult learning theory and facilitates shared learning among individuals with different professional backgrounds (Hammick, Freeth, Koppel, Reeves, & Barr, 2007; Reeves et al., 2010). In IPE, different professionals "learn from, with, and about each other" (Hammick et al., 2007). Applied to training in implementation science and practice, IPE represents a mechanism for training a range of stakeholders simultaneously in a way that takes advantage of differences. IPE has been recommended as an important strategy to address workforce shortages and improve global health (WHO|Framework for action on interprofessional education and collaborative practice, n.d.). Research on the effects of IPE is also growing (Reeves et al., 2010). In addition to positive outcomes such as improved teamwork and organizational culture, IPE in postsecondary institutions takes advantage of limited resources by reducing redundancies in training and systematizing development of trainees from different disciplines (Ho et al., 2008; Illingworth & Chelvanayagam, 2007). Participation in IPE positively influences future practitioners' attitudes toward, knowledge about, and skills for making effective use of collaboration opportunities (Hammick et al., 2007; Nisbet, Hendry, Rolls, & Field, 2008).

Specific IPE techniques are associated with more desirable outcomes. A review of techniques used to support IPE identifies use of interactive didactics (including active learning strategies such as role plays), small group discussion among individuals from different professional groups, and peer collaboration as most commonly used (Lyon, Stirman, Kerns, & Bruns, 2011). Presently, models are being established which articulate IPE approaches within behavioral science. One example is the University of Washington (UW) Interdisciplinary Workforce Initiative in the United States (Kerns et al., 2015). In this innovative IPE graduate-level course and lecture series, students from psychology, psychiatry, social work, nursing, education, and others come together in a collaborative learning environment focused on EBPs for children and adolescents. Evaluation has revealed that students across disciplines increased more than two standard deviations in the core skills associated with program delivery and reached a skill level very similar to existing professionals – and a comparable course did not need to be taught in each department (Kerns et al., 2015; Sethi, Kerns, Sanders, & Ralph, 2014). This indicates that an IPE approach may also accelerate development of core competencies.

Recommendations for Advancing Training to Address the Implementation Gap

Integrated training programs are necessary that incorporate the components described above with the goals of facilitating the development of a more integrated and collaborative EBP implementation workforce; enhancing the local relevance of implementation research questions, designs, and assessments; increasing the use of evidence-based implementation strategies and rigor in which implementation practice is planned, executed, and evaluated; and creating a context for implementation science innovation. To accomplish these goals, we recommend the development and refinement of professional training programs that (1) develop relevant didactic content, (2) train teams of diverse stakeholders, (3) train toward the development and use of efficient methodologies, (4) advance pragmatic measurement, (5) leverage knowledge about team science, and (6) apply leading models for research project development.

Recommendation 1: Develop Relevant Didactic Content

Didactic training is an essential tool for communicating basic knowledge to learners and is likely to be a critical piece of any training program. Didactic content could draw from the domains for training in implementation science outlined by Gonzales, Handley, Ackerman, and O'sullivan (2012): (a) collaborative and multidisciplinary team science; (b) careful identification of the contextual factors that inform the research and evaluation design; (c) identification of relevant theory, evidence, methods, measures, and perspectives; (d) strengthening relationships among organizational and individual stakeholders, in order to engage multiple perspectives; (e) using a comprehensive framework to integrate multiple perspectives for intervention design and research implementation; (f) evaluating the effects of the implementation activity using a variety of qualitative, quantitative, and mixed methods; and (g) communication strategies that facilitate the dissemination of information (e.g., initiative activities, evaluation results) to internal and external stakeholders and communities to maximizes their influence. Webcasts and online training platforms could be used to introduce topics such as Selecting an EBP to Optimally Fit the Context, Partnerships for Success Model of Stakeholder Engagement, Collaborative Applications of Implementation Models, Using Technology to Collect Client Outcome Data, and Effective Messaging about Project Outcomes – Techniques from the Marketing Literature.

Recommendation 2: Train Teams of Diverse Stakeholders

Leveraging IPE, training teams could be established that consist of at least one policy and/or practice leader, one intermediary, and one researcher to address limitations in the field (Fig. 12.1) and focus their learning through development and completion of a shared implementation project.

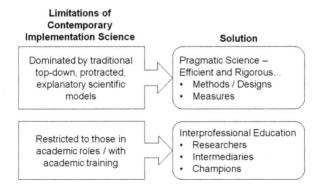

Fig. 12.1 Limitations of – and solutions for – contemporary implementation science

These are the individuals who organize, conduct, receive, or evaluate training or implementation initiatives and, as such, they represent the professionals who are most proximal to EBP implementation efforts. Ideally, training teams would be paired with mentors who also represent each of the stakeholder groups to support active mentoring and development of an implementation project. Training teams could then participate in online and in-person training events throughout their implementation project. Through IPE activities, trainees would be exposed to different stakeholder perspectives and pursue shared training project goals. Having interprofessional instructors, mentors, and peers creates a learning atmosphere that maximizes exposure to multiple perspectives and professional dialog. Existing implementation-focused meetings or conferences (e.g., the Society for Implementation Research Collaboration Biennial Conference, the Academy Health/ National Institute of Health Conference on the Science of Dissemination and Implementation, the Australasian Implementation Conference, or the Global Implementation Conference) could be leveraged to provide additional opportunities to bring training teams together.

Recommendation 3: Train Toward the Development and Use of Efficient and Pragmatic Methodologies

As described above, the dominant implementation science paradigm emphasizes experimental control and internal validity and tends to marginalize generalizable and contextually relevant methods and findings. In contrast, effective training aimed at reducing the science–practice gap in implementation should emphasize efficient methodologies that can generate practice-based implementation research while maintaining appropriate rigor (Glasgow, 2013; Glasgow et al., 2012). Key tenets of pragmatic research include (a) eligibility criteria that include potential participants regardless of their characteristics (e.g., comorbidities, training background); (b) the use of flexible interventions; (c) inclusion of all relevant practitioners in the experimental condition regardless of experimental condition practitioner expertise; (d) flexible application of usual care as the comparison intervention; (e) inclusion of all relevant practitioners in the control/comparison condition regardless of comparison condition practitioner expertise; (f) use of administrative data and other ways to ensure low follow-up burden; (g) ensuring that the primary outcomes focus on objectively measured variables that are clinically meaningful to participants; (h) unobtrusive measurement of service recipient compliance/adherence to the intervention; (i) unobtrusive measurement of service provider compliance/adherence/ fidelity; and (j) primary analyses include all patients regardless of compliance, eligibility, etc. (Thorpe et al., 2009). Encouragingly, there is evidence that the field of implementation science is beginning to recognize the importance of these types of methodologies. For instance, the theme of 2015 biennial conference of the Society for Implementation Research Collaboration (SIRC) was "Advancing Efficient

Methodologies through Community Partnerships and Team Science" (Lewis et al., 2016). Over 100 conference presentations underscored the growing emphasis on pragmatic approaches and yielded insights into ways to leverage pragmatic designs to advance implementation science (Lewis et al., 2016).

Recommendation 4: Advance Pragmatic Measurement

Efficient methods require the availability of pragmatic measures for key implementation domains. To date, implementation research has spawned a diffuse measurement literature that lacks cohesion, quality, and pragmatic relevance (Martinez et al., 2014). A comprehensive review of available implementation relevant measures for all constructs contained within two leading implementation research frameworks (Damschroder et al., 2009; Proctor et al., 2011) is currently underway, which could serve as a foundation for integrated training efforts (Lewis et al., 2014). Indeed, although the measure review is led by researchers, it is working with diverse stakeholders (e.g., organization leaders, intermediaries) to better articulate the parameters of the pragmatic measures construct and to develop an associated rating criteria (Lewis et al., 2014). New implementation-oriented training opportunities would be innovative in the extent to which they can provide state-of-the-art instruction in implementation measurement that integrates implementation science and implementation practice priorities, promoting the use of psychometrically sound and pragmatic instruments.

Recommendation 5: Leverage Knowledge About Team Science

Explicit training in the establishment of effective team science partnerships is likely to support pragmatic research and practice co-creation, the meaningful translation of research findings for both academic and nonacademic audiences, and the generation of practice-based evidence in implementation. Training should be designed to improve trainees' expertise working in their own role as well as understanding others' roles to work collaboratively using team science in their future endeavors. Such a training program could increase the capacity of policy leaders, practice leaders, and intermediary trainees and faculty to be effective consumers of implementation science and able to plan evaluation of their own implementation activities. Simultaneously, an integrated program would allow for opportunities to enhance research faculty and trainees' understanding of the community practice of implementation, which would improve the efficiency and utility of the future implementation research they conduct.

Recommendation 6: Apply Existing Models for Research Project Development

Feedback is an essential component of any improvement process, and structured feedback from experts has the potential to elevate a product while providing key learning opportunities for the feedback recipient and others in attendance. Leading models for research or project development should, therefore, be leveraged to maximize the quality of work produced by trainees. For instance, the Implementation Development Workshop (IDWs; Marriott, Rodriguez, Landes, Lewis, & Comtois, 2016) model holds great relevance for the goals of an integrated and pragmatic training program. Based on the Behavioral Research in Diabetes Group Exchange (BRIDGE) model (Behavioral Research in Diabetes Group Exchange – BRIDGE – Psychosocial Aspects of Diabetes [PSAD] Study Group, n.d.), the IDW is a group meeting that provides a unique opportunity for implementation science and practice professionals to present their "work in development" and receive expert feedback. The model emphasizes facilitated but informal discussion of research or project ideas and the preliminary or conceptual stages of a project, instead of the typical formal presentations of completed projects and results, and does not permit the use of presentation technology. Participants in meetings that have utilized this model have not only gained important research insights but also have enhanced success with funding, presentations, and publications (Behavioral Research in Diabetes Group Exchange – BRIDGE – Psychosocial Aspects of Diabetes [PSAD] Study Group, n.d.).

With the focus of improving the methodology of new and in-progress implementation research projects and building collaboration, the ultimate goal of an IDW is to enhance the likelihood that implementation science proposals are funded by external sponsors, such as federal research entities (e.g., the National Institutes of Health or Department of Veteran Affairs), or that implementation practitioners conduct effective implementations with rigorous but feasible evaluation. SIRC hosted and evaluated a series of face-to-face and online IDWs. This evaluation examined the impact of web-based IDWs compared with the more traditional in-person format. Both formats were considered acceptable and effective across presenters and attendees, with 100% of participants ($N = 38$) in both groups agreeing that they learned things they did not know before and 94.7% of participants ($N = 36$) agreeing that they felt like they could apply a lot of what they learned in their own work. Although the IDW has not yet been evaluated via a randomized trial, results indicate that more than a third (35.3%) of the projects presented were ultimately funded and 26.7% were planned for resubmission, suggesting that strong proposals have emerged from the IDW process (Marriott et al., 2016). Data from previous IDWs suggest that attendance may not only benefit the work of those receiving feedback, but that all participants substantially learn about key implementation science and practice issues (Marriott et al., 2016).

Conclusion

Training opportunities are necessary to allow policy and practice leaders to conduct and consume pragmatic research and to have an equal seat at the table with intermediaries and researchers to ensure they are well-positioned to (1) evaluate the implementation literature produced by researchers and its relevance to their setting, (2) make critical decisions about implementation strategies for EBPs in conjunction with intermediaries, and (3) determine what implementation outcomes are most appropriate for the measurement of locally relevant constructs and outcomes. Intermediaries would benefit from opportunities to (1) become fluent with research that has identified strategies that can improve the effectiveness of implementation practice; (2) work with policy and practice leaders to select and apply specific implementation strategies; and (3) collaborate with researchers to evaluate the effectiveness of their implementation strategies leading to more success of implementation practice initiatives to produce generalizable knowledge. Implementation scientists could be both challenged and inspired to ask new questions posed by the practice, policy, and intermediary stakeholders which can then provoke innovation in implementation models, measures, and methods.

Building on many of the recommendations above, SIRC is developing a training model that is designed to address the limitations of implementation science and implementation practice while promoting their integration. Because SIRC began with the recognition that there were multiple implementation researchers and practitioners working in parallel on innovative projects in behavioral health, but that formal channels for communicating and collaborating with one another were relatively unavailable (see Lewis et al., 2016, for a full description of SIRC), the organization is well-positioned to support training efforts that have relevance to a wide variety of stakeholder groups. Specifically, SIRC provides expertise to support a developing training institute – the *SIRC Training Institute for Collaborative Science (STICS)* – that is intended to harness pragmatic research, team science, and IPE and bring together researchers, intermediaries, practice leaders, and policy leaders to reduce the emerging gap between implementation science and implementation practice.

Increasing the availability of training opportunities via programs such STICS is vital for advancing the field of implementation to ensure we are not recreating the massive gap between what is known scientifically and what is done within real-world settings that originally prompted its inception. Although STICS is an approach that is currently under development, this chapter is intended to share broader recommendations about how to create novel training opportunities that simultaneously address key limitations and barriers within implementation science and practice and offer an interdisciplinary context within which innovation in implementation science can occur. Of course, the very nature of these programs may present another dilemma as they do not fit neatly into current training paradigms. The logistics involved in identifying training teams, supporting projects, and securing funding may be substantial barriers. However, the payoff is potentially crucial in the advancement of the field and enhanced integration of implementation science and practice.

References

Aarons, G. A., Hurlburt, M., & Horwitz, S. M. (2011). Advancing a conceptual model of evidence-based practice implementation in public service sectors. *Administration and Policy in Mental Health and Mental Health Services Research, 38*(1), 4–23. https://doi.org/10.1007/s10488-010-0327-7

Becker, E. M., Smith, A. M., & Jensen-Doss, A. (2013). Who's using treatment manuals? A national survey of practicing therapists. *Behaviour Research and Therapy, 51*(10), 706–710. https://doi.org/10.1016/j.brat.2013.07.008

Behavioral Research in Diabetes Group Exchange - BRIDGE - Psychosocial Aspects of Diabetes (PSAD) Study Group. (n.d.). Retrieved 24 June 2016, from http://uvtapp.uvt.nl/fsw/spits.ws.frmShowpage?v_page_id=9618214012013366

Charns, M. P., Egede, L. E., Rumsfeld, J. S., McGlynn, G. C., & Yano, E. M. (2014). Advancing partnered research in the VA healthcare system: The pursuit of increased research engagement, responsiveness, and impact. *Journal of General Internal Medicine, 29*(S4), 811–813. https://doi.org/10.1007/s11606-014-3060-1

Cook, B. G., & Odom, S. L. (2013). Evidence-based practices and implementation science in special education. *Exceptional Children, 79*(2), 135–144. https://doi.org/10.1177/001440291307900201

Damschroder, L. J., Aron, D. C., Keith, R. E., Kirsh, S. R., Alexander, J. A., & Lowery, J. C. (2009). Fostering implementation of health services research findings into practice: A consolidated framework for advancing implementation science. *Implementation Science, 4*(1), 50.

Eccles, M. P., & Mittman, B. S. (2006). Welcome to implementation science. *Implementation Science, 1*(1), 1–3.

Ehrhart, M. G., Aarons, G. A., & Farahnak, L. R. (2015). Going above and beyond for implementation: The development and validity testing of the Implementation Citizenship Behavior Scale (ICBS). *Implementation Science, 10*(1), 65.

Fedoroff, I. C., & Taylor, S. (2001). Psychological and pharmacological treatments of social phobia: A meta-analysis. *Journal of Clinical Psychopharmacology, 21*(3), 311–324.

Franks, R. P., & Bory, C. T. (2015). Who supports the successful implementation and sustainability of evidence-based practices? Defining and understanding the roles of intermediary and purveyor organizations. *New Directions for Child and Adolescent Development, 2015*(149), 41–56. https://doi.org/10.1002/cad.20112

Gaglio, B., Phillips, S. M., Heurtin-Roberts, S., Sanchez, M. A., & Glasgow, R. E. (2014). How pragmatic is it? Lessons learned using PRECIS and RE-AIM for determining pragmatic characteristics of research. *Implementation Science, 9*(1), 96.

García-Izquierdo, A. L., Aguinis, H., & Ramos-Villagrasa, P. J. (2010). Science–Practice Gap in e-Recruitment. *International Journal of Selection and Assessment, 18*(4), 432–438. https://doi.org/10.1111/j.1468-2389.2010.00525.x

Garland, A. F., Brookman-Frazee, L., Hurlburt, M. S., Accurso, E. C., Zoffness, R. J., Haine-Schlagel, R., & Ganger, W. (2010). Mental health care for children with disruptive behavior problems: A view inside therapists' offices. *Psychiatric Services, 61*(8), 788–795. https://doi.org/10.1176/ps.2010.61.8.788

Glisson, C., Landsverk, J., Schoenwald, S., Kelleher, K., Hoagwood, K. E., Mayberg, S., … Research Network on Youth Mental Health. (2008). Assessing the organizational social context (OSC) of mental health services: Implications for research and practice. *Administration and Policy in Mental Health and Mental Health Services Research, 35*(1–2), 98–113. https://doi.org/10.1007/s10488-007-0148-5

Gonzales, R., Handley, M. A., Ackerman, S., & O'sullivan, P. S. (2012). A framework for training health professionals in implementation and dissemination science. *Academic medicine: Journal of the Association of American Medical Colleges, 87*(3), 271–278.

Glasgow, R. E. (2013). What does it mean to be pragmatic? Pragmatic methods, measures, and models to facilitate research translation. *Health Education & Behavior, 40*(3), 257–265.

Glasgow, R. E., & Chambers, D. (2012). Developing robust, sustainable, implementation systems using rigorous, rapid and relevant science. *Clinical and Translational Science, 5*(1), 48–55. https://doi.org/10.1111/j.1752-8062.2011.00383.x

Glasgow, R. E., & Riley, W. T. (2013). Pragmatic measures: What they are and why we need them. *American Journal of Preventive Medicine, 45*(2), 237–243. https://doi.org/10.1016/j.amepre.2013.03.010

Glasgow, R. E., Vinson, C., Chambers, D., Khoury, M. J., Kaplan, R. M., & Hunter, C. (2012). National Institutes of Health approaches to dissemination and implementation science: Current and future directions. *American Journal of Public Health, 102*(7), 1274–1281.

Hammick, M., Freeth, D., Koppel, I., Reeves, S., & Barr, H. (2007). A best evidence systematic review of interprofessional education: BEME Guide no. 9. *Medical Teacher, 29*(8), 735–751. https://doi.org/10.1080/01421590701682576

Ho, K., Jarvis-Selinger, S., Borduas, F., Frank, B., Hall, P., Handfield-Jones, R., … Rouleau, M. (2008). Making interprofessional education work: The strategic roles of the academy. *Academic Medicine, 83*(10), 934–940. https://doi.org/10.1097/ACM.0b013e3181850a75

Illingworth, P., & Chelvanayagam, S. (2007). Benefits of interprofessional education in health care. *British Journal of Nursing, 16*(2), 121–124.

Johnston, C. A., & Moreno, J. P. (2016). Bridging the science-practice gap in obesity treatment. *American Journal of Lifestyle Medicine, 10*(2), 100–103. https://doi.org/10.1177/1559827615620381

Kazdin, A. E. (2010). Problem-solving skills training and parent management training for oppositional defiant disorder and conduct disorder. In *Evidence- based psychotherapies for children and adolescents* (pp. 211–226).

Kerns, S. E., Cevasco, M., Comtois, K. A., Dorsey, S., King, K., McMahon, R., … Trupin, E. W. (2015). An interdisciplinary university-based initiative for graduate training in evidence-based treatments for children's mental health. *Journal of Emotional and Behavioral Disorders.* https://doi.org/10.1177/1063426615583457

Kuller, A. M., Ott, B. D., Goisman, R. M., Wainwright, L. D., & Rabin, R. J. (2009). Cognitive behavioral therapy and schizophrenia: A survey of clinical practices and views on efficacy in the United States and United Kingdom. *Community Mental Health Journal, 46*(1), 2–9. https://doi.org/10.1007/s10597-009-9223-6

Lewis, C., Borntrager, C., Martinez, R., Weiner, B. J., Kim, M., Barwick, M., & Comtois, K. A. (2014). Systematic review and synthesis of dissemination and implementation science instruments: Description of a protocol to promote rigorous evaluation. *Implementation Science*, (in press).

Lewis, C. C., Weiner, B. J., Stanick, C., & Fischer, S. M. (2015). Advancing implementation science through measure development and evaluation: A study protocol. *Implementation Science, 10*, 102. https://doi.org/10.1186/s13012-015-0287-0

Lewis, C., Darnell, D., Kerns, S., Monroe-DeVita, M., Landes, S. J., Lyon, A. R., et al. (2016). Proceedings of the 3rd Biennial Conference of the Society for Implementation Research Collaboration (SIRC) 2015: Advancing efficient methodologies through community partnerships and team science. *Implementation Science, 11*(1), 1–38. https://doi.org/10.1186/s13012-016-0428-0

Lyon, A. R., Stirman, S. W., Kerns, S. E., & Bruns, E. J. (2011). Developing the mental health workforce: Review and application of training approaches from multiple disciplines. *Administration and Policy in Mental Health and Mental Health Services Research, 38*(4), 238–253.

Marriott, B. R., Rodriguez, A. L., Landes, S. J., Lewis, C. C., & Comtois, K. A. (2016). A methodology for enhancing implementation science proposals: Comparison of face-to-face versus virtual workshops. *Implementation Science, 11*, 62. https://doi.org/10.1186/s13012-016-0429-z

Martinez, R. G., Lewis, C. C., & Weiner, B. J. (2014). Instrumentation issues in implementation science. *Implementation Science, 9*(1), 118. https://doi.org/10.1186/s13012-014-0118-8

McHugh, R. K., & Barlow, D. H. (2010). The dissemination and implementation of evidence-based psychological treatments. A review of current efforts. *American Psychology, 65*(2), 73–84.

Meissner, H. I., Glasgow, R. E., Vinson, C. A., Chambers, D., Brownson, R. C., Green, L. W., ... Mittman, B. (2013). The U.S. training institute for dissemination and implementation research in health. *Implementation Science, 8*(1), 12. https://doi.org/10.1186/1748-5908-8-12

National Cancer Institute. (n.d.). Team science toolkit: About team science. Retrieved 2 June 2015, from https://www.teamsciencetoolkit.cancer.gov/public/WhatIsTS.aspx

Nisbet, G., Hendry, G. D., Rolls, G., & Field, M. J. (2008). Interprofessional learning for pre-qualification health care students: An outcomes-based evaluation. *Journal of Interprofessional Care, 22*(1), 57–68. https://doi.org/10.1080/13561820701722386

Palinkas, L. A., Aarons, G. A., Horwitz, S., Chamberlain, P., Hurlburt, M., & Landsverk, J. (2011). Mixed method designs in implementation research. *Administration and Policy in Mental Health and Mental Health Services Research, 38*(1), 44–53. https://doi.org/10.1007/s10488-010-0314-z

Powell, B. J., McMillen, J. C., Proctor, E. K., Carpenter, C. R., Griffey, R. T., Bunger, A. C., ... York, J. L. (2012). A compilation of strategies for implementing clinical innovations in health and mental health. *Medical Care Research and Review, 69*(2), 123–157.

Powell, B. J., Waltz, T. J., Chinman, M. J., Damschroder, L. J., Smith, J. L., Matthieu, M. M., ... Kirchner, J. E. (2015). A refined compilation of implementation strategies: Results from the Expert Recommendations for Implementing Change (ERIC) project. *Implementation Science, 10*(1), 21.

Proctor, E. K., & Chambers, D. A. (2016). Training in dissemination and implementation research: A field-wide perspective. *Translational Behavioral Medicine,* 1–12. https://doi.org/10.1007/s13142-016-0406-8

Proctor, E. K., Landsverk, J., Aarons, G., Chambers, D., Glisson, C., & Mittman, B. (2009). Implementation research in mental health services: An emerging science with conceptual, methodological, and training challenges. *Administration and Policy in Mental Health and Mental Health Services Research, 36*(1), 24–34. https://doi.org/10.1007/s10488-008-0197-4

Proctor, E., Silmere, H., Raghavan, R., Hovmand, P., Aarons, G., Bunger, A., ... Hensley, M. (2011). Outcomes for implementation research: Conceptual distinctions, measurement challenges, and research agenda. *Administration and Policy in Mental Health and Mental Health Services Research, 38*(2), 65–76. https://doi.org/10.1007/s10488-010-0319-7

Proctor, E. K., Landsverk, J., Baumann, A. A., Mittman, B. S., Aarons, G. A., Brownson, R. C., ... Chambers, D. (2013). The implementation research institute: Training mental health implementation researchers in the United States. *Implementation Science, 8,* 105. https://doi.org/10.1186/1748-5908-8-105

Reeves, S., Zwarenstein, M., Goldman, J., Barr, H., Freeth, D., Koppel, I., & Hammick, M. (2010). The effectiveness of interprofessional education: Key findings from a new systematic review. *Journal of Interprofessional Care, 24*(3), 230–241. https://doi.org/10.3109/13561820903163405

Selby, J. V., Beal, A. C., & Frank, L. (2012). The Patient-Centered Outcomes Research Institute (PCORI) national priorities for research and initial research agenda. *JAMA, 307*(15), 1583–1584.

Scaccia, J. P., Cook, B. S., Lamont, A., Wandersman, A., Castellow, J., Katz, J., & Beidas, R. S. (2015). A practical implementation science heuristic for organizational readiness: R = Mc2. *Journal of Community Psychology, 43*(4), 484–501. https://doi.org/10.1002/jcop.21698

Sethi, S., Kerns, S. E. U., Sanders, M. R., & Ralph, A. (2014). The international dissemination of evidence-based parenting interventions: Impact on practitioner content and process self-efficacy. *International Journal of Mental Health Promotion, 16*(2), 126–137. https://doi.org/10.1080/14623730.2014.917896

Shea, C. M., Jacobs, S. R., Esserman, D. A., Bruce, K., & Weiner, B. J. (2014). Organizational readiness for implementing change: A psychometric assessment of a new measure. *Implementation Science, 9*(7), 1–15.

Simons, A. D., Padesky, C. A., Montemarano, J., Lewis, C. C., Murakami, J., Lamb, K., ... Beck, A. T. (2010). Training and dissemination of cognitive behavior therapy for depression in adults:

A preliminary examination of therapist competence and client outcomes. *Journal of Consulting and Clinical Psychology, 78*(5), 751–756. https://doi.org/10.1037/a0020569

Stokols, D., Hall, K. L., Taylor, B. K., & Moser, R. P. (2008). The science of team science: Overview of the field and introduction to the supplement. *American Journal of Preventive Medicine, 35*(2, Supplement), S77–S89. https://doi.org/10.1016/j.amepre.2008.05.002

Stokols, D., Misra, S., Moser, R. P., Hall, K. L., & Taylor, B. K. (2008). The ecology of team science: Understanding contextual influences on transdisciplinary collaboration. *American Journal of Preventive Medicine, 35*(2, Supplement), S96–S115. https://doi.org/10.1016/j.amepre.2008.05.003

Straus, S. E., Brouwers, M., Johnson, D., Lavis, J. N., Légaré, F., Majumdar, S. R., … Grimshaw, J. (2011). Core competencies in the science and practice of knowledge translation: Description of a Canadian strategic training initiative. *Implementation Science, 6*, 127. https://doi.org/10.1186/1748-5908-6-127

Thorpe, K. E., Zwarenstein, M., Oxman, A. D., Treweek, S., Furberg, C. D., Altman, D. G., … Chalkidou, K. (2009). A pragmatic–explanatory continuum indicator summary (PRECIS): A tool to help trial designers. *Journal of Clinical Epidemiology, 62*(5), 464–475. https://doi.org/10.1016/j.jclinepi.2008.12.011

Weiner, B. J. (2009). A theory of organizational readiness for change. *Implementation Science, 4*(1), 67.

Weisz, J. R., Jensen-Doss, A., & Hawley, K. M. (2006). Evidence-based youth psychotherapies versus usual clinical care: A meta-analysis of direct comparisons. *American Psychologist, 61*(7), 671–689. https://doi.org/10.1037/0003-066X.61.7.671

Weisz, J. R., Ng, M. Y., & Bearman, S. K. (2014). Odd couple? Reenvisioning the relation between science and practice in the dissemination-implementation era. *Clinical Psychological Science, 2*(1), 58–74. https://doi.org/10.1177/2167702613501307

WHO | Framework for action on interprofessional education and collaborative practice. (n.d.). Retrieved 2 June 2015, from http://www.who.int/hrh/resources/framework_action/en/

Wuchty, S., Jones, B. F., & Uzzi, B. (2007). The increasing dominance of teams in production of knowledge. *Science, 316*(5827), 1036–1039. https://doi.org/10.1126/science.1136099

Index

© Springer Nature Switzerland AG 2020
B. Albers et al. (eds.), *Implementation Science 3.0*,
https://doi.org/10.1007/978-3-030-03874-8